MILESTONES
in MODERN

with a Foreword by

J. ENGLEBERT DUNPHY, M.D.

Professor of Surgery,
Harvard Medical School

A HOEBER-HARPER

Milestones in Modern Surgery

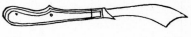

1740

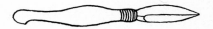

1795

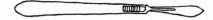

20th CENTURY

Sept. 2, 1958

To George Greenberger
With deep appreciation of
the past and sincere
best wishes for the future
Alfred Hurwitz

CONTENTS

FOREWORD

In some books all that may be gained from them is found in them. Their value is purely intrinsic. In other books, not only is the content of interest and importance, but the stimulating effect of the book on the reader is of much greater significance. Such is the case with this work of Doctor Hurwitz and Doctor Degenshein.

The rapid advances of surgery in recent years have tended to obscure the wealth of information that may be gleaned from a study of the past. Pressure to learn new ideas and new facts consumes the time of student, resident and surgeon. Yet there is not one of us who is not amazed and thrilled by the chance discovery of an early contribution to surgical thought. The authors are to be congratulated for making readily available this carefully selected collection of medical writings. There are very few who will have firsthand familiarity with all of the articles in this book and there are none who will not profit from perusing them.

Although there may be a few who will disagree with the author's choice of particular articles as "milestones," it must be remembered that a milestone has significance not only as indicating a change of direction, but also as a measure of the distance one has traveled. The development of surgery and surgical thought between the milestones depicted here is of incomparable value and interest, and this book will more than serve its purpose if it opens the reader's eyes to the fascinating and instructive scenery which lies between these milestones.

J. Englebert Dunphy

PREFACE

More progress has been made in surgery during the past seventy-five years than in all the preceding years of recorded history. A surprisingly small number of milestone advances have been responsible for this golden age of surgery. These include the development of hemostasis, anesthesia, a knowledge of fluid and electrolyte balance, the control of infection and the development of technical skills for specific diseases, viz., Billroth's gastrectomy, Halsted's radical mastectomy, Bassini's herniorrhaphy, Kocher's thyroidectomy, Graham's pneumonectomy, Souttar's commissurotomy and others.

It is our purpose in this volume to place in easily accessible form our choice of the surgical classics that have stood the test of time. In all but a few instances, we were able to fulfill the following criteria:

1. That the paper was of such importance that it represented a significant advance in surgery
2. That the paper was well written and that it demonstrated the scientific method
3. That the principle or operation described, whether in its original form or some variation thereof, is still of current value.

Although we considered many earlier articles on infection including Lister's, Reid's paper crystallizes the problem so well that, in our opinion, it is a classic. Every surgeon who reads this paper is bound to reassess his own management of the wound.

From the beginning it was obvious that an article that appeared first was not always appropriate for inclusion in this volume. We were repeatedly surprised to find that the articles often quoted as originals contained references to earlier investigators who failed to appreciate the significance of their discoveries. In many instances it was impossible to establish a definite priority. When several articles were under consideration, we chose the one that we believed to be the most informative and of greatest interest to the reader.

In many instances, discoveries went unheeded because of poor communication. Matas had used the Fell–O'Dwyer apparatus for endotracheal anesthesia in performing thoracotomies many years before Meltzer and Auer published their work, yet general acclaim followed only after the latter publication. Another disturbing observation was the long delay that occurred between a discovery and its practical application. In 1901 Carrel described an accurate method of blood-vessel anastomosis. In the article he emphasized the fact that his objective was to develop a method of transplanting organs. It is only during the past few years that transplantation of thyroid and parathyroid glands and of kidneys has been successfully performed by the technique described over fifty years ago by Carrel. Approximately twelve years elapsed between Fleming's discovery of penicillin and its application for the benefit of mankind. We are convinced that many latent milestones still lie buried in the literature.

Our original purpose in writing this volume was to fill a gap in the resident training program. With the emphasis on reading the current literature, little time is available for seeking out the significant contributions of the past. As the project developed, we found that the clinical surgeon also displayed great interest in having readily available the literature to which he had heard many references but which he had never found the time to dig out of the library stacks. In our perusal of several hundred volumes, we were surprised to learn that many were leaving the library for the first time.

Professor Ostwald, quoted by Camac, had this to say: "It is well known to what a degree a man's life is influenced by the impressions gained in youth; these are, as it were, the warp upon which the intellectual life of a man is woven. So it has been absolutely necessary for me to have free access to original literature and it has been my first concern to place this indispensable aid at the disposal of my colleagues and myself."

Since the original draft of this book was made, two anticipated milestones have become realities. Hence we have added the section "Milestones on the Horizon" in which we have included the description of an extracorporeal pump and of renal homotransplantation.

We hope that our editorial comments will prove interesting and thought-provoking. If the reader fails to come away with an appreciation of the significance of the basic principles of surgery, with a deep sense of humility and with a feeling of optimism in the fecundity of the future, then we have failed to clarify the *raison d'être* of this book.

It is always interesting to know something of the men who have made great contributions. Therefore, we have included a biographical sketch of each principal author. Our efforts to obtain photographs were well rewarded, with only one exception. Despite cooperation by a member of the Soviet Information Bureau in Moscow who provided a biographical sketch of Nikolai Eck, a photograph could not be obtained.

We have made several omissions where they would not detract from the value of an article. For example, reprinting every one of Bassini's 262 case reports would have added many pages but very little critical information. Figures that were considered unimportant were omitted. All such omissions are indicated in the text. In every instance, bibliographical references have been deleted; citations of references within the text have also been deleted.

We are indebted to Mrs. Helen McKee for her loyal efforts in carrying out an extensive correspondence and in typing the manuscript. We are indebted to Dr. Carl Wertheimer for the translations of the articles by Billroth, Wölfler and Bassini and to Dr. Isidore Cohn of New Orleans for his biographical sketch of Rudolph Matas. Paul B. Hoeber and his editors, Mrs. Eunice Stevens and George D. McKinnon, have been excellent guides throughout this adventure. We should like to thank Miss Norma Stahl for her splendid work in designing this book. We appreciate the many favors granted to us by the staff of the library at the Medical Society of the County of Kings, especially by Mrs. Mabel Camp and Mr. John Ische, and their good temper despite many trips to the obscure parts of the stacks. All the authors as well as their publishers were extremely cooperative in granting us permission to reproduce these articles. We also owe our gratitude to the many authors whose excellent articles we considered for inclusion but could not use because of limitation of space.

Finally we are indebted to the unsung heroes of any literary attempt, our families whose time we borrowed.

A. H.
G. A. D.

New York

1. Hemostasis

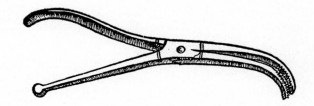

PREFATORY COMMENTS

THE LIGATURE

Ambroise Paré is considered by many historians to be the father of modern surgery. It is from his period that we may follow its development with some degree of continuity. Paracelsus, Giovanni di Vigo and many others began to break with the Galenical tradition by the elaboration of independent observations, e.g., the use of the ligature and principles of wound healing. Their writings were soon forgotten and it remained for Paré to popularize the first essential in the development of surgical technique, viz., hemostasis by ligature. His condemnation of the cauterization of wounds was based on an accidental experience when he ran short of boiling oil during a battle which produced many casualties. In desperation he concocted a salve made of egg yolk, oil of roses and turpentine which he applied to the wounds. He could not sleep that night for fear all of the wounds so treated would become poisoned and that his patients would die. To his surprise and joy, he found that these wounds fared much better than those cauterized with boiling oil. Others had undoubtedly seen this phenomenon but it remained for Paré to recognize the dangers of cauterization and to denounce its use. It was the same foresight which led him to condemn the cauterization of amputation stumps with hot irons and to develop the suture ligature. Although three hundred years were to elapse before Pasteur discovered the microbes, the seeds of antisepsis were germinating in Paré's mind.

Paré's versatility was manifest in his description of hernia trusses, prostheses and post-mortem examinations. His *Ten Books of Surgery* are delightful treatises but no more remarkable than those of some of his predecessors. His practice of putting salves on the weapon that in-

3

flicted the wound attests to his showmanship for it is doubtful that he believed in its value. Nevertheless, he was not free from superstition. One salve that he obtained only after a long pursuit had as part of its recipe two newborn puppies boiled in oil and earthworms drowned in white wine. That he knew humility is evident in his famous quotation which is inscribed on his statue: "Je le pansay, Dieu le guarit" ["I dress the wound, God heals it."] His definition of surgery is as applicable today as it was then: "Chyrurgie is an Art, which teacheth the way by reason, how by the operation of the hand we may cure, prevent and mitigate diseases which accidently happen unto us."

We have chosen to reproduce excerpts from his original description of the ligature and also the first part of his classic *Apology and Treatise*. Although he was surgeon to four French kings he was considered, nevertheless, a barber surgeon and suffered greatly at the hands of his colleagues of the "long coat." In Paré's time there were three echelons of practitioners. The physicians were learned men at the top of the profession who carried a high social status. They practiced no surgery. The intermediate group were the "surgeons of the long coat" who were members of the confraternity of St. Côme. These men did the actual surgery and prided themselves in their ability to read and write Latin. At the lowest end of the scale were the barber surgeons who evolved from the profane and vulgar. These men were employed originally in monasteries to perform the shaving of heads and also the regular bleedings prescribed by many orders. Paré started as a barber surgeon and was in constant conflict with the surgeons of the long robe. When his fame became great, he was grudgingly admitted to the Collège de St. Côme. Etienne Gourmelen, Dean of the Faculty of Medicine, attacked Paré so bitterly that he answered the attack with his famous book in which he included the humane *Journey into Divers Places*. The *Apology and Treatise,* published in 1585, contains more than a dozen references to those who had used the ligature at an earlier date. It also contains heart-warming accounts of his military experiences and vivid descriptions of his reconnaissances through enemy lines. Logan Clendenning has said: "If I had a son and he wanted to study medicine he should begin on the *Apology and Treatise* of Ambroise Paré, because there is something in that book he would find in none of his texts—there is life."

SURGICAL INSTRUMENTS

Surgery embraces a technical art and mechanical devices are essential to its progress. The hemostatic forceps has been a prime factor in the development of more meticulous surgical techniques.

Forceps were employed by the Egyptians over 5000 years ago as a depilatory. In *The Iliad,* reference was made to the use of forceps by Greek surgeons to remove missiles from the wounded. Paré's *Bec de Corbin* (crow's beak) resembles the modern hemostat closely and was used by him to obtain hemostasis in traumatic wounds. Desault introduced the first artery compression forceps with a spring device which closed the jaws and maintained their grip. In 1840 the present form of hemostat was devised by Charrière. This instrument had crossed legs which operated as a clamp. The forceps of Koeberlé and Péan were the immediate precursors of the present-day pressure forceps. Spencer Wells introduced his first forceps in 1872. After several modifications, he arrived at the hemostatic pressure forceps as we know it today. Torsion for hemostasis was in vogue at that time, but after Spencer Wells' instrument was introduced, the modern method of hemostasis rapidly made torsion obsolete. We reprint here the account of Spencer Wells' improved forceps published in his book on ovariotomy.

A few years later, Halsted introduced his finer-nosed forceps. As recently as 1880, few hospitals in New York boasted of more than six artery clamps. Halsted mentioned witnessing an operation performed by Mikulicz in Billroth's clinic in 1879 when the visiting Americans were amused at seeing a dozen hemostats hanging from a thyroid incision. They ridiculed the method as being untidy but soon became proponents of the use of multiple forceps. There is no doubt that Mikulicz's influence on Halsted paid many dividends to American surgery.

AMBROISE PARÉ (1510–1590)

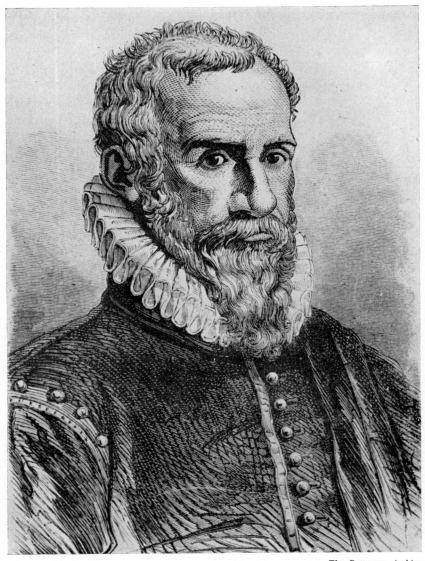

Ambroise Paré was born in Bourg–Hersent, Maine, France. His father was a servant and barber. His brother, Jehan, and brother-in-law, Gaspard Martin, were barber surgeons. He was trained at Hôtel Dieu as a "pupil dresser" and operator for three years. As an army surgeon he was beloved by troops and considered to be the equivalent of ten thousand replacements. His primary works were The Ten Books of Surgery, Apology and Treatise, and Journeys in Divers Places. He is noted for his break with Galenical tradition; the repopularization of the ligature for hemostasis; the treatment of gunshot wounds; and the development of artificial limbs. He was a humane, practical, clinical surgeon of extraordinary talent and foresight. In an age before anesthesia, he made careful and exhaustive diagnoses and he spared the knife whenever possible. He has been described as a dextrous and meticulous operator. His attitude toward the art of surgery was prophetic. In the 1575 edition of his book, Paré wrote in his dedication to the king: "God is my witness, and men are not ignorant of it, that I have labored more than forty years to throw light on the art of surgery and bring it to perfection and in this labor I have striven so hard to attain my end that the ancients have naught wherein to excel us, save the discovery of first principles; and posterity will not be able to surpass us (be it said without malice of offence) save by some additions, such as are easily made to things already discovered."

He died in December, 1590, at the age of eighty, active to the end.

THE APOLOGIE AND TREATISE, CONTAINING THE VOYAGES MADE INTO DIVERS PLACES

BY AMBROISE PARÉ

of Laval in Maine
Counsellor and cheefe Chirurgion to the King

Truely I had not put my hand to the penne, to write on such a thing, were it not that some have impudently injured, taxed, and more through particular hatred, disgraced me, than for zeale or love they beare to the publicke good; which was, concerning my manner of tying the Veines and Arteries, writing thus as followeth.

Malè igitur & nimiùm arroganter inconsultus & temerarius quidam, vasorum ustionem post emortui membri resectionem a veteribus omnibus plurimùm commendatam & semper probatam damnare ausus est, novum quendam deligandi vasa modum, contra veteres omnes medicos sine ratione, experientia & judicio docere cupiens, nec animadvertit majora multo pericula ex ipsa vasorum deligatione quam acu partem sanam profunde transfigendo administrari vult, imminere quàm ex ipsa ustione. Nam si acu nervosam aliquam partem, vel nervum ipsum pupugerit, dum ita novo & inusitato modo venam absurde conatur constringere, nova inflammatio necessariò consequetur, a qua Convulsio & a convulsione cita mors. Quorum symptematum metu Galenus non ante transversa vulnera suere audebat (quod tamen minus erat periculosum) quàm musculorum aponeuroses denudasset. Adde quòd forcipes quibus post sectionem iterum carnem dilacerat, cum retracta versus originem vasa se posse extrahere somniat, non minorem adferant dolorem quaàm ignita ferramenta admota. Quod si quis laniatum expertus incolumis evaserit, is Deo optimo maximo cuius Beneficentia crudelitate ista & carnificina liberatus est, maximas gratias habere & semper agere debet; which is thus: Ill then, and too arrogantly a certaine indiscreet and rash person would blame and condemne the cauterizing of vessells after the amputation of a rotten and corrupted member, much praised and commended and alwayes approved by the Ancients; desiring to shew and teach us without reason, judgment, and experience, a new way to tye the vessells, against the opinion of the Ancient Physitions, taking no heede, nor being well advised, that there happens farre greater perills, and accidents, through this new way of tying the vessells (which will have to be made with a needle, piercing deepely the sound part) than by the burning and ustion of the sayd vessells; for if the needle shall pricke any nervous part, yea the nerve it selfe, when he shall by this new and unaccustomed way absurdly constraine the veine by binding it, there must necessarily follow a new inflammation; from an inflammation a convulsion, from a convulsion death: for feare of which accidents, Galen never durst stitch transversall wounds, (which notwithstanding were lesse dangerous) before he had discovered the Aponeuroses of the muscles. Moreover the pincers with which after the section, the flesh is again dilacerated, while he thinkes to draw the vessells out which are drawne in toward their originall, bring no lesse paine than the cautering irons doe. And if any one having experimented this new manner of cruelty have escaped danger, he ought to render thankes to almighty God forever, through whose goodnesse he hath beene freed from such tyrannie, feeling rather his executioner than his methodicall Chirurgion.

O what sweete words are heere for one, who is sayd to be a wise and learned Doctor? he remembers not that his white beard admonisheth him, not to speake any thing unworthy of his age, and that he ought to put off and drive out of him all envie and rancor conceived against his neighbour. So now I will proove by authority, reason and experience, that the sayd Veines and Arteryes ought to be tyed.

AUTHORITIES.

As for Authorities, I will come to that of that worthy man *Hippocrates,* who wils and commands the cure of Fistula's in the fundament by ligature, as well to consume the callosity, as to avoyd hemorragie.

Galen in his method, speaking of a fluxe of blood made by an outward cause, of whom see heere the words, It is (saith he) most sure to tye the roote of the vessell, which I understand to be that which is most neere to the Liver, or the heart.

Avicen commands to tye the veine and the Arterie, after it is discovered, towards his originall.

Guido of Chauliac, speaking of the wounds of the Veines and Arteries, injoyneth the Chirurgion to make the ligature on the vessell.

Master *Hollier* speaking of a fluxe of blood, commands expressely, to tye the vessells.

Calmetheus in the chapter of the wounds in the Veines and Arteries, tells a most sure way to stay a fluxe of blood, by ligature of the vessell.

Celsus from whom the sayd Physition hath snatched the most part of his booke, chargeth expressely, to tye the vessells in a fluxe of blood happening to wounds, as a remedy most easie and most sure.

Vesalius in his Chirurgery, willeth that the vessells be tyed in a fluxe of blood.

John de Vigo treating of a hemorragie in bleeding wounds, commands to tye the Veine, and the Artery.

Tagaultius treating of the meanes to stay a fluxe of blood, commands to pinch the Veine or Artery with a Crow or Parrot's bill, then to tye it with a very strong thred.

Peter of Argillata of *Bullogne,* discoursing of a fluxe of blood, and the meanes to stoppe it, giveth a fourth way expressely, which is made by ligature of the vessells.

John Andreas a Cruce, a *Venetian,* makes mention of a method, to stay a fluxe of blood by the ligature of the vessells.

D'Alechamps commands to tye the Veines, and Arteries.

See then (my little good man) [*Ed. Note:* Here he refers to Etienne Gourmelen] the authorities which command you to tye the vessells. As for the reasons, I will debate of them.

The hemorragie (say you) is not so much to be feared in the section of the Call,[1] as in that of the Varices, and the incision of the temporall Arteries, as after the amputation of a member. Now you your selfe command, that in cutting the Varices, the fluxe of blood

[1] i.e. the omentum.

be stopped by the ligature of the vessells. You command the same speaking of the stitch, with the amputation and section of the Call, changed by the outward ayre, see heere your owne words. After that must bee considered concerning the Call for if there be any part corrupted, putrified, withered, or blackish: First having tyed, for feare of a fluxe of blood, you doe not bid afterward to have it cauterized, but to say the truth, you have your eyes shut, and all your senses dulled, when you would speake against so sure a method, and that it is not but through anger, and an ill will. For there is nothing which hath more power to drive reason from her seate, than choler and anger. Moreover when one comes to cauterize the dismembred parts, oftentimes when the eschar comes to fall off, there happens a new flux of blood: As I have seene divers times, not having yet been inspired by God, with so sure a meanes then, when I used the heate of fire. Which if you have not found, or understood this method in the bookes of the Ancients, you ought not thus to tread it under your feete, and speake unluckely of one who all his life hath preferred the profit of the Commonwealth before his owne particular. Is it not more than reasonable to bee founded upon the saying of *Hippocrates;* upon whose authority you serve your selfe, which is thus? That what the medicament cureth not, the iron doth, and what the iron doth not amend, the fire exterminateth: It is a thing which savours not of a Christian, to fall to burning at the first dash without staying for any more gentle remedies. As you your selfe write, speaking of the conditions required in a Chirurgion to cure well; which passage you borrow from some other place: for that which may bee done gently without fire, is much more commended than otherwise. Is it not a thing which all schooles hold as a Maxime, that we must alwaies begin with most easie remedies, which if they be not sufficient, we must then come to extreame, following the doctrine of *Hippocrates?* *Galen* commands in the place before alledged, to treate or dresse the diseased quickly, safely, and with the least of paine that is possible.

LET US COME NOW TO REASON.

Now so it is, that one cannot apply hot irons but with extreame and vehement paine in a sensible part, void of a Gangreene, which would be cause of a Convulsion, Feaver, yea oft times of death. Moreover, it would bee a long while afterwards before the poore patients were cured, because that by the action of the fire there is made an eschar, which proceeds from the subject flesh, which being fallen, nature must regenerate a new flesh in stead of that which hath beene burned, as also the bone remaines discovered and bare; and by this meanes, for the most part there remaines an Ulcer incurable. Moreover there is yet another accident. It happeneth that oftentimes the crust being fallen off, the flesh not being well renewed, the blood issueth out as much as it did before. But when they shall be tyed, the ligature falls not off until first the flesh have very well covered them againe: which is prooved by Galen saying, that escharoticke medicines which cause a crust or eschar, whensoever they fall off, leave the part more bare than the naturall habit requires. For the generation of a crust proceeds from the parts subject, and which are situate round about it, being also burned, as I may say: wherefore by how much the part is burnt, by so much it looseth the naturall heate. Then tell me when it is necessary to use escharoticke medicines, or cautering irons? Tis when the flux of blood is caused by erosion, or some Gangreene or putrifaction. Now is it thus? In fresh bleeding wounds there is neither Gangreene nor putrifaction. Therefore, the cauteries ought not to be there applyed. And when the Ancients commanded to apply hot irons to the mouthes of the vessells, it hath not beene onely to stay the flux of blood, but cheefely to correct the malignitie, or gangreenous putrifaction which might spoile the neighbouring parts. And it must be here noted, that if I had knowne such accidents to happen, which you have declared in your booke, in drawing and tying the vessells, I had never beene twice deceived; nor would I ever have left by my writings to posteritie, such a way of stopping a flux of blood: But I writ it after I had seene it done and did it very often, with happy successe. See then what may happen through your inconsiderate counsell, without examining, or standing upon the facility of tying the sayd vessells. For see, heere's your scope and proposition, to tye the vessells after amputation is a new remedy, say you; then it must not be used, it is an ill argument for a Doctor.

But as for that (say you) one must use fire after the amputation of members, to consume, and drie the putrification, which is a common thing in Gangreenes, and mortifications, that indeed hath no place here, because the practise is to amputate the part above that which is mortified, and corrupted; as *Celsus* writes and commands, to make the amputation upon the sound part, rather than to leave any whit of the corrupted. I would willingly aske you, if when a veine is cut transverse, and that it is very much retracted towards the originall, whether you would make no conscience to burne till that you had found the orifice of the veine, or artery; and if it be not more easie onely with a Crow bill to pinch and draw the vessell, and so tie it? In which you may openly shew your ignorance, and that you have your minde seised with much rancor and choler. We daily see the ligature of the vessells practised with happy successe after the amputation of a part, which I will now verifie by experiences and histories, of those to whom the said ligature hath beene made, and persons yet living.

EXPERIENCES.

The 16. day of *June* 1582. in the presence of Master *John Liebaud* doctor in the faculty of Physicke at *Paris, Claud Viard* sworne Chirurgion, Master *Mathurin Huron,* Chirurgion of Monsieur *de Souvray,* and I, *John Charbonell* master Barber Chirurgion of *Paris,* well understanding the *Theoricke,* and *Practicke* of Chirurgery, did with good dexterity amputate the left legge of a woman tormented the space of three yeares with extreame paine, by reason of a great *Caries* which was in the bone *Astragal, Cuboides,* great and little *focile,*[2] and through all the nervous parts, through which she felt extreame and intollerable paines night and day: she is called *Mary* of *Hostel,* aged 28 yeares, or thereabouts, wife of *Peter Herve,* Esquire of the Kitchin to the Lady *Duchesse of Uzez,* dwelling in the streete of *Verbois* on the other side Saint *Martin* in the fields, dwelling at the signe of the Saint *Johns* head; where the sayd *Charbonell* cut off the sayd legge, the breadth of foure large fingers below the Knee, and after that he had incised the flesh, and sawed the bone, hee griped the Veine with the Crow bill, then the Artery, then tyed them; from whence I protest to God (which the company that were there, can witnesse) that in all the operation which was sodainely done, there was not spilt one porrenger of blood: and I bid the sayd Charbonell to let it bleed more, following the precept of *Hippocrates,* that it is good in all wounds and also in inveterate ulcers, to let the blood runne: by this meanes, the part is lesse subject to inflammation. The sayd Charbonell continued the dressing of her, who was cured in two moneths, without any fluxe

[2] i.e. the tibia and fibula.

of blood happening unto her, or other ill accident; and she went to
see you at your lodging being perfectly cured.

Another history of late memory, of a singing man of our Ladyes
Church named master *Paulain,* [*Ed. Note:* Instead of this name the
English text has Colt] who broke both the bones of his legge which
were crusht in divers peeces, insomuch that there was no hope of cure:
to withstand a gangreene and mortification, and by consequence
death. Monsieur *Helin* Doctor, Regent in the faculty of Physicke, a
man of honour and of good knowledge, *Claud Viard,* and *Simon
Peter,* sworne Chirurgions of Paris, men well exercised in Chirurgery;
and *Balthazar of Lestre,* and *Leonard de Leschenal,* Master Barber
Chururgions, well experimented in the operations of Chirurgery were
all of opinion to withstand the accidents aforesayd to make entire amputation of the whole legge, a little above the broken & shivered bones
& the torne nerves, veines, arteries; the operation was nimbly done,
by the sayd *Viard,* and the blood stancht by the ligature of the vessells in the presence of the sayd *Helin,* and master *Tonsard* great Vicar
of our Ladyes Church, and was continually drest by the sayd *Leschenal,* and I went to see him other whiles; he was happily cured
without the application of hot irons, and walketh lustily on a woodden
legge.

ANOTHER HISTORY.

In the yeare 1583. the 10. day of *December Toussaint Posson* borne
at *Roinville,* at this present dwelling at *Beauvais* neare Dourdan, having his Legge all ulcered and all the bones cariez'd and rotten, prayed
me for the honor of God to cut off his Legge by reason of the great
paine which he could no longer endure. After his body was prepared
I caused his legge to be cut off, fowre fingers below the *rotula* of the
knee, by *Daniel Poullet* one of my servants, to teach him and to im-
bolden him in such workes; and there he readily tyed the vessells to
stay the bleeding, without application of hot irons, in the presence
of *James Guillemeau* ordinary Chirurgion to the King, and *John
Charbonell* master Barber Chirurgion of *Paris:* and during the cure
was visited by Master *Laffilé* and Master *Courtin* Doctors, Regents in
the facultie of Medicine at *Paris.* The said operation was made in the
house of *John Gohell* Inkeeper, dwelling at the signe of the white horse
in the Greve. I will not here forget to say, that the Lady Princesse of
Montpensier, knowing that he was poore, and in my hands, gave him

money to pay for his chamber and diet. He was well cured, God be praysed, and is returned home to his house with a woodden Leg.

ANOTHER HISTORY.

A Gangreene happened to halfe of the Legge to one named *Nicholas Mesnager* aged threescore and sixteene yeares, dwelling in *S. Honoré* street, at the signe of the Basket; which happened to him through an inward cause, so that wee were constrained to cut off his Legge to save his life: and it was taken off by *Anthony Renaud,* masto Barber Chirurgion of *Paris* the 16. day of *December* 1583. in the presence of Master *Le Fort,* and Master *La Nouë* sworne Chirugions of *Paris;* and the blood was stanched by the Ligature of the vessells, and hee is at this present cured and in health, walking with a woodden Leg.

HOW THE SECTION OR AMPUTATION MUST BE PERFORMED.

The first care must be of the patients strength, wherefore let him be nourished with meats of good nutriment, easie digestion, and such as generate many spirits; as with the yolkes of Egges, and bread tosted and dipped in Sacke or Muskedine. Then let him bee placed, as is fit, and drawing the muscles upwards toward the sound parts, let them be tyed with a straite ligature a little above that place of the member which is to be cut off, with a strong and broad fillet like that which women usually bind up their haire withall; This ligature hath a threefold use; the first is, that it hold the muscles drawne up together with the skin, so that retiring backe presently after the performance of the worke, they may cover the ends of the cut bones, and serve them in stead of boulsters or pillowes when they are healed up, and so suffer with lesse paine the compression in susteining the rest of the body; besides also by this meanes the wounds are the sooner healed and cicatrized; for by how much more flesh or skinne is left upon the ends of the bones, by so much they are the sooner healed and cicatrized. The second is, for that it prohibites the fluxe of blood by pressing and shutting up the veines and arteries. The third is, for that it much dulls the sense of the part by stupefying it; the animall spirits by the straite compression being hindred from passing in by the Nerves: Wherefore when you have made your ligature, cut the flesh even to the bone with a sharpe and well cutting incision knife, or with a crooked knife, such as is here expressed.

Now you must note, that there usually lyes betweene the bones, a portion of certaine muscles, which you cannot easily cut with a large incision or dismembring knife wherefore you must carefully divide it and separate it wholly from the bone, with an instrument made neately like a crooked incision knife. I thought good to advertise thee hereof; for if thou shouldst leave any thing besides the bone to bee divided by the saw, you would put the patient to excessive paine in the performance thereof; for soft things as flesh tendons and membranes, cannot be easily cut with a saw. Therefore when you shall come to the bared bone, all the other parts being wholly cut asunder and divided, you shall nimbly divide it with a little saw about some foote and three inches long, and that as near to the sound flesh as you can. And then you must smooth the front of the bone which the saw hath made rough.

HOW TO STANCH THE BLEEDING WHEN THE MEMBER IS TAKEN OFF.

When you have cut off and taken away the member, let it bleed a little according to the strength of the patient, then so the rest of the part may afterwards be lesse obnoxious to inflammation and other symptomes; Then let the Veins and Arteries be bound up as speedily and streightly as you can; that so the course of the flowing blood may be stopped and wholly stayed. Which may be done by taking hold of the vessells with your Crowes beake, whereof this is the figure.

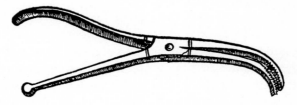

Fig. 1.—The Crowes beake fit for to draw the vessells forth of the flesh wherein they lye hid, that so they may be tyed or bound fast.

The ends of the vessells lyin hid in the flesh, must be taken hold of & drawn with this instrument forth of the muscles whereinto they presently after the amputation withdrew themselves, as all parts are still used to withdraw themselves towards their originalls. In performance of this worke, you neede take no great care, if you together with the vessells comprehend some portion of the neighbouring parts, as of the flesh, for hereof will ensue no harme; but the vessells will so bee consolidated with the more ease, than if they being bloodlesse parts should grow together by themselves. To conclude, when you have so drawne them forth, binde them with a strong double thred.

[*Ed. Note:* At a later date Paré described the suture ligature. His respect for the gentle handling of tissues is evident in the use of a "linnen ragge" to protect the skin.]

HOW YOU MUST STOPPE THE BLEEDING, IF ANY OF THE BOUND UP VESSELS CHANCE TO GET LOOSE.

The businesse hitherto being performed as we said, if peradventure it happen that any bandage of any of the vessels be unloosed; then must you againe binde the member with that kinde of Ligature which you did before the amputation thereof. Or else, which is better, more easily and lesse painefull, let your servant taking hold of the member with both his hands, pressing his fingers strait stoppe the passage of the loosed vessell, for so hee may stanch the bleeding. Then let the worke-master take a needle some foure fingers long, square, and having sharpe edges, drawing after it a three or foure doubled strong thred. With this let him binde the vessell after the following manner. Let him thrust his needle on the outside into the flesh, some halfe fingers breadth from the loosed vessell untill he come to the end thereof, then let him put it about it, and bring it backe againe, but so that there be no more than the space of a fingers bredth betweene the going in and comming forth of the needle. In this space let him put a linnen ragge three or foure times doubled, and thereupon bind somewhat straite the two ends of the thred together. For so he shall hinder the knot from hurting the flesh which lyes under it in the bindings, and also adde strength thereto. For so the bound up orifice of the vessell will in short space be agglutinated to the adjoyning flesh, and that so firmely, that there hath never beene seene, any one drop of blood to have flowed from a vessell so bound up. But if the blood which flowes forth proceede from any small vessell, you must not use this suture and ligature, nor make any such great matter thereof; for it will quickly be stanched by the only application of Astringents presently to be mentioned.

SIR THOMAS SPENCER WELLS (1818–1897)

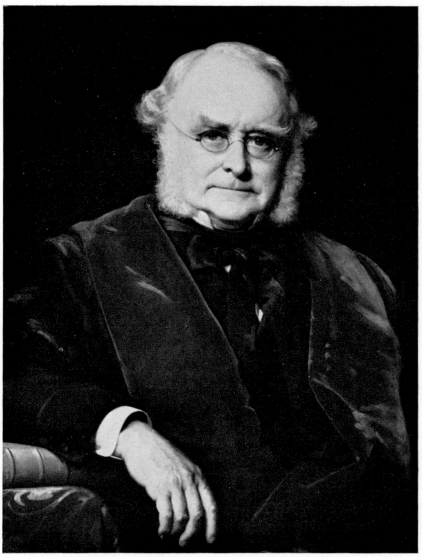

Portrait by Rudolph Lehmann, now in possession of the Royal College of Surgeons

Thomas Spencer Wells was born at St. Albans, Hertfordshire, England, on February 3, 1818. His early experience was obtained under such teachers as Stokes, Graves and Travers. He served as a Navy surgeon for six years and gained considerable experience as an army surgeon during the Crimean War. His army experience made him "much less afraid of abdominal wounds than before" when he returned to practise in London in 1856. In 1858, after several failures, he performed a successful ovariotomy. Subsequent success by his employment of rigid aseptic technique and painstaking training of assistants gave him world fame. In 1872 Wells first used his hemostatic forceps to overcome the custom of using the fingers of an assistant for compression to control bleeding. In 1880 he reported one thousand cases of ovariotomy with a low mortality. He became President of the Royal College of Surgeons in 1881 and received a baronetcy in 1883. He died near Cannes on January 31, 1897, of a cerebral hemorrhage.

SPENCER WELLS' HEMOSTATIC FORCEPS

I have for many years used forceps with long handles, which answer all the purposes of "bull-dogs," as well as of artery and torsion forceps. The catch at the handles serves to fix the instrument, and the short, roughened points stop bleeding completely, and enable the surgeon to twist the vessel if he wishes.

The forceps of Péan and Koeberlé are either curved or angular. But both have the disadvantage of a space between the blades, which admits of entanglement of one instrument with another, or of the passage of omentum or other structures. This was a fault in my own earlier instruments. It has been completely corrected in the later instruments without at all lessening the compressing power exerted on the vessel.

The handles meet without leaving any opening between them. The rings do not admit the thumb and finger too far; and the end which compresses the vessel is so bevelled, that, if it be desirable to apply a ligature, the silk will easily slip over the forceps, and not tie the blades together. Thus my instrument is not only useful in forci-pressure and in torsion, but enables the surgeon to dispense with any other kind of artery–forceps if he wish to apply a ligature.

The distal end of the larger forceps which I use for holding the pedicle in ovariotomy, or any mass of tissue in other operations where the temporary command of bleeding or oozing vessels is urgent, made

From *Abdominal Tumours* by Spencer Wells, P. Blakiston's Sons & Co., Philadelphia, 1885. Reprinted by permission.

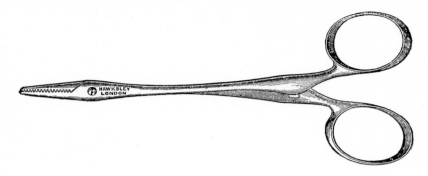

upon the same principle, is here represented of its ordinary size. The pressure in use is ascertained to be in pounds avoirdupois:

Large forceps—1½ in. fulcrum—object 1 millimetre:

First catch	Second catch	Third catch	Fourth catch
20–10	32.8	47.8	60.0

All the instruments in known numbers are placed on a table near the feet of the patient and the right hand of the operator, in shallow

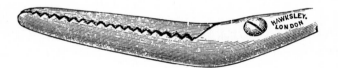

FIG. 2.

dishes, filled with a 2 per cent solution of phenol. The smaller forceps are more conveniently arranged in upright trays, to which they are returned immediately after use. A certain given number being taken and counted before the operation is begun, should also be carefully counted before the abdomen is closed.

2. *Anesthesia*

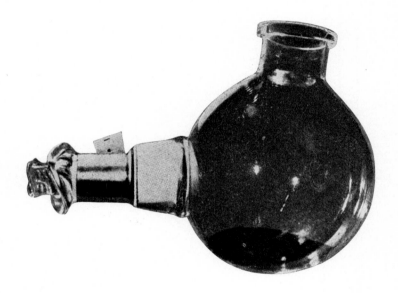

PREFATORY COMMENTS

The discovery of anesthetics was like opening the door to an endless corridor flanked on either side with countless other doors, all slightly ajar and waiting for someone to push them open to reveal their secrets. The importance of this milestone is self-evident, but the tremendous impact it had on the development not only of surgery but also of related fields was immeasurable. It marked the end of the era of stop-watch surgery, and provided the "open sesame" to a surgical attack on all organs of the body. In contradistinction to the rapid and crude operations that had to be practised in the preanesthetic era, surgery could now be refined to embrace careful hemostasis, painstaking exposure and meticulous handling of tissues.

In 1824 Hickman attempted to relieve pain by inhalation of gas. This work was negated by the Royal Society when Davy, who had also reported the analgesic properties of nitrous oxide, was president. Jackson, who first familiarized Crawford Long with the properties of ether, failed to recognize its value and its eventual impact on mankind. The ill-fated Horace Wells, who failed in his attempt to introduce nitrous oxide as an anesthetic, committed suicide. Pope actually did the first dental extraction under ether administered by Clarke, but he also was not aware of its potentialities. Crawford Long removed a tumor of the neck under ether anesthesia in 1842 but never reported the incident until 1846.

It remained for Morton to convince Dr. John C. Warren, a senior surgeon at the Massachusetts General Hospital in Boston, of the efficacy of ether as an anesthetic agent. The success of the experiment received immediate acclaim and initiated the impetus to its widespread

25

use. We decided to reproduce a letter sent by John C. Warren to the *Boston Medical and Surgical Journal* in 1846, in which he presented an authentic and thrilling account of his and his colleagues' original experience with ether anesthesia. Morton, who had given up a lucrative dental practise, then tried to patent ether under the name of Letheon. He actually received a patent but it was rescinded. Wells, Jackson and Long all filed claims to priority and the fight was carried to the United States Senate. A patent was refused after several attempts, and even the President of the United States became involved. In 1862 Morton, broken and humiliated, returned to his farm where he lived in poverty until 1868. Goaded on by a new pamphlet written by Jackson, he journeyed to New York to file suit against him and died there of a stroke a few days later. It is a paradox that a discovery which was to relieve more suffering than any other should have brought so much misery to the principals who were responsible for it. The Letheon controversy received considerable publicity and the good name of medicine suffered. Despite this, the manufacture of new anesthetic agents and of improved apparatus was inevitable.

The other advance in anesthesia which we consider a milestone is the development of the endotracheal method of administration of anesthetic agents. The history of this procedure dates back to 1543 when Vesalius experimented on a sow. In 1878 Macewen performed the first successful intubation without tracheotomy for glottic edema. The Fell-O'Dwyer apparatus, first designed for croup, was employed successfully by Matas during a thoracotomy in 1899. Because of poor communication, this work received little recognition. It remained for Meltzer and Auer in 1909 to demonstrate that respiration could be carried on without any respiratory movements at all in the presence of a bilateral pneumothorax. Their article attracted attention immediately and within a year endotracheal anesthesia with assisted controlled respiration was popularized. Their discovery is considered an important milestone because the application of endotracheal anesthesia to thoracic surgery set up a chain reaction which catapulted surgery of the esophagus, the lung and, more recently, the heart and the great vessels to unprecedented heights.

JOHN COLLINS WARREN (1778–1856)

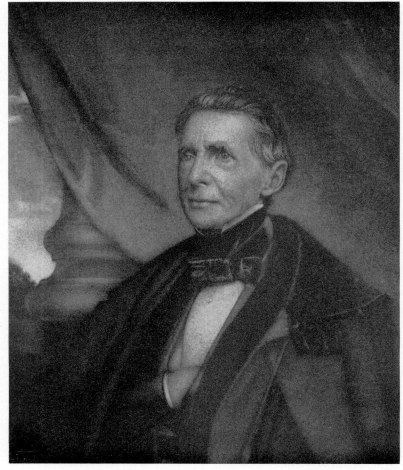

John Collins Warren was the son of John Warren, first professor of surgery of the Harvard Medical School. He studied under Sir Astley Cooper, Cuvier and Dupuytren. He was a pioneer in the excision of bones and joints and in the extirpation of tumors. In 1811, while professor of anatomy and surgery at Harvard, he founded the Massachusetts General Hospital where he made many contributions to medical education. In 1846, in his seventieth year, he removed a vascular tumor of the neck on a patient anesthetized with ether given by W. T. G. Morton. It was then that he made the famous statement: "Gentlemen, this is no humbug." It is admirable that a man of his age should have risked a fine reputation on an uncharted course. His endorsement of ether undoubtedly saved many years of delay in its acceptance. Before 1846 approximately 37 operations were performed at the Massachusetts General Hospital each year. Following the introduction of anesthesia the rate rose to 100 per year, and in 1898 more than 3700 operations were performed.

He died in May, 1856, leaving his son, J. Mason Warren, to succeed him.

INHALATION OF ETHEREAL
VAPOR FOR THE PREVENTION OF PAIN
IN SURGICAL OPERATIONS

BY JOHN C. WARREN, M.D.

Communicated for the Boston Medical and Surgical Journal

Application has been made to me by R. H. Eddy, Esq., in a letter dated November 30th, in behalf of Dr. W. T. G. Morton, to furnish an account of the operations witnessed and performed by me wherein his new discovery for preventing pain was employed. Dr. M. has also proposed to me to give him the names of such hospitals as I know of in this country, in order that he may present them with the use of his discovery. These applications, and the hope of being useful to my professional brethren, especially those concerned in the hospitals which may have the benefit of Dr. M.'s proposal, have induced me to draw up the following statement and to request that it be made public through your journal:

The discovery of a mode of preventing pain in surgical operations has been an object of strong desire among surgeons from an early period. In my surgical lectures I have almost annually alluded to it, and stated the means which I have usually adopted for the attainment of this object. I have also freely declared that, notwithstanding the use of very large doses of narcotic substances, this desideratum had never been satisfactorily obtained. The successful use of any article of the materia medica for this purpose would, therefore, be hailed by me as an important alleviation to human suffering. I have, in consequence,

From *Boston Medical and Surgical Journal* (now *New England Journal of Medicine*), Dec., 1846. Reprinted by permission.

readily admitted the trial of plans calculated to accomplish this object whenever they were free from danger.

About five weeks since, Dr. Morton, dentist of this city, informed me that he had invented an apparatus for the inhalation of a vapor, the effect of which was to produce a state of total insensibility to pain, and that he had employed it successfully in a sufficient number of cases in his practice to justify him in a belief of its efficacy. He wished for an opportunity to test its power in surgical operations, and I agreed to give him such an opportunity as soon as practicable.

Being at that time in attendance as surgeon of the Massachusetts General Hospital, a patient presented himself in that valuable institution a few days after my conversation with Dr. Morton, who required an operation for a tumor of the neck; and, agreeably to my promise, I requested the presence of Dr. M.

On October 17th the patient being prepared for the operation, the apparatus was applied to his mouth by Dr. Morton for about three minutes, at the end of which time he sank into a state of insensibility. I immediately made an incision about three inches long through the skin of the neck, and began a dissection among important nerves and blood-vessels without any expression of pain on the part of the patient. Soon after he began to speak incoherently, and appeared to be in an agitated state during the remainder of the operation. Being asked immediately afterwards whether he had suffered much, he said he had felt as if his neck had been scratched; but subsequently, when inquired of by me, his statement was that he did not experience pain at the time, although aware that the operation was proceeding.

The effect of the gaseous inhalation in neutralizing the sentiment faculty was made perfectly distinct to my mind by this experiment, although the patient, during a part of its prosecution, exhibited appearances indicative of suffering. Dr. Morton had apprized me that the influence of his application would last but a few minutes after its intermission; and as the operation was necessarily protracted, I was not disappointed that its success was only partial.

On the following day, October 18th, an operation was done by Dr. Hayward on a tumor of the arm in a female patient at the hospital. The respiration of the gas was in this case continued during the whole of the operation. There was no exhibition of pain except some occasional groans during its last stage, which she subsequently stated to have arisen from a disagreeable dream. Noticing the pulse in this patient before and after the operation, I found it to have risen from 80 to 120.

Two or three weeks after these occurrences, on meeting with Dr. Charles T. Jackson, distinguished for his philosophical spirit of inquiry, as well as for his geological and chemical science, this gentleman informed me that he first suggested to Dr. Morton the inspiration of ether as a means of preventing the pain of operations on the teeth. He did not claim the invention of the apparatus nor the practical application; for these we are indebted to Dr. Morton.

The success of this process in the prevention of pain for a certain period being quite established, I at once conceived it to be my duty to introduce the apparatus into the practice of the hospital, but was immediately arrested by learning that the proprietor intended to obtain an exclusive patent for its use. It now became a question whether, in accordance with that elevated principle long since introduced into the medical profession, which forbids its members to conceal any useful discovery, we could continue to encourage an application we were not allowed to use ourselves, and of the components of which we were ignorant. On discussing this matter with Dr. Hayward, my colleague in the hospital, we came to the conclusion that we were not justified in encouraging the further use of this new invention until we were better satisfied on these points. Dr. Hayward thereupon had a conversation with Dr. Morton, in consequence of which Dr. M. addressed to me a letter. In this he declared his willingness to make known to us the article employed, and to supply assistance to administer the inhalation whenever called upon. These stipulations he has complied with.

This being done, we thought ourselves justified in inviting Dr. Morton to continue his experiments at the hospital and elsewhere; and he, directly after, November 7th, attended at a painful and protracted operation performed by me, of the excision of a portion of the lower jaw, in which the patient's sufferings were greatly mitigated. On the same day an amputation of the thigh of a young woman was performed at the hospital by Dr. Hayward. In this case the respiration of the ethereal vapor appeared to be entirely successful in preventing the pain of the operation; the patient stating, afterwards, that she did not know that anything had been done to her.

On November 12th, an operation for the removal of a tumor from the arm of a young woman was performed by Dr. J. Mason Warren. The vapor was administered for three minutes, when the patient became unconscious; the operator then proceeded the inspiration being continued. Standing myself on one side of the patient, while the operator was on the other, so entirely tranquil was she that I was not aware the operation was begun until it was nearly completed.

On November 21st an operation was performed by Dr. J. Mason Warren on a gentleman, for the removal of a tumor, which covered nearly the half of the front of the right thigh. The patient lying upon a bed the vapor was administered by Dr. Morton, in the presence of Drs. Charles T. Jackson, Reynolds, J. V. C. Smith, Flagg, Gould, Shurtleff, Lawrence, Parsons, Briggs, and others. After he had breathed the vapor for three minutes his head fell and he ceased to respire it, but presently awakening, the inhalation was renewed till he again appeared insensible. The operation was then commenced. At the first stroke of the knife he clapped his hand on the wound, but I immediately seized and held it during the remainder of the operation, though not without some difficulty in consequence of his struggles. The operation was completed in two or three minutes, and the patient remained quietly on his back with his eyes closed. On examination the pupils were found to be dilated; the pulse was not materially affected. After he had lain about two minutes, I roused him with the inquiry, "How do you do to-day?" to which he replied, "Very well, I thank you." I then asked him what he had been doing. He said he believed he had been dreaming: he dreamed that he was at home and making some examination into his business. "Do you feel any pain?" "No." "How is that tumor of yours?" The patient raised himself in bed, looked at his thigh for a moment, and said, "It is gone, and I am glad of it." I then inquired if he had felt any pain during the operation, to which he replied in the negative. He soon recovered his natural state, experienced no inconvenience from the inhalation, was remarkably free from pain, and in three days went home into the country.

In all these cases there was a decided mitigation of pain; in most of them the patients, on the day after the operation, and at other times, stated that they had not been conscious of pain. All those who attended were, I think, satisfied of the efficacy of the application in preventing, or, at least, greatly diminishing, the suffering usual in such cases.

The phenomena presented in these operations afforded grounds for many interesting reflections, but it being my principal intention, at this time, to give a simple statement of facts, I shall not pursue the subject further, but close with two or three remarks:

First. The breathing of the ethereal vapor appears to operate directly on the cerebral system, and the consequent insensibility is proportionate to the degree of cerebral affection.

Second. Muscular power was for the time suspended in some cases; in others its loss was partial, and in one instance was scarcely sensible. The great relaxation of muscular action produced by a full dose of the application leads to the hope that it may be employed, with advantage, in cases of spasmodic affection, both by the surgeon and by the physician.

Third. The action of the heart is remarkably accelerated in some cases, but not in all.

Fourth. The respiration is sometimes stertorous, like that of apoplexy.

All these changes soon pass off without leaving any distinct traces behind them, and the ordinary state of the function returns. This has been the course of things in the cases I have witnessed, but I think it quite probable that so powerful an agent may sometimes produce other and even alarming effects. I, therefore, would recommend that it should never be employed except under the inspection of a judicious and competent person.

Let me conclude by congratulating my professional brethren on the acquisition of a mode of mitigating human suffering which may become a valuable agent, in the hands of careful and well-instructed practitioners, even if it should not prove of such general application as the imagination of sanguine persons would lead them to anticipate.

BOSTON, December 3, 1846.

SAMUEL J. MELTZER (1851–1920)

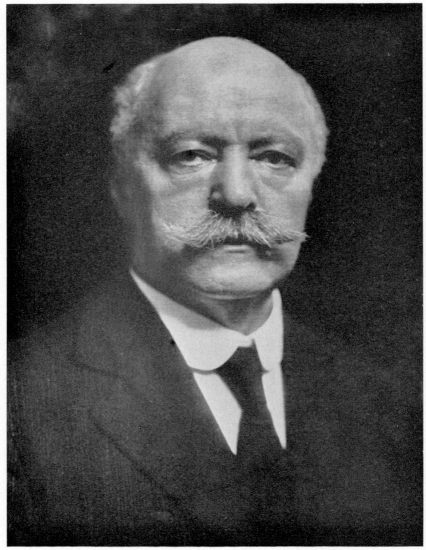

Samuel J. Meltzer was born on March 22, 1851, in Trape near Kovno, Lithuania. His early education was in a rabbinical seminary. Later he entered the University of Berlin where he studied philosophy and ultimately medicine. In 1882 he returned to Russia where he practised for a short time, and in 1883 he settled in the United States.

Dr. Meltzer did pioneer work in physiology and pharmacology and wrote more than 250 scientific articles. His work with Auer on endotracheal anesthesia won him the presidency of the American Association for Thoracic Surgery in 1919. He also did considerable work on the action of magnesium salts and developed the Meltzer–Lyon test associated with nonsurgical drainage of the gallbladder. From 1906 to 1920 he was head of the Department of Physiology and Pharmacology at the Rockefeller Institute. He was a dynamic, energetic, charming individual whose organizational ability made him president of many societies.

He died on November 7, 1920.

CONTINUOUS RESPIRATION WITHOUT RESPIRATORY MOVEMENTS

BY S. J. MELTZER AND JOHN AUER

*From the Department of Physiology and Pharmacology of
the Laboratories of the Rockefeller Institute for Medical Research*

T he object of the function of respiration is to supply the animal with oxygen and to remove carbon dioxide. To attain this object the vertebrates are provided with a complicated mechanism of which the respiratory movements are an essential feature. The respiration appears as a continuous chain of rhythmically recurring cycles, each cycle consisting of two antagonistic movements, one which carries air into the body and the other which assists its removal from the body. When the muscular activity of the body is eliminated by one cause or other and the exchange of the gases is carried on by so-called artificial respiration, again the respiration is rhythmically discontinuous and each cycle is composed of the two antagonistic movements: the inflow of air is carried on rhythmically by some external mechanism, while the return of the air is accomplished during the intermission by the elastic forces of the body. The rhythmic antagonistic movements seem thus to be inseparable from the function of respiration.

In studying recently the nature of the mechanism of the respiration in the presence of a double pneumothorax, while the animal is breathing compressed air by the Brauer method of overpressure, we discovered the fact that under certain conditions respiration can be carried on by continuous inflation of the lungs, and without any normal or

From *Journal of Experimental Medicine,* 1909, 11. Reprinted by permission.

38

artificial rhythmical respiratory movements whatever. This observation was verified by many experiments and we will describe here briefly the essential features of the experiment.

A longitudinal slit is made in the trachea of an anesthetized dog or rabbit and a glass tube introduced down to the tracheal bifurcation. The protruding end of the tube is then connected with a pressure bottle by means of a T-tube, the opening of the free branch of which is regulated by a screw clamp. The air which streams from the bottle under pressure partly escapes through the free branch of the T-tube and partly enters the trachea and reaches the bifurcation from which it returns through the space between tracheal wall and tube and escapes through the slit in the trachea and through mouth and nose. It is essential that the tube should fill out two-thirds of the lumen of the trachea, that the slit in the trachea be not too short and that the pressure of the air which enters the T-tube should amount to about fifteen to twenty millimeters of mercury. The pressure within the trachea is of course much lower than that. In the connection between the trachea and the pressure bottle are interpolated a manometer, an ether bottle and a bottle with Ringer's solution to keep the mucous membrane of the trachea moist. The essential point of the arrangement is that air is reaching the bifurcation under pressure and returns through another path than that through which it entered. When the air is thus circulating through the trachea the diaphragm descends, the thorax becomes moderately distended and the respiration mostly becomes very slow. The heart beats also frequently become dangerously slow. This danger, however, is easily obviated by an intravenous injection of one milligram of atropin: in a few seconds the pulse becomes frequent and remains so for many hours. The animal may receive now an intravenous injection of curare sufficient to completely abolish any spontaneous or reflex movements; its life is as safe as under regular artificial respiration, when the anterior thoracic wall is removed, the distended lungs are seen to be immobile while the heart continues to beat with a regular rhythm. If the above described arrangement is carried out properly the lungs retain their pink color, the heart continues to beat regularly and efficiently for many hours and the blood-pressure shows but little variation.

We have observed animals four hours and longer under these normal conditions. If the glass tube within the trachea is a little too wide or too narrow in relation to the lumen of the trachea the lungs acquire easily a slightly cyanotic appearance. But then a disconnection of the tube from the pressure bottle for two seconds, which means a momentary collapse of the lungs, restores immediately the pink color of the lungs and a repetition of this procedure once every three or four minutes is sufficient to maintain the life of the animal in a satisfactory fashion for many hours, although under these circumstances the blood-pressure is subject to frequent variations.

In another method, the tube which conveys the air to the lungs is short—a regular tracheotomy tube—and is tied in firmly in the upper part of the trachea, while another narrower tube is inserted into the trachea through a narrow opening made at a lower place. This tube reaches the bifurcation and serves for the removal of the air. This method also was found to do satisfactory service. In a third method, a long O'Dwyer tube, bent at right angles, was introduced through the mouth and inserted into the larynx. Through this tube a catheter was pushed into the trachea until it reached the bifurcation. Both tubes were then connected with the pressure bottle in such a manner as to let the air enter through the O'Dwyer tube and escape through the catheter. This arrangement, however, has failed as yet to give uniform results. The method, however, is surely capable of improvement and it is probable that it will finally give satisfactory results.

If the air is made to enter the lungs through a short tracheal tube finally tied into the trachea, the curarized animals die in a very short time from asphyxia. With this method, the spontaneous respirations of the animals are apparently indispensable for the maintenance of their life. The result is not perceptibly better even if the firmly tied-in tube reaches the bifurcation. The difficulty of this method consists mainly in the fact that the removal of the carbon dioxide has to take place against the stream of the air within the tube; while in our method the removal of the carbon dioxide is rather assisted by this stream of air.

The following three points are the essential factors in the success of our method: (1) The lungs are kept in continuous inspiratory state of distension which facilitates the exchange of the gases. (2) The fresh air reaches the lowest part of the trachea. (3) The air escapes by another path (although also through the trachea) than by the one it enters. Under these conditions the supply of oxygen and removal of carbon dioxide takes place apparently in physiological fashion without the aid of any rhythmic antagonistic movements.

Besides the direct physiological bearing of our experiments on the function of respiration the method is destined to be of methodical service in other physiological investigations, for instance in the study of the heart actions where the movement of the lungs is a disturbing factor. This method might in a certain way offer some advantages over the known methods of Langendorff and of Bock–Hering. Furthermore the method promises to be of practical service in various directions. We shall not omit to refer to two statements in the literature which can be considered as forerunners of our method. In the first place, there is the statement that Hook in 1667 maintained the life of a dog for an hour by continuous inflation of the lungs previously punctured at various places. In the second place, we have to mention Nagel's communication according to which the life of curarized pigeons was maintained by sending a continuous stream of air through the humerus which in birds is connected with the air sacs. In this case the air escaped through the trachea. In both instances the air escaped through the paths opposite to those through which it entered. In our method the air enters and escapes through the trachea, although through the separate paths within it.

3. The "Milieu Intérieur"

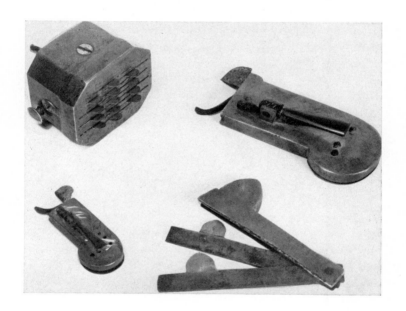

PREFATORY COMMENTS

For many centuries, blood-letting either by the use of mechanical devices or leeches was a common practice. The idea of administering blood germinated very slowly and flowered only during the past thirty years. The early days of direct transfusion have been depicted vividly by Crile and others. In 1915 Lewisohn provided the milestone advance in transfusion when he described the method of preserving blood by the addition of citrate. His pioneer spirit overcame the discouragement of a near fatality due to the experimental use of hirudin as an anticoagulant. Lewisohn's discovery made our present-day method of transfusing blood a reality. The judicious use of blood has markedly reduced the mortality of major operations and has encouraged the surgeon to embark upon more extensive procedures than his predecessors envisioned.

The development of other solutions was an outgrowth of a knowledge of fluid balance. This was not a hit-and-miss discovery but depended on controlled and carefully conducted experiments in the laboratory. A thorough understanding of fluid balance is a *sine qua non* for the well-trained surgeon.

MacCallum, Hartwell and Hoguet and Gamble showed that in the experimental animal pyloric obstruction resulted in hypochloremic alkalosis which could be combatted satisfactorily by the administration of saline solution.

We have elected to reprint MacCallum's original work which was begun in 1909 and published in 1920. He refuted the existence of a toxic substance in cases of high intestinal obstruction and maintained that replacement of chlorides could keep animals alive for long periods of time. Hayden and Orr, who also studied chemical changes in the blood, claimed that the sodium chloride was a specific antagonist of an unknown toxic substance. Unfortunately MacCallum's and Gamble's sound contributions were misinterpreted and salt solutions were given with great abandon for many unrelated conditions, with deleterious effects. It is within the scope of our recollections that patients in the early postoperative period were literally "drowned" by the administration of excessive amounts of saline solution. Finally Coller of Ann Arbor brought us to our senses with the publication of several papers emphasizing the desirability of curtailing and even abandoning salt solutions during the first few days after operation. Coller's observations should not detract from the significance of the need for chlorides which is as applicable today to the patient with pyloric obstruction as it was then. It emphasizes, however, a tendency of some to seize upon every new discovery and to apply it more widely than seemed indicated in the original description.

Although Darrow had previously stressed the importance of administering potassium to children ill with diarrhea, Lockwood and Randall first envisioned the efficacy of giving potassium to surgical patients. It became apparent that some patients showed evidence of deterioration characterized by apathy, asthenia and, in extreme cases, myasthenia, even though adequate amounts of water and salt had been administered in the early postoperative period. These authors described the dramatic response shown by such patients when ample amounts of potassium were given. When this monumental work was first published, many of us looked back on our experience and could recount deaths in patients that were completely preventable in the light of this newer knowledge. In 1949 Moore wrote a comprehensive article on the rates of absorption and the exchange of various electrolytes. His final paragraphs entitled "The need to be left alone" emphasized the fact that overzealous treatment by the enthusiast may be just as dangerous as undertreatment by the uninformed. This admonition was in keeping with the concept of the "milieu intérieur" as conceived by Claude Bernard. In our opinion, a practical approach to this problem is elucidated in the article by Randall which is reprinted here. Lack of space restricts us from reprinting the many significant contributions made by numerous authors to the study of electrolyte balance. We should be remiss in our obligation, however, if we failed to mention the voluminous and noteworthy writings of Selye of Montreal on the metabolic disorders associated with the "alarm reaction." Moore's classic description of the division of the postoperative period into four phases: first, the adrenergic-corticoid phase; second, the corticoid withdrawal phase; third, the anabolic gain; and finally, the fat-gain phase has given us a more profound understanding of how to treat a patient after he has suffered the trauma of surgery. It is for that reason that Moore's article is included as a milestone in this book.

These fundamental discoveries made it clear that the administration of parenteral fluids should be based on careful calculations of the patient's basic needs as well as his extraneous losses, made on a day-to-day basis. To ensure exact replacement of the latter losses several pharmaceutical companies have manufactured solutions that have the approximate composition of gastric secretions on the one hand and of bile, pancreatic and small-bowel losses on the other. When these and other solutions are used intelligently the patient can be maintained in a state of normal fluid and electrolyte balance.

With the advent of "tagging" with radioisotopes, there looms on the horizon the promise to acquire a more profound knowledge of fluid and electrolyte exchange.

RICHARD LEWISOHN (1875–   )

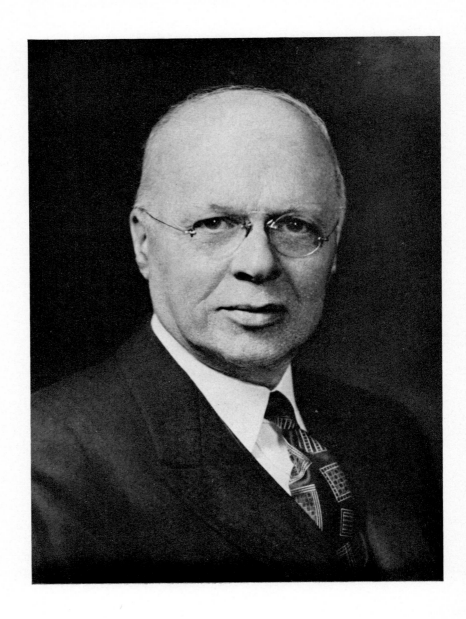

Richard Lewisohn was born in Hamburg, Germany, on July 12, 1875. He studied medicine at the following German Universities: Kiel, Strassburg, Berlin, Breslau, Freiburg. He was an assistant at the Jewish Hospital in Hamburg from 1900 to 1902, at the Senckenberg Pathological Institute under Professor Weigert from 1902 to 1904, and at the University surgical clinic in Heidelberg under Professor V. Czerny from 1904 to 1906. He came to the United States in 1906. Since 1907 he has been connected with the surgical department of Mount Sinai Hospital, New York City.

Dr. Lewisohn has written extensively on a variety of surgical subjects, particularly on blood transfusion and gastric surgery. He introduced the sodium citrate method of blood transfusion in January, 1915. He is a member of numerous surgical societies. In November, 1955, he was presented with the Karl Landsteiner Award, accompanied by the following citation: "For distinguished contribution to the field of blood-banking in discovering the use of sodium citrate as an anticoagulant which made possible the safe and effective storage of blood and the subsequent development of blood banks. A milestone in the history of medical science which has saved countless lives both in war and in peace and which has made possible further advances in the medical and surgical treatment of disease."

BLOOD TRANSFUSION BY THE CITRATE METHOD

BY RICHARD LEWISOHN, M.D.

Attending Surgeon, Beth Israel Hospital and Montefiore Home;
Associate Attending Surgeon, Mount Sinai Hospital, New York

In a preliminary communication I reported on a new method of performing blood transfusion with the aid of sodium citrate. This short report dealt mainly with the results of animal experiments. Since that time I have applied the citrate method in twenty-two blood transfusions on eighteen patients. I have thus been able to collect in a comparatively short time (about two months), partly with the kind aid of the staff of Mount Sinai Hospital, a sufficient number of cases to test the clinical value of this new and very simple method of blood transfusion. The object of this paper is to describe these clinical experiences, in the hope that the profession may be induced to give this method a trial on a larger scale and form their own opinions as to its clinical value.

HISTORY

The current idea, that transfusion of blood for therapeutic purposes dates back only a few decades, is an erroneous one. In fact, the history of blood transfusion (quoted from Amstel) takes us back as far as 1667, when Denis conceived the idea of blood transfer and used it successfully on the human being. The first one to make use of blood transfusion on a larger scale was Blundell, who reported four

From *Surgery, Gynecology and Obstetrics*, 21:37, 1915. Reprinted by permission of *Surgery, Gynecology and Obstetrics*.
Sixteen case reports have been omitted.

cases; two of these ended fatally, but the other two were successful. The largest amount of blood used in these cases was 480 cubic centimeters. It is interesting to note that the use of blood transfusion in puerperal fever dates back as far as 1829, although it has recently been again suggested by different authors. It would go far beyond the scope of this paper to give a detailed review of the extensive work in this field in the nineteenth century, although it is a most interesting study. Transfusion was used over fifty years ago in carbon monoxide-poisoning, eclampsia, leukaemia, etc. Toward the end of the last century it was gradually abandoned in favor of saline infusion. It is only since Carrel's masterful work in blood-vessel surgery that transfusion was taken up again on a large scale, especially in this country. The reason that Carrel's work was such a great step forward is that his method afforded for the first time a safe way of transferring blood from donor to recipient without the risks and dangers of coagulation. The artery-to-vein anastomosis was for a great many years the method of choice in blood transfusions. Its great technical difficulties were obviated to some extent by the use of certain cannulas (Crile, Elsberg, etc.). Later vein-to-vein anastomosis for transfusion was substituted as a more simple and quite as satisfactory a method as artery-to-vein anastomosis.

The greatest objection to the method of direct transfusion, as the anastomosis method is usually called, is not its minute and rather cumbersome technique, but the impossibility of ascertaining the exact amount of the transfused blood. It is obvious that this is a serious objection. That is one of the reasons why in such a short time the syringe method of Lindeman become so popular that it practically did away with all the different direct methods. It might be of historical interest to state here that practically this same method was used by Ziemssen about twenty years ago. It never became popular, however, and was almost forgotten, until Lindeman revived it. There can be no doubt that the syringe method gives excellent results in the hands of experts. It is not a method, however, which can be used by any physician, or for that matter any surgeon, without strict observance of a great many technical details. The syringe method requires for its proper execution three or four people, who must work together with great precision. Furthermore, the method is an expensive one. The usual set consists of twelve twenty-cubic-centimeter record syringes; and if not handled very carefully they break easily, especially during the process of boiling.

The best proof that the method is not an ideal one lies in the fact that since Lindeman's publication several other methods have been devised which modify it. Modifications always tend to show that the original method is not perfect, for nobody will try to improve upon a method which is perfectly satisfactory in everybody's hands. Unger has lately constructed a very ingenious apparatus, which is an improvement on Lindeman's technique. Its essential feature is that the aspiration and injection of the blood is regulated by a double-way stop-cock. In this manner the team-work between the two men working on the donor's arm and the recipient's arm respectively is replaced by a piece of machinery and the prompt working of aspiration and injection of the blood is assured.

Kimpton advised the use of large paraffin-coated glass cylinders (150 to 250 ccm.); after the collection of the blood the cylinder is attached to the recipient's vein and the blood injected with the aid of rubber bulb. Satterlee and Hooker used weak solutions of hirudin, to rinse out their cannulas and glass cylinders, minimizing the danger of coagulation of the blood during transfer.

The fundamental difference between all methods of transfusion heretofore suggested and the citrate method which shall be described in detail in this paper is based on the following considerations: All the older methods consider the coagulation time of the blood, which normally occurs in about five minutes after the blood has left the vessels, as a *noli me tangere*. They all tried to adapt their methods to this well-known fact. That is the reason why the vessel anastomosis met with success. The adaptation of endothelium to endothelium is, as we all know, a safe way of preventing coagulation. The danger of coagulation makes the use of a set of small syringes (20 ccm.) imperative for the syringe method, instead of one or two large syringes (200 to 300 ccm.), and thus complicates the method materially.

Any transfusion, in which the normal coagulation time of the blood is considered as an unalterable factor, is apt to be difficult and apt to require a great deal of personel experience and skill. Must we accept this coagulation time as an unchangeable law? Might it not be possible to inhibit the danger of the clotting of the blood during its transfer without diminishing the clinical value of the transferred blood for the recipient? This was the problem to be worked out, and it seemed to me that this problem would be worth a thorough and careful investigation. If solved, blood transfusion, which so far has given only good results in the hands of a limited number, would be changed from a very complicated and difficult method to one of greatest simplicity. Special clinical skill and experience for this work would not longer be required, no haste would be necessary in the performance of transfusion; in short, blood transfusion would be technically as easy as an ordinary saline infusion.

EXPERIMENTS

The problem, then, was to find a chemical substance which would retard the coagulation of the blood for at least thirty minutes, so as to guarantee a safe transfer of the blood without any haste. Furthermore, this substance had to be conditionally atoxic, so that large transfusions of blood (up to 1500 ccm.) could be performed with perfect safety.

Several anticoagulating substances are well known in physiological chemistry and have been used extensively in the laboratories: hirudin (leech extract), sodium citrate, sodium oxalate, peptone, glucose, etc.

My work was commenced by testing hirudin. Hirudin has been used quite extensively in Germany in the treatment of eclampsia. Engelmann reported 14 cases, in which he used up to 0.3 grams of hirudin intravenously without any toxic symptoms. We know from the work of Friedrich that 0.1 gram of hirudin prevents 750 ccm. of blood from coagulating. From a series of experiments on blood received from patients, where a phlebotomy was indicated, it became apparent that the smallest dose of hirudin applicable for our purpose was 0.03 grams of hirudin to 200 cubic centimeters of blood. For the average transfusion of 1000 cubic centimeters we would then use 0.15 grams of hirudin, only half of the dose injected by Engelmann in eclampsia. Preliminary to using hirudin on the human being, I injected up to 0.1 gram of hirudin intravenously into some medium-sized dogs. One dog died four hours after the injection, but we thought this might be due to an overfilling of the circulatory system, as we had diluted 0.1 gram of hirudin with 100 cubic centimeters of saline solution. The other dogs (0.1 gram of hirudin diluted in 20 cubic centimeters of solution) showed no ill effects (after having been observed five days). I then used hirudin on a patient who had an inoperable carcinoma of the stomach (exploratory laparotomy). As she needed a saline infusion the day following the operation, I added 0.1 gram of hirudin (Sachsse) to 500 ccm. of saline solution. The symptoms following this infusion were most alarming; cyanosis and precordial pain set in immediately, followed by a severe chill. Her pulse became almost imperceptible; she was in a precarious condition for over thirty-six hours and recovered only very slowly from this severe reaction.

This experience naturally ended further trials with hirudin. Engelmann's reports might induce other investigators to use comparatively large doses of hirudin for different diseases, and it is just this possibility which has induced me, although the results were negative, to embody in my paper these tests with hirudin as a warning against its use.

After the failure of my experiments with hirudin I took up experiments with sodium citrate to test its possible usefulness for our purpose. When I began my experiments with the citrate method I looked over the current literature, but was unable to find any reference to any work done along these lines. After my work had come to a successful conclusion I found that a paper published by Hustin in May, 1914, had escaped my notice. It appears from this paper that the priority, not only for taking up this problem in a series of animal experiments, but in applying it successfully in a case of human blood transfusion, belongs to Hustin, though his method, as we shall see later, limited its usefulness to small transfusions.

Again, as in my experiments with hirudin, the first series of investigations was carried out with the object of finding the smallest dose of sodium citrate required to keep the blood from clotting for thirty minutes. We took ten test tubes containing 0.1, 0.2, 0.3, etc., up to one cubic centimeter of a 10 per cent solution of sodium citrate. A dog was narcotized and 10 cubic centimeters of blood, taken from his jugular vein, poured into each of the test tubes; another test tube, not containing any citrate, was filled with 10 ccm. of blood. The blood in the first test tube, containing 0.01 sodium citrate to 10 ccm. of blood, clotted just as quickly as the blood in the control; namely, in about five minutes. The blood in the next tube (0.2 per cent) did not clot for two days. On the third day this tube, as well as the next one (0.3 per cent), showed a soft clot, whereas the rest of them (0.4, 0.5 per cent, etc.) were still fluid. These experiments were repeated at different times, always with the same results. The interesting fact elicited from these experiments was that sodium citrate mixed at the rate of 0.1 per cent does not change the coagulation time of blood, but that a mixture of the sodium citrate with blood at the ratio of 0.2 per cent prevents the blood in the test tubes from clotting for three days. The quantity of citrate needed for this object lies just below 0.15 per cent, but in order to be on the safe side it seems advisable to fix the ratio needed for our purpose as 0.2 per cent. Exactly the same rulings were proved to hold good for human blood.

The next question to be answered was in reference to the toxicity of sodium citrate. If the citrate method was to compete with the older transfusion methods, it had to be applicable to transfusions as large as 1,500 ccm. It was not sufficient to prove that small quantities of blood (that is 200 ccm.) could be transfused with this method without risk to the patient. I am sure that hirudin would have answered the problem if we had expected to transfuse only small quantities. In a great many cases, however—in fact, in the great majority of blood transfusions—it is necessary to transfuse 700 to 1,000 cubic centimeters and sometimes more. The whole method would have only a limited field of usefulness, if we could not use it for large transfusions with perfect safety to the patient.

Sodium citrate can be used with perfect safety at the ratio of 0.2 per cent. Three hundred cubic centimeters of blood were removed from a dog's carotid artery, mixed with sodium citrate (0.06 gram) and reinjected into the jugular vein of the same dog. No ill effect was noticed during the observation time (two weeks). This experiment was repeated a few times with exactly the same result.

On the other hand, sodium citrate is only conditionally atoxic, which means that we cannot inject any unlimited quantity of sodium citrate into the vascular system without running a great risk. This is proved by the following experiments, which differed from those just described only in so far as the dose of citrate was increased. I took a dog weighing 11 pounds and mixed the blood with 15 ccm. of a 10 per cent solution of sodium citrate. The dog died almost instantaneously. This experiment was repeated twice with exactly the same fatal result. It follows that we have to consider 1.5 grams of sodium citrate as a fatal dose for a dog weighing eleven pounds. Fifteen grams would then be a fatal dose for a patient weighing one hundred and ten pounds. As even 10 grams would nearly reach the fatal limit, it would be utterly impossible to apply this method, if the 1 per cent ratio, as suggested by Weil, would really present the smallest dose of sodium citrate necessary for our purpose. The whole method would then be applicable only for small transfusions (Weil has injected 250 ccm. of blood mixed with 2.5 grams of sodium citrate), and would thus have a rather limited field of usefulness. Hustin also thought, that 0.2 per cent was too small a dose to keep the blood from clotting, and therefore mixed the citrated blood with the same amount of saline solution, adding some glucose, which is a well-known means of retarding coagulation. Here again the adding of an equal amount of saline solution to a given quantity of blood would limit its application to small transfusions (Hustin transfused only 150 ccm. in the one case referred to above); it would not be practical from a clinical standpoint to add 1,000 ccm. of saline solution to a blood transfusion of 1,000 ccm.

The third point of interest, in addition to the questions of dose and toxicity, is the question of the coagulation time of the recipient's blood after the transfusion. We have seen that blood mixed with 0.2 per cent sodium citrate does not clot outside the body in two to three days. If this fact would hold good after the injection of the citrated blood into the recipient, the older, though more complicated methods, would have clinically such an advantage over this method that this paper need not have been written. However, confirming a statement made by Weil at the New York Academy of Medicine, animal experiments and experience in human blood transfusions show, the most interesting fact, that the same citrated blood which does not coagulate outside the body in two days, does not retard the coagulation of the general blood volume. On the contrary, the coagulation seems to be temporarily hastened. Three hundred cubic centimeters of blood were taken from a dog, mixed with citrate (0.2 per cent) and reinjected. The time for the coagulation of the normal blood taken before the experiment was started was five minutes. Blood taken from the same dog three minutes after the reinjection of the citrated blood showed that coagulation occurred after only ten seconds. A third test taken three minutes later showed the same result as the second.

This question certainly would lend itself to a further and more detailed investigation. We have not been able to find in our human blood transfusions any marked changes of the coagulation. The marked hastening of the coagulation of the blood, which we found in the dog experiment, does not seem to hold good, at least not to that extent, for human blood. And if it does, it is of such a short duration that it escaped our notice, as most of our coagulation time tests were taken a few hours or the day after the transfusion. There certainly does not exist, however, any marked retarding of the coagulation after a citrate transfusion, a fact which is of the utmost importance for the question of blood transfusion by the citrate method.

TECHNIQUE

Before describing the technique of blood transfusion by the citrate method, I would like to say a few words about the donor, as I consider the proper selection of a suitable donor of the greatest importance. The donor ought to be a strong, husky individual with prominent veins. It is not advisable as a rule to use members of the patient's family, as they are, often, naturally very excited about the condition of the patient and do not stand the loss of blood as well as a professional donor, who offers his blood for a monetary consideration and has no personal interest at stake. I have seen donors who have given up large quantities of blood for transfusion at short intervals— ten to twelve times inside of twelve months. Though no fixed laws can be laid down, it is advisable to refuse donors who have been repeatedly used. It is needless to say that all the preliminary tests (Wassermann, agglutination, haemolysis, etc.) must be done just as well with the citrate method as with other methods. There is no doubt that the procuring of a donor and the necessary blood tests make transfusion impossible, when needed on the spur of the moment. In exceptional cases (see Case 16) transfusion may be done without the tests; as a rule it is certainly wise to wait for the tests, which can be done in a few hours.

The technique of the citrate method is so simple that it can be dealt with in a few words. The donor is put on a table, a tourniquet applied to the arm, and the vein punctured with a cannula. The blood is received in a sterile graduated glass jar (500 ccm.) containing 25 cubic centimeters of a 2 per cent sterile solution of sodium citrate at the bottom. While the blood is running into the glass receptacle, it is well mixed with the citrate solution by means of a glass rod. After 250 cubic centimeters of blood have been taken another 25 cubic centimeters of citrate solution are added. If less than 500 cubic centimeters of blood are taken (i.e., in infants), the amount of citrate solution added to the blood is reduced accordingly. In cases where we expect to take more than 500 cubic centimeters of blood we have another glass container (500 ccm.) ready to be used in exactly the same manner. The glass jar containing the blood is then put aside and covered with a towel to safeguard against contamination. I have not found it necessary to immerse it in hot water or surround the jar with an asbestos covering. The blood is then taken either into the recipient's room or the recipient is brought into the operating room. I consider it a great advantage that this method does not require donor and recipient to be in the same room; this lessens the physical shock of the whole procedure for the patient. In fact the donor's blood may be collected in the laboratory or office and carried to the patient's bedside (Kaliski).

Another very great advantage of the citrate method is that as there is no connection between the donor and recipient the donor is safeguarded against contagion of any disease or infection which the patient may have.

The recipient's vein is then punctured or exposed by a small incision; the cannula is introduced and attached to a salvarsan flask or a glass funnel. It is advisable to fill the rubber tubing connection between flask and cannula with some saline solution, so as to prevent air from getting into the circulation. After the connection is made the blood is poured into the salvarsan apparatus. In order to prevent sudden overloading of the circulation it is advisable (especially in larger transfusions) to stop the flow of blood from time to time by compressing the rubber tubing. After the blood has been injected the cannula is removed and the transfusion is thus ended. The whole procedure can be performed with the greatest ease and without any hurry, because the citrated blood, as we have seen above, can be kept for two or three days in the glass jar without danger or clotting.

It is rather immaterial what size needle we use for the injection of the blood; in children, for instance, we can use a very fine Goldenberg or Schreiber needle. But it is of the greatest importance for the successful application of the citrate method that we use a large size cannula in taking the donor's blood. I have lately punctured the vein with a Kaliski cannula (gauge 11, B. & S.), and thus collected 500 cubic centimeters of blood in less than five minutes. The shape and construction of the needle (Linderman, Kaliski, Unger, etc.) are immaterial so long as one uses one of large caliber. I would like to warn against the use of needles of smaller caliber (for instance, 14 or 16), because if the blood does not shoot out of the vein, and comes out only drop by drop, the blood is apt to clot in the glass jar. I suppose that Zingher, who has lately published a paper, advising a combination of the Lindeman and the citrate method, did not use needles of sufficiently large caliber. For if we use needles of sufficiently large caliber, we do not need syringes, which only complicate this method, and certainly are not to be considered as an improvement in the technique.

The 2 per cent citrate solution can be sterilized and resterilized without losing its efficiency. I selected a 2 per cent solution because it simplifies the calculation (30 solution to 300 blood). By varying the percentage one can easily reduce the quantity of solution to be added to the blood. It might be just as advisable, for instance, to add 50 ccm. of a 4 per cent solution to 1,000 ccm. of blood. I have had made up sterile glass tubes (like those for saline solution) containing 50 ccm. of the 2 per cent solution ready for immediate use.

[*Ed. Note:* Eighteen cases are reported. Two illustrative cases are presented.]

CASE 7. B. F., Mount Sinai Hospital. Diagnosis: Carcinoma of the stomach; Virchow node present. Patient had had a Satterlee-Hooker transfusion a few weeks before, followed by a very severe reaction (temperature of 104°, chills, etc.). Haemoglobin 23 per cent. January 24: Transfusion of 700 ccm. of blood. Haemoglobin after transfusion 27 per cent. January 25: Haemoglobin 34 per cent. No rise in temperature followed this transfusion, no reaction in any way. Immediately after the transfusion the supraclavicular lymph-node was removed under local anaesthesia by Dr. Lilienthal. Microscopical report: Carcinoma. January 26: Haemoglobin 39 per cent. January 28: Haemoglobin 34 per cent. January 29: Patient left the hospital.

This case was interesting mainly in so far as when the node was removed immediately after the transfusion, there was very little bleeding. This case and other cases in this series tend to show that one can safely operate immediately after the citrate transfusion, which is in accord with the experimental findings.

CASE 10. M. S., age 22, Roosevelt Hospital. Diagnosis: Adenocarcinoma of rectum.

February 11: Transfusion of 800 ccm. of blood. Haemoglobin before transfusion 38 per cent; erythrocytes 3,600,000. Haemoglobin after transfusion 50 per cent; erythrocytes 4,300,000. February 12: Haemoglobin 55 per cent. February 16: Exploratory operation was done. The tumor was found to be inoperable.

The indication for transfusion preliminary to a major operation seems to be a very good one, especially when the patients are cachectic. They thus have a much better chance to stand a major surgical operation.

CONCLUSIONS

I have intentionally given a rather detailed account of the cases in order that the reader may be enabled to form his own opinion concerning the merits of the citrate method. I have embodied in this list only those cases in which the transfusion was performed by me and which I had occasion to follow up after the transfusion. I have not included half a dozen cases done by others of which I have personal knowledge; the results of this new method seem to have been just as satisfactory in the hands of others as in my own. They all seem to welcome the easy and safe way with which transfusion can be performed.

The clinical material of this review of 22 citrate transfusions in 18 cases is comprised of the following cases: Inoperable carcinoma, 3 cases; preoperative transfusions, 3 cases; purpura haemorrhagica and allied conditions, 5 cases; lymphatic leukaemia, 1 case; severe anaemia, 2 cases; gastric haemorrhage, 2 cases; actinomycosis, 1 case; puerperal sepsis, 1 case. Out of these 18 cases 4 were transfused twice within short intervals.

All the points of clinical interest have been discussed in the records of the cases. However, I would like to dwell on some which are of importance, not only in regard to the citrate method but in reference to any human blood transfusion.

Some of the cases showed a rather marked polyuria lasting twenty-four hours, though I must say that this increased excretion of urine appeared only in a small percentage; none of the cases showed any macroscopical or microscopical changes in the urine. A marked rise of temperature was noted in 5 cases, 3 of which were accompanied by a chill after the transfusion. It is possible that some rises in temperature escaped our notice, as the patients were running septic temperatures before the transfusions. It is a well-known fact that chills following transfusion, or even simple saline infusions, occur rather frequently (Lindeman had 22 chills in a series of 62 cases). In our series chills were observed in three cases out of twenty-two transfusions.

A good indicator of an effective transfusion of blood is the automatic rise of the haemoglobin after the transfusion. For instance, by a transfusion we raise the haemoglobin of the patient from 20 per cent to 40 per cent, and we notice during the following week that the haemoglobin goes up automatically another 10 to 12 per cent. This rise of the haemoglobin was noticed in a large number of our cases and is a proof of the good clinical value of the citrated blood.

The question of the coagulation time has been discussed above. If the hastening of coagulation after the injection of citrated blood, as apparent from animal experiments and some experiences on the human being, were to last any length of time, it would be of the greatest value in different haemorrhagic conditions (especially haemophilia). The shortening of the coagulation time is, however, of such transitory nature, the clinical conditions existing before the transfusions are reëstablished so quickly, that we cannot expect any greater help for these diseases from the citrate method than from any other method of transfusion.

It would be very tempting to enter upon the broad question of the indications calling for blood transfusions. This paper, however, was written mainly to advocate a new method of transfusion, and a thorough investigation of these indications would go beyond its scope. Furthermore, Ottenberg and Libman have taken up this subject in an admirable paper on "Blood Transfusions, Indications, Results, General Management," which will be published in the near future. Their paper, based on experiences in 212 cases of blood transfusions, dwells upon all the interesting factors of this subject. It must be considered as one of the most valuable publications in this field.

Transfusion of blood, as we have seen above, had a very varied career in our medical armamentarium. Though practically forgotten for nearly a century, it has been revived in the last decade, and on account of great improvements in the technique (uppermost among them the blood tests for agglutination and haemolysis) transfusion is now to be considered a safe method, yielding excellent results in properly selected cases. The success of transfusions is most striking in profuse haemorrhage (ulcer of the stomach and duodenum, ectopic pregnancy, typhoid and cholaemic haemorrhages, etc.), in different forms of poisoning, and in some haemorrhagic conditions. It produces excellent and lasting results in cases of primary and secondary anaemia, whereas improvements following transfusions in different forms of leukaemia and pernicious anaemia are not as a rule of a lasting character. I think transfusion ought to be practiced much more than heretofore as a preparatory step in cachectic patients who are to undergo extensive operations. Operative shock seems to be a promising field, though the experiences of Ottenberg and Libman are not very encouraging. Though a great deal has been written on this subject in the last year, some of the indications for transfusion in sepsis and tuberculosis are still very questionable. If we approach the question of transfusion without too great an optimism on the one hand and without being overskeptical on the other hand, we are sure to make progress in this most interesting field. Transfusion is not a panacea for every disease, but it certainly has a wide field of usefulness.

I am well aware that this new method of transfusion has to be tested on a much larger scale before definite judgment can be passed upon it. However, I think that the reports given above are sufficiently encouraging to induce the profession to give this method a fair trial. I feel assured that the citrate method has come to stay. Clinically, it appears to be as good as any of the older methods, and at the same time it has the advantage of the utmost simplicity.

WILLIAM GEORGE MacCALLUM (1874–1944)

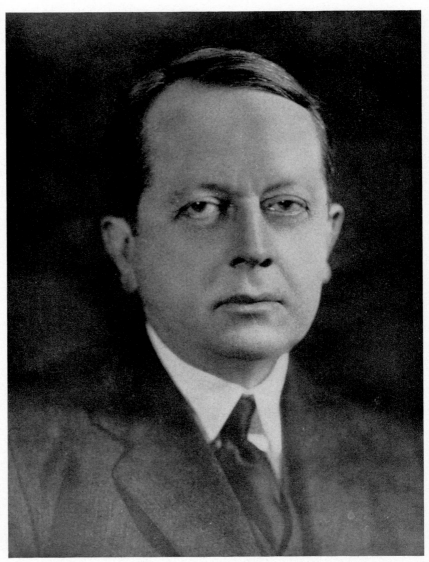

William George MacCallum was born in Dunnville, Ontario, on April 18, 1874. He was graduated from the University of Toronto and took his early medical training at Johns Hopkins. He ultimately became Director of Pathology at Johns Hopkins and except for a stay at Columbia from 1909–1917, did most of his work in Baltimore. His textbook on pathology, published in 1916, was used as a standard text in many schools. He did pioneer work on malaria, pancreatic glycosuria, cirrhosis of the liver, virus infections and parathyroid physiology. His work on pyloric obstruction was published in 1920, eight years after the Hartwell and Hoguet report. However, his experiments began in 1909, and his data were more complete.

He died on February 3, 1944.

THE EFFECT OF PYLORIC
OBSTRUCTION IN
RELATION TO GASTRIC TETANY[1]

BY W. G. MacCALLUM, JOSEPH LINTZ,
H. N. VERMILYE, T. H. LEGGETT,
AND E. BOAS

*From the Pathological Departments of Columbia University
and The Johns Hopkins University*

The nature of gastric tetany has long been a matter of interest and the theories already advanced to account for it are quite unsatisfactory. According to one it is due to desiccation of the tissues, whereas another ascribes it to the absorption of toxic materials from the stagnating contents of the dilated stomach. It is known that if a communication be established between the stomach and the intestine by a gastroenterostomy so that the contents of the stomach can once more pass into the intestine, the symptoms disappear at once. It was with the desire of determining the nature of the changes produced by pyloric obstruction that the following experiments were carried out. But, although

[1] These experiments were begun in 1909 in Baltimore, where all the effects of pyloric obstruction and of the administration of chlorides and hydrochloric acid were observed. They were resumed later with more accurate quantitative measurements in New York.

They were described, practically as they now appear, at the meeting of the American Society for Experimental Pathology held in New York with the Federation of Biological Associations at Cornell University Medical School in January, 1917, but various circumstances connected with my leaving New York for Baltimore and the press of work during the war have delayed their publication up to the present. In the meanwhile a paper by W. S. McCann has appeared in the *Journal of Biological Chemistry*, 1918, xxxv, 553, which describes quite similar experiments and results but with a somewhat different interpretation. (W. G. M.)

From the *Bulletin of The Johns Hopkins Hospital*, January, 1920. Reprinted by permission.

they give clear evidence that a certain chain of events follows such an obstruction, they do not necessarily give an explanation of gastric tetany in the human being, and we have had no opportunity to make the same observations on man.

It was observed long ago (1909) by one of us (MacCallum) that when the pylorus was completely obstructed and the stomach frequently washed out, an animal wasted rapidly and died in a few days, usually with violent convulsions which were not precisely of the same character as the twitchings seen in parathyroid tetany.

We held the idea at that time that, since nothing was absorbed from the stomach, while water was given abundantly through the intestine, the older explanations offered for gastric tetany were faulty and that the convulsions must be due to loss of hydrochloric acid in the gastric juice. Later experiments have supported this view and we have tried to work out the nature of the whole disturbance.

Although many different methods have been employed from time to time in the attempt to obstruct the pylorus partially or completely we finally returned to the simplest, which consists in cutting through the stomach just above the pylorus and closing it off with sutures so that it becomes a blind sac on the end of the oesophagus. The pyloric end with the duodenum was then brought into the abdominal wound and sutured there. Through it food and water were given, but in the later experiments, in order to eliminate all intake of chlorides and to prevent loss of bile and intestinal contents, the opening was closed except for a tube through which distilled water was introduced. The food which could be given in this way always contained chlorides and when it was given the symptoms following pyloric obstruction appeared only slowly so that the animal lived about a week. When nothing but water was given, convulsions appeared in about 48 hours and death soon followed. Such a result could not be due to starvation, because a dog will live a long time without food.

It is unfortunate that our observations upon the daily intake and output of chlorides are not more complete, but they are sufficient to show that under the conditions of the operation, even when no chlorides are given in the food, the obstructed stomach continues to secrete hydrochloric acid. Estimation of the chlorides in the stomach washings show that a considerable amount is lost to the body and this must be sufficient, in the absence of any intake, to lower the chlorides of the body rapidly. Indeed it is difficult to devise any other way in which such an abstraction of chlorides could be attained since the tissues ordinarily hold tenaciously to their chloride content when the intake is decreased. It seems that the gastric mucosa can still exercise its function of secreting hydrochloric acid even when the plasma chlorides are diminished.

6709. Pylorus obstructed May 6, 1909. Animal fed through intestinal fistula with sugar and beef together with distilled water. Six days later, May 12, violent twitching and stiffness, flexor spasm of fore feet and rigid clinching of jaws. Toward the end of the experiment sodium chloride was injected intravenously and relieved the twitching. Chlorides estimated in the washings from the stomach as follows:

6709 Chlorides as NaCl	6	7	8	May 9	10	11	12	13
Gastric fluid	...	1.56	3.0	3.3	.42	...	...	...
Urine	...	.27	.56	.22	1.6	.65	1.9	...

6909. Pylorus obstructed May 18, 1909. Animal fed as above with washed beef, sugar and water. Well until May 23, when there was violent twitching of all the muscles. Was given calcium lactate intravenously which diminished the twitching.

6909 Chlorides as NaCl	18	19	May 20	21	22	23
Gastric fluid	...	5.37	4.8	2.7	2.6	...
Urine	...	....	2.2	1.6	.72	3.2

6309. Pylorus obstructed April 22, 1909. Fed with capsules of dried washed beef (chloride free) and water. Slight twitching beginning April 27. Was given sodium chloride intravenously. Died late next night.

6309 Chlorides as NaCl	22	23	April 24	25	26	27
Gastric fluid	...	...	1.7	3.07	3.1	1.4
Urine	...	...	2.7	.6	...	...

These observations show that the loss of chlorides from the stomach was continued for days after the operation. The excretion in the urine tended to decrease day by day after the operation. Later when we had found that the analysis of the blood plasma showed more directly and more precisely the changes in the chlorides, we made these determinations every day and ceased to analyze stomach washings and excreta for chlorides.

Since the chloride lost in the gastric juice is in the form of free hydrochloric acid, it seemed probable that the sodium ion would be retained in the circulating fluids and that the alkali reserve of the blood might be increased.

In the next series of experiments, therefore, we studied the changes in the plasma chlorides, the alkali reserve as determined by Van Slyke's method and the electrical excitability of the nerves.

In brief we found that, especially in those cases in which no chlorides were given by the intestinal fistula, the recognizable chlorides in the plasma dropped rapidly. The average course taken from 12 cases was as follows, beginning with the day of the operation: 6.6, 6.4, 5.1, 4.6, 3.9, but in some cases the chloride content of the plasma fell to 2.5 or 2.8.

The carbon dioxide combining power was found to rise as the chlorides decreased. Averaging once more eight cases in which this is tabulated we find that the change proceeds as follows, beginning with the day of operation: 46.2, 42.4, 55.2, 61.1, 66.6, 71.9, 74.7, 80 (volume in c. c. per 100 c. c. blood). It is hardly possible to average the records of the electrical excitability, but an approximation was made in six cases by adding the figures KC, KO, AC and AO into one figure for each observation. Then if these figures be averaged for the series of animals beginning with the day of operation they run as follows: 7.6, 7.1, 4.5, 2.8, in which of course the lowest number represents the lowest current necessary and therefore the highest excitability.

The following are illustrative protocols:

1605. Pylorus obstructed October 30, 1916. Animal fed through the intestinal fistula with milk and eggs; developed distinct tetany-like twitchings on November 6, followed by violent convulsions and death. During this time the dog's weight sank from 7630 grams to 6210 grams. Electrical excitability was very distinctly heightened. The plasma chlorides sank.

| 1605 | October | | November | | | | | |
	30	31	1	2	3	4	5	6
	Operation						Tetany	
Electrical excitability ⌈KC	......	0.2	....	0.2	...	0.05	......	0.05
⎸KO	......	Neg. 5	....	Neg. 5	...	Neg. 5	......	1.2
⎸AC	......	1.0	....	0.4	...	0.4	......	0.4
⌊AO	......	1.0	....	1.2	...	1.2	......	0.4
Plasma chlorides	......	......	6.41	5.67	...	5.67	......	4.10

1609. Pylorus obstructed November 24, 1916. Fed through fistula with milk and eggs. On November 27, distinct tetanic twitchings were developed with high electrical excitability. An intravenous injection of 35 c. c. of 10% NaCl was given which relieved the twitchings but these reappeared the next day and the dog died.

| 1609 | November | | | | | |
	23	24	25	26	27	28
		Pyloric obstruction			NaCl ↓	
Electrical excitability ⌈KC	0.3	....	0.2	....	0.15 0.3 0.4	0.3
⎸KO	Neg. 5	....	Neg. 5	....	1.4 3.6 2.2	1.8
⎸AC	1.2	....	0.8	....	0.8 0.7 1.3	0.8
⌊AO	1.4	....	1.6	...	0.4 1.2 2.5	1.2
Plasma chlorides	7.4	....	......	5.43	4.9 6.4 5.8	5.3
Total NaCl intake	1.20	1.24	1.31	1.33	3.95 ...	Neg. Bal.
Total NaCl output	2.11	1.30	5.33	2.81	2.92 ...	5.44

1612. After a preliminary operation to establish an intestinal fistula on Dec. 2, 1916, the pylorus was obstructed on December 8. The dog lived until Dec. 14. There was nothing resembling tetany but observations on

| 1612 | December | | | | | | | |
	7	8	9	10	11	12	13	14
Electrical excitability ⌈KC	....	0.2	0.3	0.3	0.2	0.3	0.3	0.2
⎸KO	....	Neg. 5	Neg. 5	Neg. 5	Neg. 5	Neg. 5	Neg. 5	3.0
⎸AC	....	1.2	1.4	1.4	1.0	1.2	1.2	1.0
⌊AO	....	2.6	2.8	2.4	2.0	2.0	1.8	1.0
Plasma chlorides	6.6	6.7	6.8	5.7	5.4	4.7	4.3	2.5
CO_2 combining power (vols. in c. c. per 100 c. c. of blood)	....	49.0	58.6	62.4	61.4	63.3	74.9	80
Total NaCl intake	1.43	1.27	1.34	1.28	1.1	1.1	1.06	
Total NaCl output	1.48	0.75	3.09	0.2	1.48	....	2.14	

the chlorides and the alkali reserve are recorded. The animal was fed with milk, eggs and sugar.

1618. Pyloric obstruction December 14, 1916. Given distilled water only through intestinal fistula; developed distinct and continuous twitchings on December 16 and died.

1618		December 14	15	16
Electrical excitability	KC	....	0.2	0.2	0.2
	KO	....	Neg. 5	Neg. 5	1.8
	AC	....	0.8	1.0	0.6
	AO	....	1.4	1.8	1.0
Plasma chlorides		6.6	6.7	5.5	4.4
CO_2 combining power		46.7	39.1	43.0	33.1

1620. Pylorus obstructed December 17, 1916. Dog given distilled water only through intestine. Violent convulsion with opisthotonos on December 19. Electrical excitability greatly increased, plasma chlorides diminished. Alkali reserve not greatly heightened. Given 50 c. c. of 1% HCl intravenously. This lowered the alkali reserve but scarcely affected the electrical excitability. Died about four hours later.

1620		17	18	December 19			
				Convulsion		HCl	
Electrical excitability	KC	0.2	0.2	0.2	0.1 ↓	0.3	0.4
	KO	Neg. 5	Neg. 5	1.0	1.2	1.6	1.8
	AC	1.0	1.0	0.8	0.6	0.6	1.2
	AO	1.4	0.4	0.8	1.2	0.8	0.8
Plasma chlorides		......	7.2	5.63	5.22	....	
CO_2 combining power		4.15	38.2	57.3	50.7	47.5	

1621. Pylorus obstructed December 18, 1916. Given only distilled water through intestinal fistula. On December 20 extremely weak and apathetic. No twitching but occasional convulsive stretching into a position of

1621		18	19	December 20		21	22	23
				NaCl injected				
Electrical excitability	KC	....	0.1	0.1	0.1 ↓ 0.2	0.1	0.1	
	KO	....	Neg. 5	1.6	2.2	5.0	2.4	4.4
	AC	....	1.0	0.4	0.4	1.6	0.8	0.8
	AO	....	1.0	1.2	1.0	1.2	1.2	1.6
Plasma chlorides		6.9	7.7	5.8	3.8	6.0	5.6	4.5	4.2
CO_2 combining power		43.4	41.4	49.3	64.5	61.2	61.7	50.7	74.7

opisthotonos. Given 50 c. c. 2 M. NaCl intravenously. Much improved and lived for three days longer with gradual reproduction of the same condition.

1622. Pylorus obstructed December 18, 1916. Animal given only distilled water through the intestinal fistula. The dog lived five days during which the plasma chlorides became greatly diminished and the alkali reserve increased. An attempt to introduce $\frac{N}{10}$ HCl in dilute solution ended fatally.

1622			December					
		18	19	20	21	22	23	
							$\frac{N}{10}$ HCl	
Electrical excitability	KC	....	0.1	0.1	0.3	0.3	0.1 ↓	0.3
	KO	....	Neg. 5	5.0	Neg. 5	Neg. 5	Neg. 5	Neg. 5
	AC	....	1.0	1.2	1.5	1.6	1.0	1.6
	AO	....	2.4	1.6	2.6	2.8	2.0	2.8
Plasma chlorides		7.03	6.99	....	4.48	3.54	2.79	
CO_2 combining power		32.1	35.7	53.2	71.1	78.0	78.4	67.3

1704. Pylorus obstructed January 20, 1917, and animal given only distilled water through the intestinal fistula. The electrical excitability rose and on January 22 the dog had a violent convulsion lasting one minute. An hour later was given 50 c. c. 2 M. NaCl intravenously. Electrical excitability remained high but the dog was quiet and fairly well. On January 26, 50 c. c. 2 M. NaCl were again given intravenously. The dog remained alive until January 29 and there was no further twitching.

1704		20	21	January 22	23	24	25	26	27	28	29
				NaCl				NaCl			
Electrical excitability	KC	....	....	0.05 ↓ 0.10	0.05	0.05	0.05	0.2 ↓ 0.05	0.1	0.1	
	KO	....	....	1.6	Neg. 5	1.6	2.8	2.8 2.6	Neg. 5	Neg. 5	2.8
	AC	....	....	0.5	1.0	0.4	0.8	0.8 0.6	1.2	0.8	0.2
	AO	....	....	0.9	1.6	1.0	1.2	1.0 0.8	1.6	1.0	1.0
Plasma chlorides		6.1	5.7	4.1	4.1	4.6	4.6	3.6 2.5	4.1	3.7	....
CO_2 combining power		44.7	38.1	43.0	44.0	47.3	68.6	69.1 82.7	70.0	71.5	94.

1705. Pylorus obstructed January 21, 1917. Given only distilled water by intestinal fistula. No symptoms on January 22 and 23, but on the morning of January 24 the dog was found in convulsions or "tetany." This was slower and more deliberate, less clonic than parathyroid tetany. There were no fibrillary tremors of the tongue. The convulsions were severe, stretching the animal into opisthotonos with attempts at vomiting. They were rather more like the convulsions of ammonia poisoning than those of parathyroid tetany. On January 24, after the convulsion had lasted four hours, the animal was given 50 c. c. 2 M. NaCl solution intravenously. The convulsions disappeared and the animal lived until January 27 without any further attack.

					January			
1705		*21*	*22*	*23*	*24*	*25*	*26*	*27*
					NaCl			
	KC	....	0.2	0.05	0.2 ↓ 0.6	0.6	0.4	0.4
Electrical	KO	....	Neg. 5	Neg. 5	Neg. 5 Neg. 5	Neg. 5	Neg. 5	3.8
excitability	AC	....	1.2	1.0	1.4 1.6	1.6	1.0	0.8
	AO	....	2.2	2.2	2.6 2.8	4.0	2.0	1.2
Plasma chlorides		5.7	5.6	4.4	3.2		4.0	3.2	3.0
CO₂ combining power		53.7	43.	47.3	... 63.5	65.3	71.5	34.5

1707. Pylorus obstructed January 26, 1917. As usual, the stomach was washed out twice daily and found to contain 300–500 c. c. fluid. No symptoms until January 29, when there were violent convulsions. The mouth was opened wide and there were retching and salivation. No convulsions on January 30, but the animal was very stuporous and appeared to be dying. Given intravenously 100 c. c. 2 M. NaCl. January 31, very apathetic. Given 300 c. c. 2 M. NaCl intravenously, seemed rather improved but died in the afternoon. This was of course an extreme dose of sodium chloride amounting to 41 grams. It raised the plasma chlorides above the normal figure but only when the dog was moribund.

					January			
1707		*26*	*27*	*28*	*29*	*30*	*31*	
					Con-vulsions	NaCl	NaCl	
	KC	0.4	0.4	0.1	0.1	0.2	0.2	0.6
Electrical	KO	Neg. 5	Neg. 5	Neg. 5	Neg. 5	Neg. 5	Neg. 5	4.0
excitability	AC	1.2	2.0	1.0	0.8	0.8	1.2	1.4
	AO	2.0	3.8	2.4	2.4	2.3	3.0	1.4
Plasma chlorides		6.2	6.1	5.2	4.5	3.6	4.7	10.0
CO₂ combining power		60.0	45.0	58.0	64.0	74.9	65.3	24.2

1714. Pylorus obstructed March 6, 1917. Given only distilled water by intestinal fistula. No symptoms until March 9 when violent convulsions with much frothing at the mouth occurred. In this case practically no change in electrical excitability was observed, although characteristic alterations in the plasma chlorides and alkali were present.

		March		
1714	*6*	*7*	*8*	*9*
Electrical excitability {KC	0.3	0.2	0.2	0.2
KO	Neg. 5	Neg. 5	Neg. 5	Neg. 5
AC	1.2	1.0	0.7	1.0
AO	1.8	1.6	1.0	1.8
Plasma chlorides	7.4	5.4	5.0	4.1
CO_2 combining power	46.0	48.0	60.0	72.0

From these experiments it is seen that a peculiar condition accompanied by convulsions appears whenever the pylorus is obstructed so that the acid gastric juice is all removed and no chlorides are given in the food. It must be recognized that the condition is not the same as that produced by parathyroidectomy. The muscular rigidity with vibrating clonic twitchings and extreme tachypnoea are lacking. Instead the rather apathetic animal usually lies quiet until seized with a violent universal convulsion which throws the body into extreme and rigid opisthotonos with attempts at vomiting and abundant salivation. After this is over he sinks into a kind of coma with slow, deep respirations. Rigid respirations of great volume often precede the onset of the convulsion. The electrical excitability is heightened definitely and up to the time of the convulsions it increases but never to a point comparable with that seen in parathyroid tetany, and even during the most violent twitching, stiffness and clenching of the jaws the KO reaches only 1.8 or 1.6, whereas in parathyroid tetany it is not unusual to have it 0.6 or 0.4.

The rapid diminution in the plasma chlorides with the corresponding rise in the alkali reserve as measured by van Slyke's method was constant. We, therefore, thought that the condition might be relieved by the replacement of the chlorides, and as a matter of fact injections of sodium chloride into the blood stream when the symptoms were well developed regularly caused the disappearance of the convulsions and a general improvement in the condition, and lowered for a time the electrical excitability.

When a dog otherwise treated in the same way, that is by obstruction of the pylorus and washing out of the stomach, was given distilled water with the addition of 10 grams of sodium chloride daily, it lived for a week or more without symptoms, maintained a constant proportion of plasma chlorides and a constant alkaline reserve as measured by the carbon dioxide combining power. Moreover, the electrical excitability of the nerves remained normal.

1711. Pylorus obstructed February 22, 1917. Given distilled water with 10 grams NaCl through intestinal fistula. Remained quiet; no twitching or convulsions. Walked about apparently well until February 27 when it was found dead. The wound had been torn open and there was an acute pleuritis.

1711		February					
		22	23	24	25	26	27
Electrical excitability	KC	0.2	0.2	0.1	0.4	0.8	
	KO	Neg. 5	Neg. 5	Neg. 5	Neg. 5	Neg. 5	
	AC	1.2	0.8	0.7	1.2	2.2	
	AO	1.2	0.8	0.8	1.2	2.8	
Plasma chlorides		6.8	6.6	6.4	7.0	8.0	
CO_2 combining power		43.8	50.4	52.2	50.1	49.0	

1712. Pylorus obstructed February 26. Given distilled water with sodium chloride as before. Remained well until March 2 when he was apathetic and there were attempts at vomiting. Died on March 4 without infection or other obvious cause of death.

1712		February				March		
		26	27	28	1	2	3	4
Electrical excitability	KC	0.1	0.1	0.1	0.1	0.3	0.6	
	KO	Neg. 5	Neg. 5	Neg. 5	Neg. 5	Neg. 5	Neg. 5	
	AC	0.8	0.8	0.8	0.6	1.6	2.2	
	AO	1.2	1.6	2.2	1.8	2.6	Neg. 5	
Plasma chlorides		6.7	7.0	7.0	7.5	8.2	8.2	8.3
CO_2 combining power		35.0	49.0	46.2	49.2	30.9	42.8	35.0

We had of course regarded the whole alteration as due to loss of hydrochloric acid with the result that an excess of base had been left in the circulating fluids, so that the natural experiment would be the replacement of the chlorine ion by the introduction of hydrochloric acid. This was done several times but without much success (1620, 1622, 1709 and others), whereas the introduction of sodium chloride has a life saving effect and the administration of sodium chloride continuously after the operation prevented the development of changes in the electrical excitability, disturbances of the alkali reserves or symptoms. The fate of the Na ion requires explanation since it appears that so long as the Cl ion is supplied there is no heightened alkali reserve.

The prompt effect of calcium salts in stopping parathyroid tetany led to their trial in some of these cases. The injection of calcium lactate, although it exerts a temporary effect in stopping the twitchings or modifying the convulsions, has no such controlling influence, as is seen in the tetany following parathyroidectomy after which an animal can be kept perfectly well for a long time by the proper administration of calcium.

We had started with the idea that the loss of chlorides might throw out of function soluble calcium in the plasma or even actually precipitate it and we made numerous analyses of the blood to determine the changes in the proportion of calcium. The analyses were made (not to show the absolute, but the relative, amount of calcium in the plasma) by dialyzing 10 c. c. of blood received in 1 c. c. of 15% sodium citrate solution for 24 hours at 4° C. in a fish bladder sac against 100 c. c. of a solution containing 0.8% of sodium chloride and 0.3% sodium citrate. The clear colorless dialysate was boiled, acidulated and precipitated with oxalate after the method of McCrudden. Titrations were made against $\frac{N}{100}$ potassium permanganate. Controls were made by estimating the calcium in the residue in the sac and by analyzing the dialysate after known amounts of calcium chloride had been added to the blood and they show that a proportional amount of calcium appears in the dialysate. All that we venture to say from these studies is that there appears to be no characteristic change in the proportion of calcium in the blood from the time before the operation until the death of the animal. (As for the method, although it is probably open to many objections, it has the advantage of eliminating many difficulties in the analysis of blood for calcium and of giving accurate proportional results, which was all we required.)

It is clear, however, that there is a distinct change in the acid base equilibrium in favor of the alkali reserve and it seemed possible that this might be reproduced temporarily by the injection of sodium carbonate or bicarbonate which was done with the following results:

1614. Blood studied before injection: From 4.20 p. m. to 5.10 p. m. a gradual injection was made of 2 M. Na_2CO_3, 100 c. c. in all being run into the vein. The electrical excitability became greatly heightened temporarily. No convulsions were produced and there were no further effects.

1614		December 21								
		4	4.20	4.40	5	5.20	5.40	6	6.20
Electrical excitability	KC	0.1	...	0.05	...	0.05	...	...	0.1
	KO	Neg. 5	...	Neg. 5	...	1.8	...	...	Neg. 5
	AC	0.6	...	0.6	...	0.4	...	...	0.6
	AO	1.0	...	1.4	...	0.6	...	...	1.4
Plasma chlorides		6.8	...	......	...	6.4	...	...	7.2
CO_2 combining power		50.4	...	......	...	119.6	...	...	74.0

1623. Blood studied before injection. From 4.50 to 5.15, 160 c. c. 2 M. Na_2CO_3 run into the vein. No marked symptoms, recovery prompt.

1623				December 22					
		4.20	5.20	6.20	7.20	8.20	9.20	10.20	
		Na_2CO_3							
Electrical excitability	KC	0.2	0.1	0.1	...	...	...	0.1	
	KO	Neg. 5	0.8	1.0	...	...	...	Neg. 5	
	AC	0.8	0.5	0.6	...	...	...	1.2	
	AO	1.4	0.2	0.4	...	...	...	1.2	
CO_2 combining power		47.0	138.6	...	...	...	...		

1624. After normal electric reactions had been determined the injection of 10% Na_2CO_3 into a vein was begun at 4 p. m. and continued to 5 p. m., 240 c. c. being run in. The animal became stiff with twitching and fibrillation of the tongue. Electrical excitability much heightened. Recovery complete.

1624				January 6		
		3.30	4.00	4.30	5.00	5.30
				Na_2CO_3		
Electrical excitability	KC	0.5	...	0.3	0.4	0.2
	KO	Neg. 5	...	...	2.6	1.0
	AC	1.6	...	1.6	2.4	1.0
	AO	1.6	...	0.6	0.6	0.4
CO_2 combining power		.....	...	...	...	

1701. Injection of 2 M. Na_2CO_3 begun at 3 and continued to 4.15 p. m. during which time 150 c. c. were run in. After this the electrical reactions disappeared and no contraction could be elicited. At 3.45 dog became stiff and stretched out. At 4 p. m. a violent convulsion occurred with twitching of the whole body.

1701		2.30	2.45	3.00	November 30 3.15	3.30	3.45	4.00	4.15
			Na$_2$CO$_3$				Convulsions Na$_2$CO$_3$		
Electrical excitability	KC	...	0.1	...	0.2	0.1	0.5	0.5	Neg.
	KO	...	Neg. 5	...	Neg. 5	Neg. 5	Neg. 5	Neg. 5	Neg.
	AC	...	0.6	...	0.6	0.6	0.6	0.6	Neg.
	AO	...	0.9	...	0.5	0.3	0.2	0.4	Neg.

1702. Injection of 1 M. NaHCO$_3$ begun at 3.15 and continued until 4.30 p. m., when 250 c. c. had been run in. Vomiting at 3.50. Generalized twitchings at 4.10. Slight convulsion at 4.30. Prolonged and continuous convulsions at 4.50, after which all electric responses failed. Died at 5.15.

1702		3	3.15	3.30	3.45	December 1 4	4.15	4.30	4.45	5	5.15
		NaHCO$_3$							Convulsions		
Electrical excita- bility	KC	0.4	...	0.2	0.3	0.2	0.2	0.2	...	Neg.	Died
	KO	Neg. 5	...	Neg. 5	Neg. 5	Neg. 5	Neg. 5	Neg. 5	...	Neg.	
	AC	1.4	...	1.5	1.5	0.9	1.0	0.8	...	Neg.	
	AO	2.8	...	1.7	1.0	0.8	1.0	0.7	...	Neg.	

1704. Three c. c. per kilo of 1 M. Na$_2$CO$_3$ were injected intravenously every 15 minutes. Weight of animal 11.45 kilos. This was begun at 10 a. m. and continued till 12.15, at which time 340 c. c. had been injected. The dog died shortly afterward. (Observations made by the students in experimental pathology under Dr. Admont Clark.)

1704		10	10.15	10.30	10.45	February 7 11	11.15	11.30	11.45	12	12.15
		Na$_2$CO$_3$									
Electrical excita- bility	KC	0.8	....	0.6	....	0.5	....	0.6	.....	0.5	0.4
	KO	Neg. 5	....	Neg. 5	....	Neg. 5	....	Neg. 5	.....	1.6	1.0
	AC	1.2	....	2.0	....	2.0	....	2.2	.....	1.6	1.0
	AO	2.6	....	2.4	....	1.4	....	0.9	.....	1.0	0.5
CO$_2$ combining power		46.6	55.1	69.1	73.9	83.3	87.6	96.4	104.4	112.0	121.3
Alveolar CO$_2$ (Marriott)		34.	33.	38.	38.	42.	40.	43.	43.	44.	45.

From these experiments it seems that practically the same symptoms, twitching, convulsions, opisthotonos, etc., can be produced by excessive injections of sodium carbonate or bicarbonate solutions as by the removal of the chlorides. The preponderance of the alkali over the acids is on a higher plane since there has been no loss of acid, but the relations are similar. The alterations of the electrical excitability parallel with those of the alkali reserve are just the same in the two cases. In both the increase of excitability is moderate and rather irregular. Sometimes it seems not to occur, while in other cases it is very definite.

An explanation of such phenomena usually means an interpretation in terms of simpler phenomena. Here we find that convulsions and heightened electrical excitability of the nerve muscle apparatus coincide with an excess of alkali. The same results are produced by the withdrawal of acid which could possibly disturb the relations of sodium, potassium, magnesium and calcium in the body.

It is possible that the disturbed equilibrium of acids and bases in itself is the cause of the symptoms. It is well known that the buffer qualities of the blood are such as to prevent any change in the actual pH value without extreme interference with the alkaline reserve. The addition of acids lessens the alkaline reserve, but until it is used up there is compensated acidosis. Similarly the increase in the alkali content of the blood must be resisted to maintain the normal hydrogen ion concentration until an excessive amount of alkali is added. (This is not by retention of CO_2 because the alveolar CO_2 is increased.) A great excess of alkali must ultimately produce a marked change in the pH of the blood.

The papers of Wilson, Stearns and Janney dealing with the condition of alkalosis in tetany following parathyroidectomy state that it may develop, but later on is neutralized by the acid products formed by the muscular activities incident to tetany. This result was reached by the study of the values of the dissociation constant of oxyhaemoglobin, the alveolar CO_2 pressure and the hydrogen ion concentration of the blood. McCann confirms this by observations on two cases made by Van Slyke's method. In his first case he administered magnesium sulphate and calcium chloride and there is no way of telling the relation of the changes in alkali reserve to these procedures or to the tetany. In the second case he also removed the stomach contents at intervals, which would have its own effect. None of these writers records the chemical changes in time relation to changes in electrical excitability which are so important in the diagnosis of the condition of tetany. We ourselves in a few observations have found no change in the alkali reserve in the direction of alkalosis during tetany of parathyroid origin.

1617. Parathyroidectomy December 9, 1917. Tetany beginning December 11. On December 12, the dog was found in violent tetany. Given bicarbonate intravenously which did not relieve the tetany but appeared to add its own influence. No heightening of alkali reserve during the parathyroid tetany.

				December		
1617		9	10	11	12	
					NaHCo₃	
Electrical excitability	KC	....	0.05	0.05	0.05 ↓	0.05
	KO	....	Neg. 5	1.0	0.6	0.6
	AC	....	0.3	0.2	0.3	0.4
	AO	....	0.8	0.8	0.4	0.4
Plasma chlorides		....	6.9	6.8	6.78	6.38
CO₂ combining power		32.8	45.4	39.8	36.5	74.9

1705. Parathyroidectomy December 18, 1917. On December 19 the dog was well. On December 20 there was violent tetany and death at 3 p. m. There was no increase in the alkaline reserve.

			December	
1705		18	19	20
Electrical excitability	KC	0.1	0.2	0.05
	KO	Neg. 5	Neg. 5	1.4
	AC	1.2	1.0	0.4
	AO	1.8	1.2	1.0
Plasma chlorides		......	......	
CO₂ combining power		61.7	60.7	40.5

CONCLUSIONS

When the pylorus is obstructed and the gastric juice with its hydrochloric acid is constantly removed, there ensues a decrease in the chlorine of the plasma.

There is a consequent increase in the alkali reserve which becomes extreme.

The electrical excitability of the nerves is in general heightened and there are spontaneous twitchings and in most cases violent convulsions which lead to death.

All of this can be prevented by constantly furnishing a large supply of chlorides. It is less easy to cure the condition by the administration of chlorides.

The convulsive movements are not exactly like the twitchings of the tetany of parathyroidectomy in which we have found no heightened alkali reserve, but they can be produced by the injection of sodium carbonate or bicarbonate.

Since these convulsions can be stopped or prevented by sodium chloride, it remains a problem as to what becomes of the excessive base sodium and as to the specific need of the chlorine ion. Further experiments are contemplated to settle these points.

HENRY T. RANDALL (1914–)

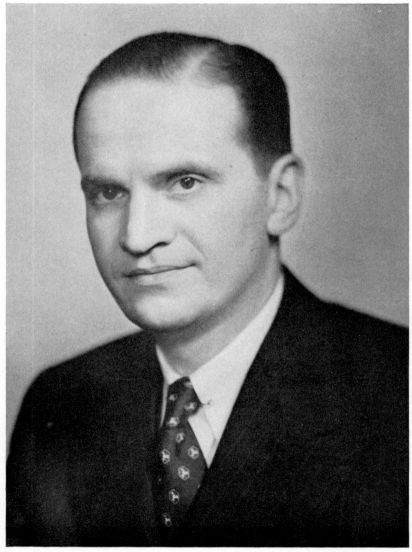

Fabian Bachrach

Henry T. Randall was born in New York on August 29, 1914. He received his preliminary education at Princeton and was graduated from Columbia University College of Physicians and Surgeons in 1941. He then served in the armed forces and attained the rank of Lieutenant Colonel. He was active at Presbyterian Hospital and held teaching appointments at Columbia and Cornell. In 1951, at the age of 37, he became Clinical Director and Chairman of the Department of Surgery at Memorial Hospital in New York. In 1955 he became Professor of Surgery at Cornell.

Dr. Randall has done outstanding work in the study of fluid and electrolyte balance and has published numerous original articles dealing with that subject. He has also carried out considerable investigative work on malignancy. He is the guiding force in a laboratory which is destined to enrich clinical surgery.

WATER AND ELECTROLYTE BALANCE IN SURGERY

BY HENRY T. RANDALL, M.D., M.Sc.D.

Clinical Director and Chief of Surgery, Memorial Center;
Associate Professor of Surgery, Cornell University Medical College, New York

The past ten years have seen a phenomenal growth in knowledge of the physiology of water and electrolyte balance in man, and with this has developed an increasing body of clinically useful information which is of such value to the surgeon that a working knowledge of it is essential to care adequately for the major or complicated surgical case. New terms have been introduced, new technics developed, and routine postoperative orders for fluids have been superseded by the quantitative approach in the preservation of body economy. The purpose of this article is to present an approach to the problem of the management of fluid and electrolyte balance in surgical patients in the light of recent developments of knowledge.[1]

A DEFINITION OF TERMS

When most of the salts of which the body's nonskeletal inorganic structure is composed are placed in water, they separate partly or com-

[1] While the basic concepts represent the ideas and work of many distinguished investigators in the field of Medicine, Biochemistry and Physiology, a long list to which a limited bibliography can give but most inadequate credit, the particular approach and much of the material presented here represents work done in the Surgical Metabolic Unit of the Department of Surgery, Columbus University and Presbyterian Hospital, New York. It was the author's good fortune to work as a member of this unit with Dr. D. V. Habif and Dr. S. C. Werner from its founding in 1948 by the late Dr. John S. Lockwood until July 1951. The work was supported in large part by research grants from the U. S. Public Health Service.

From *Surgical Clinics of North America*, April, 1952. Reprinted by permission.

pletely into positively and negatively charged particles which are called
ions. Salts of sodium, potassium and magnesium which compose by far
the largest portion of the extraskeletal electrolyte structure separate or
dissociate almost completely in solution. Positively charged ions are
termed cations, and the negatively charged ones, anions. For example,
$NaCl \rightarrow [Na]^+$ and $[Cl]^-$ in solution.
$\underset{cation}{} \underset{anion}{}$

If cations and anions existed in the body in the proportions in which
they are found as salts in bottles on the laboratory shelf, it might be

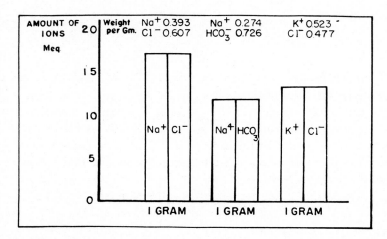

FIG. 151.—The amount and weight of ions in one gram of three
common salts. Due to differences in molecular weights of ions none
of the three are equivalent ionically.

proper to speak of them in terms of so many grams of salt per liter of
plasma. While there is always an equal total number of cations and
anions in a solution, a particular concentration of any cation is not
matched by an equivalent amount of any particular anion in either
plasma, interstitial or intracellular fluid.

In addition, neither various salts nor different cations and anions
are equal gram for gram to each other. For example, 1 gram of NaCl
is not equivalent to 1 gram of $NaHCO_3$ in either the amount of positive and negative charges or even the amount of sodium by weight.
This is illustrated graphically by Figure 151.

MILLIEQUIVALENT. It is apparent that the concentrations of ions must be expressed in terms in which one ion is equivalent to another, and that the amount of ions in a given weight of a material must be able to be calculated. The term Equivalent (Eq.) and Milliequivalent (mEq.) satisfy these requirements and have superseded older terms of weight as a salt. An equivalent of any ion is that amount which carries the same amount of electrical charge as 1 gram of hydrogen ion $[H]^+$.[1] One equivalent is equal to the molecular weight of the atom or molecule, divided by its valence or number of charges per molecule. Table 1 gives the molecular weight of the major ions in biological fluids.

$$1 \text{ Eq.} = \frac{\text{molecular weight in grams}}{\text{valence}}$$

A milliequivalent is 1/1000 of this and is the usual term for expressing biological concentrations.

$$1 \text{ mEq.} = \frac{\text{molecular weight in milligrams}}{\text{valence}}$$

For example: How many milliequivalents of Na^+ and Cl^- in 1000 cc. of 0.9 per cent NaCl?

Molecular weight Na $= 23$
$\phantom{\text{Molecular weight }}$Cl $= 35.5$
Molecular wt. NaCl $= 58.5$ gm.
Valence Na^+ and Cl^- $= 1$ each

$$\text{and } 1 \text{ mEq. of Na and Cl}^- = \frac{58.5}{1} \text{ mg.} = 58.5 \text{ mg.}$$

$$0.9\% \text{ NaCl} = 9.0 \text{ gm./L. or 9000 mg./L.}$$

$$\frac{9000 \text{ mg.}}{58.5 \text{ mg.}} = 154 \text{ mEq./L.}$$

Hence there are 154 mEq. of Na^+ and 154 mEq. of Cl^- in 1000 cc. of 0.9% NaCl

Tradition has provided for the survival of the expression of volumes per cent in expressing the amount of CO_2 released from plasma on the addition of an acid. Since CO_2 exists almost entirely as the ion $(HCO_3)^-$ and its ionic effect depends upon its negative charge, it too

---

[1] Actually 1.008 grams since $O_2 = 16$ and the combining weight of hydrogen ion is 1.008.

TABLE 1. MOLECULAR WEIGHTS AND VALENCES OF SOME
BIOLOGICALLY IMPORTANT IONS

	Molecular weight*	Valence	Equivalent weight
Cations			
H+	1	1	1
Na+	23	1	23
K+	39	1	39
Ca++	40	2	20
Mg++	24	2	12
Anions			
Cl-	35.5	1	35.5
(HCO₃)-	61	1	61
(HPO₄)--	96	2	48
(SO₄)--	96	2	48
Plasma protein	Gm./100 cc. × 2.43 = mEq. plasma protein		

*Decimal fractions of molecular weights are omitted except for chloride.

can be expressed as milliequivalents per liter by the following simple formula:

$$\frac{\text{Vol. } \% \ CO_2}{2.2} = \text{mEq. per liter } (HCO)_3^-$$

Certain substances in the plasma, interstitial and cell fluids do not dissociate into ions, but remain as intact molecules—the commonest of these nonelectrolytes are glucose (molecular weight 180) and urea (molecular weight 60). These have an osmotic but not an electrical charge effect, whereas the electrolyte ions individually exert both a charge and an osmotic effect according to their concentration.

THE FUNCTIONAL DIVISIONS OF BODY FLUID: NORMAL VOLUMES AND CONCENTRATIONS

In considering water and electrolyte balance it is important to know the normal distribution of water and electrolytes and the size of the major fluid compartments.

TOTAL BODY WATER. Body water has been variously estimated at from 50.3 to 75 per cent of body weight with an average of 65 to 70 per cent in the older literature. However, more recent studies using heavy water and antipyrine have shown in the adult that water measurable with these substances ranges from an average of 50.3 per cent to 61.8 per cent of body weight. Schloerb and associates reported that heavy water dilution showed an average of 51.9 per cent of body weight as water in normal adult women and 61.8 per cent in normal adult men. The closest correlation of body water was with body surface area, with an average of 23.6 liters per square meter in males, and 18.3 liters per square meter in females, each with a coefficient of variation of 4.4 per cent.

In infants and children, Friis-Hansen and associates employed simultaneously the heavy water and antipyrine methods and reported values for total water ranging from 70 to 83 per cent of body weight in newborn infants. They reported a gradual decrease in the percentage of body weight of water during the first six months; and, from six months to eleven years of age, values ranging between 53 and 63 per cent of body weight were found with no correlation as to age or sex.

THE SIZE OF FLUID COMPARTMENTS. Body fluid may be divided into two major parts, the extracellular fluid space and the intracellular fluid space. The extracellular fluid is further divisible into intravascular (plasma) and extravascular (interstitial) fluid. The size of the extracellular fluid space depends somewhat on the methods used in measurement, but is generally regarded as being approximately 20 per cent of the body weight. Crandall and associates, using sodium thiocyanate, described the normal extracellular space in males as 24.2 per cent of the body weight. Kalterider showed a sodium space of 24.8 per cent of body weight at three hours in the adult using radioactive sodium, while in the newborn infants, Flexner found an average extracellular space as measured by radioactive sodium of 43.5 per cent of the body weight. Schwartz, using inulin which is probably the most impermeable to cells of all substances used to estimate extracellular fluid space, found in 7 normal adult males an inulin extracellular fluid space of 14 to 18 per cent of body weight with an average of 16.2 per cent. Simultaneous sodium spaces averaged 26.7 per cent and thiocyanate space 25.9 per cent in some of the same group.

For practical purposes it is adequate to consider the extracellular fluid as 20 per cent of the body weight. Of this the plasma is 4.5 to 5 per cent of the body weight and the interstitial fluid 15 per cent of the body weight. The intracellular fluid by difference is 35 to 45 per cent of the body weight. The relationship of volume size of these compartments is illustrated in the accompanying diagram (Fig. 152).

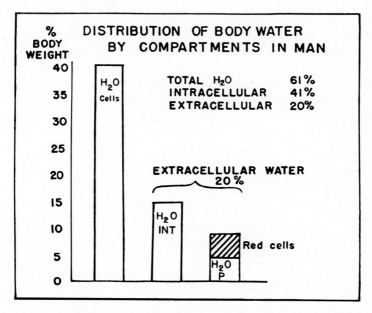

Fig. 152.—From data by Schloerb *et al.* for total body water. *H₂O Int.* is interstitial fluid and *H₂O P* plasma water. The water in red cells is considered intracellular water.

CONCENTRATION OF ELECTROLYTES. By far the most easily analyzed of the body fluid compartments is the plasma because of its availability for biopsy by venipuncture. The accompanying table prepared from the literature gives the average concentration and the range of the various major electrolyte ions of the plasma (Table 2).

TABLE 2. NORMAL PLASMA ELECTROLYTE VALUES
IN MILLIEQUIVALENTS PER LITER

	Average value	Range of normal
Na^+	142.0	135–150*
K^+	4.5	3.6–5.5
Ca^{++}	5.3	4.7–5.8
Mg^{++}	2.1	1.5–2.5
$(HCO_3)^-$	26.7	24.6–28.8
Cl^-	102.6	100–105
$(SO_4)^{--}$	1.15	1.0–1.3
$(HPO_4)^{--}$	2.0	1.5–2.5

(Compiled from the literature)

* See text.

The major difference between the plasma electrolyte concentrations and those of the interstitial fluid is illustrated by the accompanying chart modified from Gamble (Fig. 153), which also illustrates the approximate composition of the intracellular fluid as represented by skeletal muscle. According to Darrow, skeletal muscle contains approximately 70 per cent of the total intracellular water and so these concentrations can be considered fairly representative of intracellular

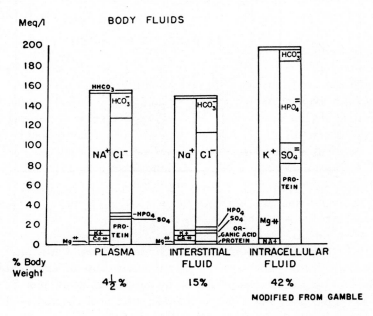

Fig. 153.—The concentration of electrolytes in plasma interstitial fluid and intracellular fluid shows the contrast between cells and extracellular fluid in chemical compositions. (From Gamble with modifications.)

fluid as a whole. The striking difference between the intracellular and the extracellular electrolyte concentrations is illustrated. In the plasma and interstitial fluid the dominant cation is sodium, with small amounts of potassium, magnesium and calcium. The anions are bicarbonate, chloride, and in the plasma, a significant amount of protein. In the interstitial fluid the only major difference is that the sodium concentration is approximately 5 per cent lower, and the chloride concentration 5 per cent higher in accordance with Donnan's law of equilibrium, since the protein concentration is much lower. The intracellular fluid, however, shows a marked contrast with the dominant cations potassium and magnesium, while the anions are phosphate, sulfate and protein with a small amount of bicarbonate and virtually no chloride. According to Darrow, the average intracellular sodium of muscle is 7 mEq. per liter. There is considerably more sodium in the cells of connective tissue, skin and bowel. Radioactive sodium dilution studies, reported by Forbes and Perley, showed that the total exchangeable body sodium averaged 41.9 mEq. per kilogram in males and 39.5 mEq. per kilogram in females as measured at eighteen to twenty-four hours. There is a considerable range in both male and female groups. In children, the total body sodium measured at eighteen to twenty-four hours, reported by the same workers, showed an average sodium of 76.4 mEq. per kilogram in infants and a gradual decline from this level to the adult value as growth and weight progressed. They estimated that approximately 82 per cent of the total body sodium was measured by the isotope exchange method and therefore total body sodium (including that in bone) would be in the range of 50 mEq. per kilogram in the adult.

Total body potassium has been measured by the radioactive isotope dilution method by Corsa and associates. They found the exchangeable potassium content of 29 healthy young males to vary from 37 to 57.1 mEq. per kilogram with a mean of 46.3 mEq. Thus, there are approximately the same number of milliequivalents of exchangeable sodium and exchangeable potassium in the human body, most of the sodium being extracellular or in bone, and most of the potassium intracellular in metabolically active tissues.

Before undertaking major surgery it is often wise to determine what the particular patient's normal electrolyte values are because of the extent of the range of some of the normal values. It is my experience that, in the case of serum sodium, the range of normal is not higher than 145 mEq. per liter. A thorough understanding of normal averages and ranges is essential to evaluate properly changes in the patient's status pre- or postoperatively, and figures in this table, particularly those for sodium, potassium, bicarbonate and chloride should be a part of the working knowledge of every surgeon.

THE GENERAL CONSIDERATIONS OF FLUID BALANCE

The term "balance" implies an equilibrium among two or more different things. Maintaining fluid and electrolyte balance requires an understanding of the normal daily intake and output of water and of the major electrolytes required for body economy. In addition, abnormal losses and their electrolyte content, and deficiencies acquired before treatment begins must be considered. The problem may be divided into three parts. The first of these, baseline, answers the question. "What do I have to give the patient if he is wholly or partially deprived of oral intake, but is otherwise in normal or relatively normal condition?" The second, dynamic loss, answers the question, "What losses does the patient have as the result of his disease, operative procedures or both that are abnormal and that are going on under observation, and what is required to replace these losses?" The third category, static debt, answers the question, "What deficiencies or excesses does the patient have in water, electrolytes and blood volume at the time when I begin to treat him?" The total daily intake of water and electrolytes required will be the sum of the baseline requirements, plus the dynamic loss, plus a proportion of the deficiencies in water, electrolytes and blood volume. A daily or more frequent evaluation of the status of the baseline and dynamic loss and a critical evaluation of deficiencies at the beginning of therapy enable the surgeon to evaluate the problems of maintaining a normal or nearly normal intra- and extracellular fluid structure for a patient before, during and after a traumatic experience.

BASELINE REQUIREMENTS

In considering baseline requirements for patients on parenteral fluids it is perhaps best to approach the problem from an analysis of the types of losses which normally occur each day, and, by adding these normal losses together, to approximate the amount and type of fluids which are required to maintain balance. These losses consist of urine, the loss which occurs as the result of the evaporation of water from respiratory epithelium in the process of breathing, and loss by direct evaporation of water from the surface of the skin. Frank sweating, as such, is not a consideration in baseline losses in the normal individual. In general, and particularly in the postoperative period, the surgeon likes to see a urinary volume in excess of 1000 cc. in each twenty-four hour period. Under ideal circumstances, according to Gamble, the kidneys are capable of excreting a urine whose concentration of solutes is 1.4 osmoles per liter or approximately four times the normal plasma concentration. However, in the postoperative period renal function cannot be assumed to be of normal or maximum efficiency, and, furthermore, most patients who have to undergo major surgical procedures are sufficiently advanced in years so that their renal function is diminished by a process of attrition involving arteriosclerosis and a reduction of functional nephrons. While, with maximum concentration, all of the necessary products of metabolism per day could be excreted in between 400 cc. and 500 cc. of urine, it is better to provide for a liter to 1200 cc. per twenty-four hours in the 70 kilogram adult. In addition, allocation must be made for respiratory loss and for loss by evaporation from the surface of the skin.

Studies conducted in the Presbyterian Hospital Metabolic Unit have confirmed observations that an intake of 800 to 1000 cc. per day is necessary to provide for these insensible losses. More detailed studies by Burch have shown that the mean rate of insensible loss in twelve normal males was 20.5 grams per square meter per hour. In the normal size adult of 1.73 square meter surface area and 70 kilogram weight (154 pounds), this represents a surface loss and respiratory evaporation loss of 35.5 grams per hour, or 852 grams per day of which 93 per cent or 800 cc. is water. Of this, 52 per cent is estimated as the mean loss by respiratory evaporation or approximately 420 cc. and the remainder or 380 cc. is loss by evaporation from skin surface. There is a variation up to 50 per cent among individuals.

Another source of water in the semistarving patient is performed water present in tissues destroyed to provide calories, and water of oxidation formed by the combustion of these tissues and of administered calories. Water of oxidation averages 12 cc. per 100 calories burned, or 200 to 300 cc. per day, and additional preformed water loss of approximately the same amount occurs when minimal carbohydrate is provided. Thus, in effect, about 400 cc. of water is added to the intake and output, and is reflected by weight loss.

TOTAL WATER REQUIREMENT. If one assumes a total insensible loss of 800 to 1000 cc. in each day, it is apparent that the total baseline water intake must be between 1800 and 2500 cc. to prevent dehydration and to insure water balance.

ELECTROLYTE REQUIREMENT: NaCl. In addition to water in baseline, minimum requirements of electrolytes must be considered. An analysis of 35 diet weeks of patient-selected diet in 28 preoperative patients from the Surgical Metabolic Unit of Presbyterian Hospital revealed the data shown in Table 3. The diet and the amount of seasoning NaCl taken by the patients was of their selection, with the exception of restriction to 30 to 40 calories per kilogram and 85 grams of protein in each twenty-four hour period. The data show that the average sodium intake was approximately 100 mEq., that of chloride 115 mEq., and the potassium intake, higher than is usually realized, 77 mEq. per day. In terms of salt as sodium chloride, the sodium intake represents approximately 6 grams per day. The individual patient variation in selection of the amount of salt used for seasoning is indicated by the wide range exhibited by these cases. The potassium variation was considerably less due to the limitation of the diet as far as total protein intake was concerned.

TABLE 3. DIETARY SODIUM, POTASSIUM AND CHLORIDE
(Average of 35 Diet Weeks in 28 Patients)
Average weight of patients—61.94 kg. (42–93).
Average caloric intake—34.36 calories per kg.
Protein intake—85 grams per day (81–94).

Intake	Average per 24 hours	Range 2/3 cases
Na	98.86 mEq.	76–120
K	77.39 mEq.	65–88
Cl	113.99 mEq.	85–145

Since an average of 5 to perhaps 10 grams per day of sodium chloride added to and included in the food is a normal dietary intake, and since it has been well demonstrated that patients immediately postoperatively are incapable of excreting large loads of sodium and chloride ions, the baseline postoperative intake of sodium and chloride ions is best limited to approximately two-thirds of the normal daily intake as a maximum. Such an intake is well satisfied by giving a maximum of 500 cc. of isotonic sodium chloride solution (0.9%) for each twenty-four hours. This is a part of a total baseline allocation of 1500 to 2500 cc. per day, and the remainder of this fluid requirement is made up of nonelectrolyte-containing solutions. There are numerous reasons for decreasing the amount of sodium chloride provided in the daily baseline. Since sweating and other losses are otherwise provided for as abnormal losses, it should be increased only when deficits are known to exist.

GLUCOSE REQUIREMENT. It has been shown that 100 grams of glucose in each twenty-four hour period diminished the amount of nitrogen lost in the starving patient by 50 per cent. In addition, this glucose diminished withdrawal of body water, and decreased the renal excretion load. Therefore, 100 grams of glucose are an essential part of the baseline requirements of each patient. An increase in the amount of glucose administered from 100 to 200 grams in a postoperative series reported by Elman, diminished the nitrogen loss insignificantly. High concentrations require a long infusion time if marked glycosuria and a dehydrating diuresis are to be avoided.

Studies reported by Werner and associates have shown that in relatively less severe major surgical procedures, such as a cholecystectomy, it is possible to completely avoid nitrogen loss by the parenteral administration of solutions containing 30 to 35 calories per kilogram of body weight per day. Such a caloric intake requires the administration of between 3000 and 5000 cc. of mixtures of 10 per cent dextrose and 10 per cent amino acids with added electrolytes, or a combination of dextrose, amino acids and alcohol in a minimum volume of approximately 3500 cc. as proposed by Rice. Frequently such a fluid load in the absence of other losses is more than that which is required or desired in the postoperative patient. With hypertonic solutions such as 10 per cent dextrose or 10 per cent amino acids, and these solutions reinforced with the necessary minimum electrolytes, many hours are required for administration. Glucose is not utilized when administered faster than 0.5 to 0.7 grams per kilogram per hour, and rapid administration of amino acids and alcohol results in undesirable side reactions.

OTHER IONS. The administration of ions other than sodium and chloride is assuming increasing importance as metabolic studies illustrate their importance in body economy. One ion which has recently been shown to be essential is potassium. It has become increasingly apparent that the prophylactic administration of approximately one-half of the normal daily potassium intake will prevent potassium deficiencies which have been previously encountered in surgical patients. One-half of the normal daily intake of potassium is from 30 to 40 mEq. of potassium ion. This is easily accomplished by the administration of solutions containing potassium as KCl. Included in the baseline therefore should be between 30 and 40 mEq. of potassium in each twenty-four hour period. There are certain definite and positive contraindications to the administration of potassium and these are discussed under static debt.

A summary of baseline requirements is illustrated in Table 4.

TABLE 4. BASELINE FLUID REQUIREMENTS FOR 70 KILOGRAM ADULT

Output to be replaced, H_2O:
Insensible Loss	800 to 1000
Urine	800 to 1500
	1600 to 2500 cc.

Electrolytes
  With no abnormal losses or major deficits:
  Na^+ 76 mEq. and Cl^- 76 mEq. (500 cc. of 0.9% NaCl) maximum, plus 30 to 40 mEq. of K^+ (2 to 3 gm. of KCl).
Calories
  100 grams glucose per day minimum.
  Added calories, amino acids if desired, or indicated.
Vitamins
  B complex, C, sometimes K.

Certain factors alter baseline requirements. In general those that increase the metabolic rate raise the requirements while those that depress oxygen consumption decrease requirements (Table 5).

TABLE 5. FACTORS ALTERING BASELINE REQUIREMENTS

Increase	*Decrease*
Size (large)	Size (small except infants)
Youth	Old age
BMR↑	BMR↓
Fever	Cardiac failure
	Renal oliguria

In adults the average baseline water requirement is 35 to 45 cc. per kilogram per day; in children this increases slightly; and in infants the requirement rises to 150 cc. per kilogram per day as the result of small size and much increased metabolic rate. Fever increases the insensible loss by evaporation from the respiratory tract, and increases the metabolic rate.

Two special considerations decrease baseline requirements. The first is a generalized overexpansion of extracellular fluid as is seen in cardiac failure, where salt and water restrictions are the rule, and the second is acute renal failure with marked oliguria as is seen following prolonged hypotension or incompatible blood transfusion. In the latter case baseline must be reduced to insensible loss levels and electrolytes and urine H_2O replaced quantitatively in both the oliguric and diuretic phases.

DYNAMIC LOSS: EXTERNAL LOSSES AND INTERNAL FLUID SHIFTS

The second major category of fluid balance is dynamic loss. This includes both external abnormal losses of water and electrolytes, and those temporary functional losses which result from a shift of fluids within the body. These processes take place during treatment, are measured in drainage bottles or reflected in the patient's changing status, as contrasted with pre-existing deficiencies which are separately considered.

RESPONSE TO OPERATION. As the result of a traumatic experience, operation and anesthesia, a chain of events is set in action which has been described by Selye under the general classification of the alarm reaction. Those that are of the greatest immediate importance to the surgeon are: intracompartmental fluid shifts, transitory water retention accompanied by a longer retention of sodium and chloride ions, and a marked excess of loss of potassium and nitrogen with potassium lost in excess of its intracellular ratio to nitrogen. The increase of the extracellular fluid space is initiated at the time of operation and appears to reach its zenith about the second or third postoperative day. It consisted, in patients observed on the Surgical Metabolic Unit at the Presbyterian Hospital, of an expansion of between 2 and 3 liters of the extracellular fluid space as measured by inulin. In some patients there appeared also to be an increase above balance in the readily exchangeable sodium as measured by sodium 24. Lyons and associates reported a 15 per cent increased thiocyanate space and plasma volume with a drop in serum chloride by the third postoperative day as a normal postoperative response.

The extracellular fluid space expansion begins to resolve by the third or fourth postoperative day in relatively minor surgical procedures, as judged by the sodium balance and urinary output, and may persist for a week or more following major procedures, particularly if there are postoperative complications. It is the postoperative retention of sodium which was observed to be responsible for an overexpansion of the extracellular fluid space with edema formation in patients who were given large quantities of sodium chloride above losses in the immediate postoperative period. This led to the reports by Coller, and many others subsequently, that patients postoperatively were intolerant to the administration of sodium chloride.

GASTROINTESTINAL TRACT LOSSES. The major external fluid losses which are of concern to the surgeon are those from the gastrointestinal tract. Table 6, modified from Abbott, indicates the normal volumes of secretion into the gastrointestinal tract in a twenty-four hour period. Total gastrointestinal tract secretions are approximately four times the normal fluid intake. In pathologic states these volumes may be exceeded. It is not uncommon to observe as much as 1500 to 1800 cc. of bile drainage immediately postoperatively from a freshly decom-

TABLE 6. SECRETIONS OF THE GASTROINTESTINAL TRACT PER DAY

Type	Volume	Character
Saliva	1000–1500	Hypotonic—alkaline
Gastric juice	2500	a. Highly acid
		b. Neutral, mucoid
Bile	700–1000	Isotonic, alkaline
Pancreatic juice	1000+	Isotonic, very alkaline
Small bowel	3000>	Slightly hypotonic, increasing base > chloride toward ileum
	8000–10000	

pressed common duct, and we have observed drainage from a pancreatic fistula in the order of 2000 cc. per day.

Not only does gastrointestinal fluid represent a loss in water which must be replaced volume for volume, but also a loss in electrolytes. The characteristics of the electrolyte losses of the gastrointestinal tract have been the subject of much study. Previous observations have indicated that gastrointestinal tract secretions were approximately isotonic, and gave rise to the idea that the logical replacement for them was isotonic sodium chloride. This serves well enough if renal function is good and the kidneys can discriminate among the ions necessary for replacement and excrete hypertonic urine. Unfortunately, in the critically ill patient both before and after operation, this renal selectivtity is often much impaired, and as a result a more quantitative replacement of gastrointestinal tract drainage is necessary.

GASTROINTESTINAL TRACT DRAINAGE CONCENTRATION. Analysis of drainages from the gastrointestinal tracts of surgical patients, utilizing previously described technics, have demonstrated that the average gastrointestinal tract drainage is not isotonic but is hypotonic, insofar as sodium and chloride are concerned. The marked differences in type of electrolytes lost depending upon the location of the drainage point within the gastrointestinal tract were shown. Table 7 gives the electrolyte concentrations found in specimens from the gastrointestinal tract from surgical patients. This report presents a continuation of the

TABLE 7. GASTROINTESTINAL TRACT LOSSES, MILLIEQUIVALENTS PER LITER

		Na	K	Cl
Gastric	Average	59.0	9.3	89.0
(Fasting)	Range	6.0–157	0.5–65.0	13.2–167.2
130 specimens	⅔ Cases	31.0–90.0	4.3–12.0	52–124
Small bowel	Average	104.9	5.1	98.9
(Miller-Abbott suction)	Range	20.1–157.0	1.0–11.0	43.0–156.1
89 specimens	⅔ Cases	72–128	3.5–6.8	69–127
Ileum	Average	116.7	5.0	105.8
(Miller-Abbott suction)	Range	82–147	2.3–8.0	60.7–137.0
17 specimens	⅔ Cases	91–140	3.0–7.5	82–125
7 patients				
Ileostomy	Average	129.5	16.2	109.7
(Recent)	Range	92–146	3.8–98.0	66–136
25 specimens	⅔ Cases	112–142	4.5–14.0	93–122
7 patients				
Cecostomy	Average	79.6	20.6	48.2
20 specimens	Range	45–135	3.7–47.3	18–88.5
9 patients	⅔ Cases	48–116	11.1–28.3	35–70

work previously reported by Lockwood and Randall with a much larger series of specimens.

The range of electrolyte concentration in gastric juice varies widely. The more hypotonic secretions were found in elderly patients with an anacidity and in these sodium nearly equaled chloride, while in patients with duodenal ulcers and pyloric obstruction, chloride exceeded sodium by 2 or even 3 to 1, and high levels of chloride were found. In the latter group the use of ammonium chloride solutions for replacement, as advocated by Zintel, has proved useful to avoid excessive sodium administration. When there is marked small bowel regurgitation, the gastric losses are more nearly like upper small bowel in their electrolyte pattern.

Upper small bowel content was slightly alkaline and was a little more than two-thirds isotonic in its average concentration. There was a considerable range of variation from patient to patient but less so than in gastric juice. Both medical ileostomies with Miller-Abbott tubes, and surgical ileostomies showed that in the ileum there was a greater difference in concentration between base and chloride than in upper small bowel. Potassium losses were moderate from the gastrointestinal tract. There was an average of 9 mEq. per liter in gastric juice and this was even higher in the lower small bowel and cecum, where values of 15 to 20 mEq. per liter were not uncommon. These potassium losses may assume considerable significance if the volume of loss is large.

Table 8 illustrates concentrations of electrolytes found in specimens

TABLE 8. GASTROINTESTINAL TRACT LOSSES, MILLIEQUIVALENTS PER LITER

		Na	*K*	*Cl*
Bile	Average	145.3	5.2	99.9
22 specimens	Range	122–164	3.2–9.7	77–127
12 patients	2/3 Cases	134–156	3.9–6.3	83–110
Pancreas	Average	141.1	4.6	76.6
3 patients	Range	113–153	2.6–7.4	54.1–95.2

from the biliary tract and from pancreatic fistulas. Bile was approximately equivalent to plasma in its electrolyte concentrations insofar as sodium, potassium and chloride are concerned, and the ratio of sodium to chloride was almost 3 to 2. On the other hand, pancreatic juice with its high alkalinity demonstrated a sodium to chloride ratio of approximately 2 to 1, and the sodium concentration of pancreatic juice may be higher than that normally found in plasma. Potassium losses from bile and pancreatic juice were approximately of the order in which potassium is found in plasma. The high potassium concentration specimens in bile were probably due to the presence of a considerable amount of purulent exudate.

An understanding of the different types of electrolyte losses from the gastrointestinal tract is essential to their adequate replacement. It is not necessary to quantitate replacement when drainage from the gastrointestinal tract is small, in the order of 500 to perhaps 1000 cc. per day, and of short duration, no more than one or two days. It is usually sufficient, as has been the general clinical experience, simply to provide an equivalent volume of isotonic sodium chloride. However, in patients who are seriously ill and in those in whom gastrointestinal tract drainages are large in volume or persist over many days, a more quantitative replacement is necessary. The result of large volumes of sodium chloride in replacement of drainage from a fresh ileostomy, for example, is likely to be a chloride acidosis as the result of the excessive loss of sodium as compared to chloride. On the other hand, the use of sodium chloride solution in isotonic form to replace a one-third isotonic gastric juice draining from a patient with an achlor-

TABLE 9. Proportions of Parenteral Fluids for Semiquantitative Replacement of Gastrointestinal Fluid Losses

	Dextrose in water	Dextrose in saline	M/6 sodium lactate	0.75% Ammonium chloride
Gastric average	33%	67%		
Ulcer	20%	30%		50%
Low acidity	67%	33%		
Small intestine	20%	70%	10%	
Ileostomy	10%	75%	15%	
Bile		67%	33%	
Pancreas		50%	50%	

Above solutions employed for volume-for-volume replacement of losses.
Potassium chloride 10 mEq. per liter to be added.

hydria is sufficient to provide for the storage of large volumes of sodium chloride and a consequent overexpansion of the extracellular fluid space.

If laboratory facilities are available and the quantities of gastrointestinal tract drainages are large, analysis of their content and quantitative replacement is in order. If not, then a practical guide to the replacement of gastrointestinal tract losses is illustrated in Table 9, which gives a "rule of thumb" for the replacement of gastrointestinal tract volumes according to their nearest round figure equivalents in four replacement fluids. This figure is modified from an earlier one by Lockwood and Randall. The addition of ammonium chloride 0.75 per cent enables the replacement of a high chloride gastric loss without the administration of a large amount of sodium. It has been shown that a persistently alkaline urine may result in damage to the kidney tubules, although in all probability simultaneous dehydration is necessary, and of course sodium may not be excreted by the immediately postoperative patient. In cases of diarrhea, the more copious the volume of fluid lost the more nearly the diarrheal fluid comes to resemble terminal ileal juice in its electrolyte content.

OTHER EXTERNAL LOSSES. *Open Wounds.* Water and electrolytes may be lost from the body by routes other than the gastrointestinal tract. The commonest causes of these losses are large open wounds and excessive sweating. The material which is lost from the surface of wounds is similar to plasma in its composition and it has been demonstrated by Moore and his associates that, following slough separation in burns, an average of 45 per cent of the daily sodium loss occurred through wound surfaces and in some patients as high as 90 per cent. It is a common experience following an abdominoperineal resection to have the packing placed in the perineal wound saturated with material which is quite similar to plasma in its composition, and 500 cc. or more of this material may be lost per day in the first few days postoperatively. Replacements required for losses from major wounds are water, volume for volume, and a plasma concentration of electrolytes. Hartman's solution is about ideal for this loss. In addition it may be necessary if there is an extensive loss of plasma protein to replace this protein intravascularly.

Excessive Sweating. Sweat loss is exceedingly variable both in amount and electrolyte concentration. In hot humid weather from 2000 cc. to 4000 cc. or more can be lost per day. Sweat contains from 30 to 70 mEq. each of sodium and chloride ions per liter and is thus hypotonic. As the volume of sweat rises, electrolyte concentration tends to increase. Sweat loss is best estimated, as indeed is over-all water balance, by daily or more frequently weighing of the patient, and sweat should in general be replaced parenterally with one-third to one-half volume of 0.9 per cent sodium chloride and the remainder as nonelectrolyte-containing fluid either parenterally or orally. Postoperatively, sweat may contain even less salt than usual, as was shown by Johnson.

INTERNAL FLUID SHIFTS. Water and electrolytes may be effectively lost to the circulation and extracellular fluid space without actually leaving the body itself. One of the best examples of this situation is in the case of the *burn*. In the burned area there is very rapidly accumulated a large amount of edema fluid which contains electrolytes essentially those of extracellular fluid composition together with such protein as leaks through damaged capillary walls. The area of injury contains large volumes of fluid, but this fluid is unavailable to the rest of the body. An area of acute infection, particularly within serous cavities, behaves in much the same fashion. The patient with acute peritonitis or empyema has an area of injury which corresponds very closely to the type seen with burns. Fluid accumulated within the body, yet unavailable to it, amounts to the creation of a third fluid space, if one considers intracellular fluid as one and extracellular fluid as the second normal physiological compartment. This third space, be it the result of burn, trauma or infection, depletes both the extracellular and intracellular compartments to satisfy the demands for its own creation.

Since the composition of third space fluid is essentially that of extracellular fluid, and since it results in internal dehydration, the replacement which is required is in terms of the composition of extracellular fluid and frequently, if protein loss is high, of plasma. Several formulas have been proposed in the case of burns for the amount and type of fluid necessary to maintain an adequate circulating volume. The recommendations of Evans for 1 cc. of plasma or plasma substitute, and 1 cc. of normal saline solution per 1 per cent body burn per kilogram of weight is the most recent. This volume of fluid, but not over 4000 cc. of each is required in the first twenty-four hours and approximately one-half as much of both plasma and saline for the second twenty-four hours. Whole blood for one-half of the plasma fraction is recommended in burns of more than 20 per cent. Also required is a baseline intake of approximately 2000 cc. of dextrose and water per day which may be taken by mouth. An acute widespread peritonitis behaves like a 15 to 20 per cent burn and requires similar treatment.

At the end of forty-eight to seventy-two hours in the case of the burn and in a variable period, usually longer in the case of infections and crush injury, the third space begins to resolve. When this occurs replacement of electrolytes and water must be stopped, for the patient obtains an autoinfusion of water and extracellular electrolytes from the resolving third place. The patient may have some difficulty in disposing of what has now become an overexpanded total extracellular fluid space. Intake at this point must be reverted back to baseline, and

electrolyte intake must be curtailed while the patient undergoes a diuresis to dispose of the fluid returning from the third space. Fluid
pooled in the gut in ileus results in internal dehydration. Electrolyte
concentration of this fluid is that of small bowel. During the acute
phase, partial replacement of fluid lost into the gut is necessary in
order to maintain circulating volume and extracellular fluid space at

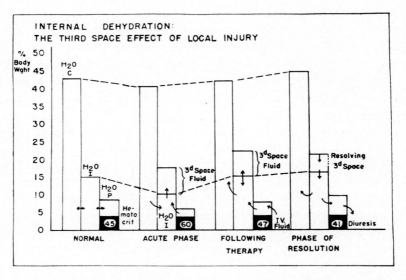

Fig. 154.—Illustrating the effects of internal dehydration by injury
or ileus with the creation of a third fluid space of unavailable fluid
which dehydrates plasma and cells and diminishes available interstitial
fluid. Replacement therapy restores normal volumes, and subsequent
resolution of third space may overexpand available extracellular fluid.
H_2O C is cell water, H_2O I, interstitial fluid and H_2O P plasma water.

a functioning level. Two to three thousand cubic centimeters of fluid
may be accumulated within the bowel in a case of marked ileus. If the
fluid is subsequently drained it becomes an external loss; if not, as the
bowel recovers the fluid will be reabsorbed and provide the same type
of return of fluid and electrolyte as is seen in the resolving phase of the
patient with a burn. The accompanying diagram, Figure 154, illustrates the various phases of the third space effect in terms of intracellular water, interstitial fluid and plasma volume.

STATIC DEBT: DEFICIENCIES OF WATER, ELECTROLYTES AND BLOOD VOLUME

When the patient is first seen and treatment is begun there may well be deficiencies or excesses in body water, in intra- and extracellular electrolytes, and in blood volume. Excesses are usually the result of previous overenthusiastic treatment, but they may be due to disease processes as well, as for example, the excess of extracellular fluid present, in cardiac failure, the nephrotic stage of nephritis, or in the cirrhotic.

DEHYDRATION. The effect of dehydration depends upon the amount of water lost, the rate at which the loss occurs, and the amount and type of electrolytes lost. In slow dehydration, such as would be seen in a patient with obstruction of the sigmoid colon and slowly increasing distention, the loss of water and electrolyte is proportionate to volume among the plasma, interstitial fluid and intracellular fluid. While the total volume of water lost may be quite large, the effect on the patient is not as profound as is seen with more rapid dehydration. The patient appears clinically moderately dehydrated; the urine specific gravity is usually high; skin turgor is lost; and the hematocrit, if no pre-existing anemia is present, shows a mild to moderate elevation.

In rapid dehydration the loss of fluid and electrolytes is largely from the plasma and interstitial fluid. This is the case in acute small intestinal obstruction with vomiting, where the patient may become acutely dehydrated with a markedly elevated hematocrit and diminshed circulating blood volume in a period of twenty-four hours. The most rapid form of dehydration is the direct loss of circulating volume as a result of hemorrhage. The various types of dehydration and the source of the fluid involved are well illustrated in Figure 155, by Moore. This shows not only the effect of slow, rapid and hemorrhage dehydration, but also illustrates the effect of the creation of a third space in burns or trauma.

Another important aspect of dehydration is the relative rate of loss of water and electrolytes. If water is lost more rapidly than electrolyte as is the case with simple thirsting, insensible loss of water results in a concentration of extracellular fluid electrolytes. There follows a transfer of cell water to the extracellular fluid space, and the secretion of a hypertonic urine containing a high concentration of extracellular fluid electrolytes to restore osmotic balance. In most surgical conditions, however, the loss of electrolyte is likely to be more rapid than the loss of water. This is well illustrated in a patient with diarrhea who drinks large volumes of water, but does not replace the electrolyte lost. Such a patient, in a relatively short time, will develop a state of acute electrolyte deficiency, with dehydration and a deficient plasma concentration of sodium and chloride ions; collapse with hypotension quickly follows.

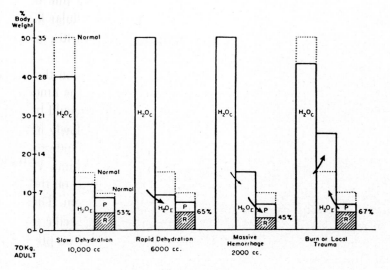

Fig. 155.—The effect of rate of dehydration on type of fluid lost. H_2O_c is cell water, H_2O_E, interstitial fluid and P, plasma. (From Moore, F. D.: *J.A.M.A. 141:646*, 1949.)

A similar situation exists in small intestinal obstruction where the patient vomits very large quantities of somewhat hypotonic gastrointestinal tract juices and drinks sufficient water between vomiting episodes to allow replacement of part of the water lost. The type of dehydration most likely to produce shock, as demonstrated by Elkinton, Winkler and Danowski, is this hypotonic type in which there is a depletion of both water and electrolytes with electrolyte loss predominating. This results in a diminished extracellular fluid space with lowered concentration of electrolytes in the remaining fluid.

The composition of replacement fluids required in dehydration depends upon the rate of dehydration and the extent of the electrolyte depletion in remaining fluids. In slow dehydration, it is obvious that a large proportion of the water loss is from the intracellular compartment. Replacement requires water, potassium and possibly phosphate for restoration, and a relatively small amount of sodium chloride and bicarbonate for the extracellular fluid component. More rapid dehydration is largely extracellular fluid in its character and here the replacement required is water and electrolytes according to the proportions in which they exist in the extracellular fluid. For straightforward expansion of the extracellular fluid space, either Hartman's solution or a proportion of two-thirds isotonic sodium chloride and one-third sodium bicarbonate or one-sixth molar sodium lactate is better than the administration of normal saline alone. However, with vomiting, chloride loss is often in excess of sodium, and saline is the fluid of choice.

Losses from the circulating blood volume require replacement in kind, in either whole blood or plasma as the case may be. A pre-existing anemia may be masked by a relative degree of dehydration to give normal values for red count, hemoglobin and hematocrit and still leave a considerably diminished blood volume. This situation was described by Clark and his associates as "chronic shock," and it is found to exist in many cases of patients suffering from debilitating diseases or chronic infection. Of 100 unselected patients admitted for truly major surgery to the General Surgical Service at Presbyterian Hospital, blood volume determinations revealed that 65 of these required one or more transfusions to restore blood volume to normal. Of this group of 65 approximately 40 per cent had normal hemoglobin, normal hematocrit and normal red blood counts. The technic of determining blood volumes has been extensively investigated and while subject to some errors is still a far better method of estimating deficiencies of blood volumes than are standard measurements of blood count and concentrations of hemoglobin.

POTASSIUM DEFICIENCY. Muscular weakness, apathy, lethargy, abdominal distention, adynamic ileus, tachycardia and infrequently skeletal muscle paralysis have been described by several different observers, in the postoperative period and occasionally preoperatively in patients who have had a diminished intake and increased losses of potassium. This syndrome usually occurs between the fourth and sixth or seventh postoperative day in patients who have been maintained on parenteral and oral fluids which do not contain potassium in significant quantities. The clinical syndrome is accompanied by an alkalosis and a hypochloremia usually with an acid urine. The fixed alkalosis and its response to potassium were described in 1946 by Darrow, following diarrhea in infants. This syndrome is unresponsive to the administration of sodium chloride but responds readily to the administration of potassium salts parenterally and somewhat more slowly to potassium intake by mouth. It is accompanied by a low serum potassium level with levels in the range of 3 mEq. per liter or less, and presents in addition certain definite electrocardiographic changes which help in diagnosis.

Treatment consists of the administration of potassium chloride or potassium phosphate intravenously with the potassium administered in concentrations not to exceed 40 mEq. per liter in infusion fluids. As much as 150 mEq. of potassium per twenty-four hours may be required in a severe case.

The majority of these cases may be prevented by the prophylactic administration of from 30 to 40 mEq. of potassium per day in baseline fluids, together with an additional 10 mEq. of potassium for each liter of gastrointestinal tract fluid aspirated. Potassium should *not* be given (1) in patients who are acutely dehydrated until rehydration is well under way, hematocrit falling and urine volume rising; (2) in patients with any degree of renal failure, particularly marked oliguria or elevated nonprotein nitrogen unless the serum potassium level is known to be low, and (3) potassium should not be given the day of operation or the first twenty-four hours postoperatively, again unless the level is known to be low.

PRIMARY CHLORIDE DEFICIENCY. This usually results from the vomiting or aspiration of large volumes of fluid from the stomach in patients with a high gastric acidity with a primary chloride loss in excess of sodium. The acute manifestation of primary chloride deficiency is likely to be tetany as the result of the alkalosis which develops with the loss of chloride. A diagnosis usually can be made from the clinical history and laboratory examination of the plasma which shows a high bicarbonate and low chloride with a normal or slightly elevated blood urea nitrogen. Patients usually respond to the administration of sodium chloride. In those patients in which there is reduction of excretion of sodium by the kidneys, and particularly in the immediately postoperative period, the administration of part of the requirement as ammonium chloride intravenously is preferred in correction. The failure of primary chloride deficiency to respond to ammonium and sodium chloride therapy should immediately arouse suspicion of potassium deficiency, as Darrow has shown that potassium deficiency can result from alkalosis.

TABLE 10. THE ELECTROLYTE CONTENT OF 1 LITER OF INFUSION FLUIDS (mEQ)

	Na	K	Cl	Effective HCO₂
Sodium chloride 0.9%	154	0	154	0
M/6 sodium lactate	167	0	0	167
Sodium bicarbonate 1.2%	143	0	0	143
Ammonium chloride 0.75%	0	0	140	0
Dextrose in water	0	0	0	0
Potassium chloride ampules (1.59 gm.) in 10 cc.	0	20	20	0
Special Solutions				
Hartman's solution *	136	5.3	112	33
Darrow's solution	120	35	105	50
Sodium chloride-potassium chloride (Mudge)	110	30	140	0
Potassium chloride (2.23 gm.) 5% dextrose in water	0	30	30	0

* Ca^{++} 3.6 mEq.

PARENTERAL FLUIDS. Two concepts must constantly be kept in mind in selecting parenteral fluids, volume and concentration. If the extracellular fluid space is larger than normal, sodium and chloride concentrations may be low as is the case postoperatively, and in cardiac failure and cirrhosis, yet the total sodium and chloride present are likely to be normal or high. Efforts to restore a normal concentration by the addition of more electrolyte is likely only to expand further an already overexpanded space, particularly if there is water and sodium retention as there is likely to be in these cases.

On the other hand, when the total extracellular fluid space is decreased, as in dehydration or a third space formation, then electrolyte must be given with water or the needed expansion cannot be achieved.

Critically low levels of electrolytes in plasma require replacement. Serum sodium is seriously low in most surgical patients if it is below 125 mEq. per liter, and shock is likely at levels below 120 mEq. per liter. Much depends on the rate of fall. If it is rapid, shock is more likely than if it is slow, and patients on prolonged sodium restriction may have serum levels in the range of 110 to 120 mEq. per liter without symptoms. Serum chloride requires replacement in most surgical patients when the level falls to 85 mEq. per liter, and bicarbonate when it is below 15 mEq. per liter (33 volumes per cent), while potassium levels below 3.4 mEq. per liter are suspect and below 3.0 mEq. require replacement.

Flame photometers for the direct measurement of sodium and potassium concentration in biological fluids have proved to be most valuable and are now essential for the management of complicated cases.

The selection of the proper parenteral fluid or combination of fluids is necessary to replace adequately dynamic losses and static debts. Table 10 gives the composition of various types of fluids commonly used.

It should be remembered that parenteral replacement is always a temporary and inadequate substitute for the gastrointestinal tract, and oral intake should be resumed as soon as returning function permits, supplementing parenterally until oral intake is adequate in water, electrolytes and calories.

FRANCIS DANIELS MOORE (1913–)

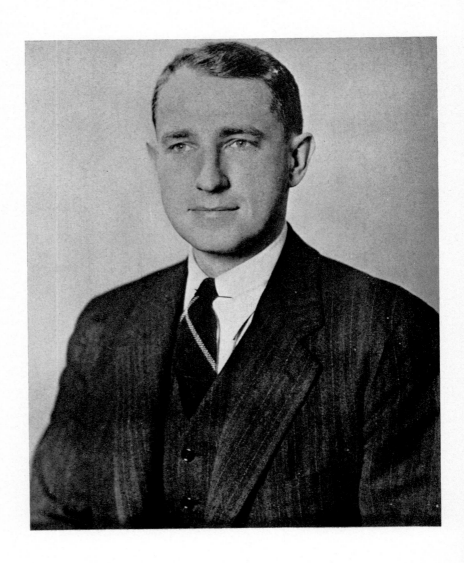

Francis Daniels Moore was born in Evanston, Illinois, on August 17, 1913. He was trained at the Harvard Medical School and the Massachusetts General Hospital.

Soon after his residency, Dr. Moore became interested in the biochemical and metabolic approach to the study of surgical patients. His work with isotopes has opened new vistas in the understanding of body composition. In 1953 Dr. Moore reported his milestone article outlining a "working theory of convalescence" in which the endocrine, metabolic and compositional changes exhibited by the surgical patient were classified.

In 1948 Dr. Moore was appointed Moseley Professor of Surgery at Harvard Medical School and Surgeon-in-Chief at the Peter Bent Brigham Hospital. He is a past president of the Society of University Surgeons and holds numerous organizational and governmental honors.

BODILY CHANGES IN SURGICAL CONVALESCENCE[1]

I—The Normal Sequence—Observations and Interpretations

BY FRANCIS D. MOORE, M.D.

*From the Peter Bent Brigham Hospital,
Harvard Medical School, Boston, Massachusetts*

I. INTRODUCTION

Surgical convalescence—the process of recovery—is initiated by the injury itself and it is maintained by the action of positive biological forces. Many years of work will pass and many more studies are needed before a complete picture of convalescence can be drawn. When such an understanding is available, we will be able to appreciate accurately the interplay of these strong forces—some directed at restoring homeostasis for the emergency, some directed at healing the wound, and still others devoted to returning the organism to its normal composition, activity and reproduction.

Despite large gaps, enough data are at hand to piece together a preliminary account of some of the clinical appearances and biochemical changes which occur and to designate these bodily changes as a normal sequence in convalescence. Secondly, it is possible to advance a tentative theory as to the forces which produce these bodily changes. Thirdly, it is justifiable to offer an interpretation of the meaning of

[1] The Seventh Annual Edward D. Churchill Lecture of the Excelsior Surgical Society, delivered at Pittsburgh, Pa., October 24, 1952. This work has been supported throughout by a grant from the Atomic Energy Commission through the Peter Bent Brigham Hospital. Submitted for publication December, 1952.

From *Annals of Surgery, 137:289,* 1953. Reprinted by permission.

these forces in the healing of the wound and in the recovery of the patient. Such are the purposes of this paper.

The significance of normal convalescence as a guide to surgical care, and the importance of understanding the normal as a basis for definition and treatment of the abnormal need no elaboration. Yet, neither therapy nor abnormality should properly become a part of the description of normal metabolism, and for this reason, they are omitted here. We will consider clinical metabolism, an illustrative case, endocrinology and teleology in that order.

II. THE FOUR PHASES OF CONVALESCENCE

Clinical Metabolism

Four phases of convalescence seem to appear in distinct sequence in normal post-trauma metabolism as we have seen it in the study of our patients. These phases are:

Phase I   —The Adrenergic-Corticoid Phase
Phase II —The Corticoid Withdrawal Phase
Phase III—The Spontaneous Anabolic Phase
Phase IV—The Fat Gain Phase[2]

It must be emphasized at the outset that the duration of each of these four phases varies with the magnitude of the trauma and the previous nutritional state of the patient. General average figures are presented for the duration of each phase after "moderately extensive" (scale 6–7) trauma.[3]

Many of the observations, calculations and correlations presented are based on facts previously reported from these and other laboratories. Other data are based on quantitative information on destruction and synthesis of fat and lean tissue, which have been obtained by studies in our laboratory and not previously published. Although the entire set of observations needed to construct this picture of convalescence can be made in a single patient, such extensive studies of a

---

[2] These four phases have been given names which are *descriptive* of the clinical and metabolic picture. Mechanisms are obscure, and the names selected should not prejudice the reader as to detailed mechanisms.

[3] By this figure is indicated an approximate scale of the severity of trauma. This scale runs from 1 to 10. Pneumonectomy, total gastrectomy, multivisceral cancer operations are examples of trauma in the range of scales 7, 8 and 9.

single person surely will be rare. The illustrative case presentation is, therefore, a synthesis based on observations made on many patients and at different times.

The metabolic balance data are based on observed averages of intake by diet and intravenous feedings, and total output by all routes. Balances of nitrogen, potassium and sodium are shown, since only for these elements do we have enough available data to construct averages or show an illustrative case. Eosinophile counts, body weights and urinary steroid hormone analyses are presented and discussed. The latter are based on available information concerning 17-ketosteroid excretion after ordinary surgical trauma, and in this area of study, we are basing our presentation on extremely fragmentary information. Data on excretion of other steroids are sorely needed. Caloric intake is indicated, based on observed averages.

Plasma concentrations of sodium and potassium are discussed because of their significance in cell permeability changes after trauma. In the well-nourished individual given adequate water and spared excessive salt loads, we have not seen significant changes in blood urea, serum protein concentration, carbon dioxide combining power or hematocrit (providing blood loss is replaced). Such changes may occur: systematic alterations have not been documented as a part of the *normal* recovery process and will not be discussed further here. Alterations in channels of protein metabolism (creatine, creatinine, urea, ammonia) and intermediary carbohydrate metabolism (lactate pyruvate) are of great interest,[4] but we are not able as yet to place them accurately in reference to other metabolic changes, and will omit them from further consideration.

Total body water is indicated, as it forms the basis for the calculation of fat oxidation rates. Other "space" measurements such as plasma volume, red cell mass and extracellular fluid are omitted because of insufficient data based on the *normal* surgical patient and carried out by acceptable methods.

The experience on which this account is based consists of the study of metabolism following trauma in 75 cases studied carefully by these

[4] Data on early changes in some of these fractions are available in the recent article by Hardy and Ravdin (Hardy, James D., and I. S. Ravdin: Some Physiologic Aspects of Surgical Trauma. *Ann. Surg. 136:*345, 1952), and in the work of Hayes and Brandt (Hayes, Mark. A., and R. L. Brandt: Carbohydrate Metabolism in the Immediate Postoperative Period. *Surgery. 32:*819, 1952).

technics, fragmentary metabolic observations in about 100 others, and clinical care of many patients in general surgery.

PREOPERATIVE

1. CLINICAL. We are considering the normal course of events in metabolically normal persons. Therefore, the preoperative period presents the clinical appearances of a hospitalized patient harboring disease which has not produced starvation, previous trauma, chronic infection or severe recent pain.[5] Any such abnormalities—however common—are of the greatest importance in modifying normal convalescence; they properly do not enter into a description of the normal process. Barring these common abnormalities, the clinical events to consider are the apprehension which normally precedes surgery, and the reduction of diet which precedes elective gastro-intestinal operation.

2. METABOLIC. A normal adult, neither gaining nor losing weight, is in zero balance of nitrogen, potassium and sodium. On the evening prior to an operation, it is not uncommon to find a reduction in nitrogen intake due to dietary restriction, with a resultant small negative balance for the 24 hours prior to surgery. It is also not unusual to find the eosinophiles dropping prior to surgery, presumably on the basis of anxiety as mentioned above. We have not regarded either of these phenomena as being of clinical significance, although they alter the metabolic picture. It may be of great value for the patient's gastrointestinal tract to be empty at the time of surgery, and an eosinophile drop a few hours before surgery indicates only the begining of convalescent metabolic changes prior to, rather than at surgery.

PHASE I—THE ADRENERGIC-CORTICOID PHASE

1. CLINICAL. As the patient goes to the operating room and anesthesia is induced, trauma is suffered and convalescence begins. The clinical appearances of the patient at this time are chiefly characterized by evidences of adrenal medullary activity; an increase in pulse rate, a narrowing of the pulse pressure, peripheral vasoconstriction—with or without sweating—and a rise in blood sugar. These are often associated with apprehension alone, or the excitement stage of ether

---

[5] Examples are cholelithiasis, duodenal ulcer, early prostatic obstruction, early carcinoma of the lung, asymptomatic carcinoma of the gastro-intestinal tract, etc.

anesthesia; but as the patient goes into the deeper planes of anesthesia for the duration of his procedure, he may show essentially normal findings in all of these regards as his circulatory dynamics assume a stable pattern, and providing traumatic or surgical shock does not occur. Spinal anesthesia, intravenous barbiturates and drugs which interfere with normal autonomic transmission produce differences with regard to the adrenal-medullary phase, either decreasing its intensity by dampening an excitement phase, or procrastinating it. Trauma in the unanesthetized individual produces intense adrenal-medullary activity, so apparent in the wounded soldier.

We are assuming here that blood lost at the operation is quantitatively replaced by immediate transfusion and that there is no over-transfusion nor incompatibility, and that the whole blood used is fresh. Although simple bleeding alone excites metabolic changes, this bleeding with immediate replacement does not alter the massive convalescent response which is now starting.

As the patient returns to the ward after an operation of two to four hours' duration, he arouses soon from his anesthesia and complains of incisional pain. He is listless and usually shows little desire to do anything. He has to be asked to turn over in bed, whereas a few hours earlier preoperatively he may have been restless and hyperactive. Auscultation of the abdomen may show some peristaltic activity, particularly if the peritoneal cavity is free of any retained blood or contamination. Within 12 to 24 hours this peristalsis quite characteristically ceases.

After an operation of approximately scale 6–7, such as a major anastomotic gastrointestinal operation involving removal of viscera, this phase of listlessness and inactivity with lack of interest in conversation, the printed page, and any contact with the outside environment lasts for approximately three to five days.[6] After very simple surgery (hernia, appendix) this clinical phase lasts only one to two days; after extensive wounds or burns, it may last a week or more.

During this phase, the patient has no hunger. If his temperature is

---

[6] Lest there be misunderstanding on this point, it should be emphasized that in elderly people or those depleted with disease, this adrenergic-corticoid phase is of much shorter duration and lesser magnitude than it is in younger individuals in good health. It is not uncommon in elderly depleted people, on the day following operation, that they are sitting up in bed, "as if nothing had happened" and they show metabolic changes in miniature, accordingly. This is an abnormal variant of normal convalescence and is not under discussion in this paper.

taken carefully by rectum, it will be found that there is a slight elevation of temperature in these first two or three days, returning to normal at about the third day. Temperatures taken by mouth, and more especially temperatures taken by axilla (where skin vasoconstriction may completely obliterate these alterations) will often fail to show this phenomenon. If the patient has atelectasis or some other source of an infectious or inflammatory process, this normal thermal response is, of course, distorted upwards. He may continue to show some adrenergic activity (such as elevated pulse rate) during this phase, but it is of short duration (lasting less than 24 hours) if pain is not severe.

There is relative oliguria (500 to 750 cc.) the day of operation unless the patient is the recipient of excessive water infusions. During the following days, outputs of 1000 to 2000 cc. are not unusual.

In summary, the clinical picture of the adrenergic-corticoid phase is that of a patient whose vascular responses have been stimulated but who has no ambition, strength or appetite. The first clinical evidences of the end of the corticoid phase are a return of peristalsis, the expelling of flatus by rectum, the onset of hunger, which is not marked, but which is a distinct change, and a gradually returning interest in the outside world, a desire to see visitors, to read the newspaper and resume contact with the environment.

2. THE WOUND. During this phase the tensile strength of the wound is reliant upon the sutures. If the wound must be reopened, it falls apart easily without the use of a sharp instrument. The microanatomic changes which occur provide a framework for subsequent fibrous union, but during this first phase, fibrous tissue proliferation is not prominent. Characteristic of this early phase are the formation of a fibrin coagulum in an accumulation of extracellular fluid and blood cells, and the accumulation of phagocytic cells around foreign material, tissue debris or bacteria. There is a polymorphonuclear leucocytosis, whether or not infection actually occurs.

3. METABOLIC.

A. *Weight*. Weight drops rapidly, and to an extent greater than that predicted from changes in nitrogen balance or extracellular water or both. This suggests the rapid utilization of body fat.

B. *Nitrogen*. After an operation of considerable magnitude it is typical, with no nitrogen intake, for the urinary nitrogen excretion to be larger than it was preoperatively on basal diet. This quantitative increase in urinary nitrogen excretion is characteristic of the response to more extensive trauma, whereas after a lesser trauma, the absolute urinary nitrogen excretion rate may be quite moderate (5 Gm. or less). Since there is characteristically no nitrogen intake during this first phase, the source of this nitrogen is presumed to be the general body protein, and since most of this protein is in skeletal muscle, that is considered to be the source. This rate of nitrogen excretion decreases stepwise during the succeeding days of the adrenergic-corticoid phase. One occasionally observes a so-called "delayed peak" nitrogen excretion, but in our experience, it is the exception rather than the rule. In either event, since there is little or no nitrogen intake in this phase, a negative balance results.

C. *Potassium.* Potassium excretion shows the characteristic loss on the operative day of about 70 mEq., thereafter reducing itself to about 40 mEq. per day for two or three days and then, in a stepwise fashion, reducing itself further. Again since intake is ordinarily zero at this time, there is a negative balance. The potassium:nitrogen ratio of the negative balance of the adrenergic-corticoid phase is characteristically 5 mEq. per Gm. or more, indicating a mobilization of cell water and electrolyte disproportionate to cell matrix.

D. *Sodium.* The sodium excretion on the day of operation is reduced almost to zero if the patient is given no sodium.[7] The net metabolic effect is that of no total flux with the environment. There may be a tiny excretion of 5 to 15 mEq. which, in the face of no intake, results in a miniature negative balance, but its total magnitude is inconsequential. The loss of sodium in the sweat is likewise small after trauma.

E. *Calories.* During these days, caloric intake by mouth is usually quite low or zero. Approximately 150 to 400 calories a day may be supplied by dextrose in ordinary concentrations used intravenously, or more calories may be supplied by other materials (alcohol, fat), the utility of which, in this early period, remains to be proven.

---

[7] This refers to the normal situation. Alkalosis, saline infusion, excess water infusions and possibly malnutrition may increase postoperative renal sodium excretion. These alterations are not dealt with here, though they may account for some of the postoperative sodium excretions reported by Snyder (Snyder, H. E., C. D. Snyder, and L. D. Bunch: Urinary Excretion of Electrolytes and Water Before, During and After Surgery. *Arch. Surg.* 65:578, 1952).

F. *Eosinophile Count and Steroid Excretion.* By the indices under consideration here, the first outward evidence of the convalescent response is a drop in the eosinophile count which may start preoperatively, proceeds during anesthesia and is often at zero or close to zero by the time operation is completed. Further study is necessary before we can ascribe the differences in eosinophile fall to different types of anesthesia or to different preoperative psychological settings, although such would appear to be the logical explanation for these variations. The eosinophile count may remain low (near zero) for two to five days, depending upon the magnitude of the operation, the continuance of postoperative pain or the superimposition of abnormalities such as infection. If there are no complications of a major sort, the eosinophile count starts upward about the third or fourth day and by the sixth day postoperatively, may quite regularly be found to be higher than it was to begin with (the "backswing overshoot"), a characteristic of the second phase of convalescence (see below). Just as the fall in eosinophiles heralded the onset of the adrenergic-corticoid phase, so their rise and backswing overshoot heralds its conclusion.

Urinary steroid excretion shows a sharp rise on the day of operation. This, however, may last only one day. Thereafter, the excretion of 17-ketosteroids returns to a below-normal level.[8]

G. *Blood Chemistry.* The concentration of sodium in the plasma shows a distinct drop during this phase. A drop from a normal level of 140 to 143 mEq. per liter to a value of 137 to 139 would be expected for a moderate degree of trauma (scale 3–5). For more extensive injury (scale 6–7) the plasma sodium may fall to 134 to 137 mEq. per liter. This drop does not in any way endanger the survival of the patient, nor is it harmful in itself. Yet it indicates an alteration which is of great theoretical interest and of extreme practical significance in severely ill patients with concomitant extra-renal losses, heart or renal disease, where it is tremendously exaggerated. It must be recalled that this lowering of plasma sodium occurs in the face of extreme renal sodium conservation and in the presence of potassium losses averaging 125 to 150 mEq. in the first three days after moderately severe (scale

---

[8] Again to avoid misconception, it is important to emphasize the very commonly observed fact that in elderly people with advanced cancer or depleting disease, there may be no increases in 17-ketosteroid excretion whatsoever after trauma. This, again, is an abnormality of convalescence associated with previous depletion and is not the subject of this discussion.

6–7) injury. In the normal patient there is no rise in plasma potassium concentration despite the apparent mobilization from cells into extracellular fluid.

H. *Total Body Water and Fat.* During this phase, total body water changes only slightly, the direction depending upon the degree of hydration maintained by administration of fluids orally, rectally or parenterally.[9] This fact, together with the disproportionate weight loss, is the basis for the calculation of the rate of endogenous fat oxidation which is found to be significantly increased over the starvation rate.

K. *The End of Phase I.* The clinical appearances already mentioned, the rise of eosinophiles to a high level and lowering of urinary nitrogen excretion signalize the end of phase I.

PHASE II—THE CORTICOID WITHDRAWAL PHASE

I. CLINICAL. This phase of convalescence begins about the fourth day and lasts two to three days after extensive surgery, occupying the period from about the fifth to the seventh or eighth day.

During this time, two sets of clinical happenings are of outstanding interest. The first has already been mentioned, namely the increase in peristalsis, passage of flatus, increase in appetite, increase in spontaneous physical activity and an increasing interest in the surroundings. These need no further comment save to point out that the patient quite characteristically shows an interest in doing things which are greater than his ability to follow through. This second phase may be described as a phase of convalescence when the patient is "ambitious but weak"; a characteristic happening is that the patient seeks the newspaper with great interest but after reading it a little, he puts it aside and falls asleep. Or he may make a telephone call to his home or office only to find, after a few moments' conversation, that he is no longer interested and it is simply tiring him. This is the phase of convalescence when an excess of chatty visitors is most disturbing and tiring to the patient.

The second set of happenings relate to a water diuresis which is readily observed if daily urinary outputs are measured. It is not uncommon during this phase to see the water output actually exceed the

---

[9] The administration of large quantities of water or saline during the adrenergic-corticoid phase will result in sudden massive increases in total body water and may completely obliterate the normal loss of weight observed. This is a pathological variant as is the associated weight gain.

intake for a day or two. There may be a further sharp weight loss during such a water diuresis but, as will be pointed out below, this weight loss is accompanied by a different metabolic picture and has a very different interpretation from that encountered during the adrenergic-corticoid phase.

2. THE WOUND. During this period the wound usually becomes free of acute pain, although strain on the wound may still be painful. The wound at this phase shows the tissue hiatus to be filled with fibroblasts and there is considerable fibroblastic proliferation going on. Intercellular substance is now laid down; presumably collagen. Tensile strength increases and after extensive trauma may be great enough to permit suture removal by the sixth to eighth day in primarily incised wounds. By the end of this phase, reopening the wound requires the use of a scalpel. Epithelization occurs; the line of a primarily sutured wound remains red.

3. METABOLIC.

A. *Weight.* There is a further weight loss in phase II, but it bears a closer correlation to water and lean tissue changes, and fat utilization is much less prominent.

B. *Nitrogen.* During this time the nitrogen excretion rate in the urine is definitely lower than it has been during the adrenergic-corticoid phase, yet since oral intake of diet may not have restored the nitrogen intake to normal, one does not commonly see a strongly positive nitrogen balance during this phase. There is instead a net zero balance with a gradual trend to positivity. It is, therefore, not the balance but the sharply decreased urinary nitrogen excretion rate which is the key to this metabolic alteration of phase II. Whether or not nitrogen is supplied, the loss rate is reduced. This change may be dramatic as, for example, in cases where, in a period of 48 hours, the urinary nitrogen excretion rate is reduced from 15 to 5 Gm. per day in the face of unchanged nitrogen intakes, urine outputs and blood urea. This alteration indicates relative cessation of lean tissue destruction and a readiness to start anabolism, the initiation of which, by provision of exogenous (dietary) calories and nitrogen, ushers in phase III (see below).

C. *Potassium.* As small potassium intakes are commenced, associated with "early" liquids and soft solids, the urinary potassium excretion rate (like the nitrogen excretion rate) is sharply reduced to a low figure, occasionally the lowest figure that one ever sees in surgical patients with normal urine outputs (as low as 5 to 15 mEq. per day). The result (with even small liquid intakes) is a marked positive potassium balance—in contrast to nitrogen, where positive balance is slower to occur. The K:N ratio of the negative balance in the adrenergic-corticoid phase has been high, and here we see the reverse of this phenomenon, namely a positive potassium balance during a zero or only weakly positive nitrogen balance. After but two or three days of this phenomenon, potassium excretion is again increased as intake increases until, characteristically at the end of this phase, the patient is only in weakly positive potassium balance again. The result of this interesting phase is to restore to the body most of the potassium initially lost "in excess" of nitrogen.

D. *Sodium.* The sodium picture is the inverse of potassium. As the sodium intake is progressively increased as a result of increasing oral diet, the sodium excretion is disproportionately increased, resulting in a diuresis of sodium, the extent of which is directly proportional to previous sodium loading. Where excess sodium has not been given during the adrenergic-corticoid phase, the subsequent net loss is, by the same token, small.

E. *Calories.* The caloric intake characteristically increases in a step-wise fashion during this phase. As the patient has more interest in food, he increases his diet, but during phase II it usually does not return to normal.

F. *Eosinophile Count and Steroid Excretion.* The eosinophile count, as previously mentioned, backswings to a level above its starting value. This is a characteristic finding of the early corticoid withdrawal phase. It is interesting that this backswing overshoot may last only one day or a fraction of a day, and then the eosinophiles gradually start back down to normal. After extremely extensive trauma, where the eosinophiles have been low for several days or weeks (as in burns), it has been our impression that the backswing overshoot lasts for a much longer time and goes to higher levels. This is a healthy phenomenon which carries a good prognosis.[10]

G. *Blood Studies.* Blood chemical findings during this time are

---

[10] We have seen instances where the high eosinophile count in this phase is insensitive to further trauma—or may even rise with trauma—although there is no convincing collateral evidence of adrenal insufficiency.

characterized by a return of the sodium concentration in the blood to normal, despite an increased sodium excretion in the urine.

H. *Total Body Water and Fat.* There is a minor drop of total body water associated with any diuresis which may occur (depending on previous loading). However, the change in body weight correlates well with nitrogen and extracellular phase changes, and body fat utilization no longer looms as a large source of calories.

K. *End of Phase II.* The cessation of rapid potassium loading and sodium diuresis a day or two after the backswing overshoot of the eosinophiles indicates that phase II is over and phase III is "ready to begin." A normal third phase can only begin if diet is resumed; if diet is not increasing rapidly towards normal at this time, convalescence is "stalled." This abnormality of the convalescent process will be dealt with elsewhere; it is characterized by a failure to gain weight, strength and vigor. It is noteworthy that wound healing commonly proceeds to completion despite prolonged dietary interruption and despite negative nitrogen balance on the basis of postoperative starvation. Return of strength and clinical recovery do not occur under such circumstances, however, and convalescence is incomplete. Up to this point, diet is not needed for convalescence or wound healing; now it becomes essential for survival.

PHASE III—SPONTANEOUS ANABOLIC PHASE

I. CLINICAL. This phase is initiated by—and can only occur with —adequate oral diet. After major peritoneal injury, it commences about the seventh to tenth day.

During this period the patient has increasing strength. He becomes very hungry and soon finds himself eating a normal diet or a diet larger than his normal average. He is "ambitious and stronger." During this time he picks up the paper and reads it completely from cover to cover, observing many little details in the newspaper to which he never ordinarily devotes any attention; he may even do the cross-word puzzle. He is bored. If he has a telephone at his bedside, he calls up people and engages in prolonged and wordy conversations. Visitors come to see him and he coaxes them to stay longer. He begins to wonder when he is going to go home, and during the middle of his spontaneous anabolic phase, he is discharged home. However, when he arrives home from the protected hospital environment, he finds his strength is less than he thought, and that there is some resumption still to do—which he proceeds to do during the next few weeks, at the end of which time he returns to work. Sexual function is not vigorous; normal menses do not return during the early part of this phase and may not return until it is completed.

There are few laboratory findings by ordinary methods which are particularly significant during this time. Blood chemistry appears to be normal, as is urine output.

2. THE WOUND. Tensile strength has now increased towards normal. Some consciousness of the presence of a wound—if not actual pain—persists. The wound remains red and grows above the surrounding tissue, and a primarily sutured wound is palpable as a red raised line. The small suture marks gradually disappear. That the wound still carries a high biologic priority even at this late time is evidenced by the common occurrence of complete healing in the absence of dietary intake, as mentioned above. The local activity in the wound is apparently related to deposition of intercellular substance such as collagen and bone matrix.

3. METABOLIC.

A. *Weight.* There is a weight gain which correlates perfectly with that predicted from nitrogen balance, indicating that fat gain is not prominent.

B. *Nitrogen.* The characteristic and controlling feature of this phase is a steady, sustained, positive nitrogen balance in the range of 3 to 5 Gm. nitrogen per day per 70 kg. body weight. This is the convalescent anabolic norm, and in our experience it cannot be increased by forced feeding or any form of hormone therapy now available. The caloric intake (see below) must be at a high level to sustain this nitrogen anabolism, and indeed calories:nitrogen ratios[11] of 150 or higher are of vital importance. Sustained positive nitrogen balance cannot occur without balanced diet, including an adequate supply of vitamins. For this reason, a normal phase III cannot commence until diet begins. Anabolism is ready to begin after a few days of phase II. Diet "lets it start." The role of diet here is *permissive,* not *initiative.*

C. *Potassium.* There is a potassium balance which is only weakly positive, yet adequate to account for a normal intramuscular K:N

---

[11] The calorie:nitrogen ratio is the ratio of nonprotein calories to nitrogen in the diet.

ratio of about 2.7 mEq. per Gm. nitrogen. By ordinary methods, this positive potassium balance is scarcely discernible, and is much smaller than the spectacular positive potassium balance seen during the corticoid withdrawal phase.

D. *Sodium.* Zero sodium balance is encountered. It is important to note that in measuring sodium balances, there are wide daily swings. However, the average for any period of a few days will be close to zero.

E. *Calories.* Caloric intake, as mentioned above, must be sustained in the region of 2000 to 3000 calories per day in order to sustain the maximum rate of protein synthesis. This synthesis presumably occurs in skeletal muscle which has been the site of the previously lost nitrogen.

F. *Eosinophiles and Steroid Excretion.* The eosinophile count is normal during this period. The excretion of 17-ketosteroids remains at a low level. This is of signal interest in the face of nitrogen anabolism, and suggests that endocrine forces, other than anabolic steroids, are at work.

G. *Blood Chemistry.* There are no characteristic changes in blood chemistry during this period.

H. *Total Body Water and Fat.* Total body water increases during this time in an amount commensurate with the lean tissue being synthesized, assuming that this tissue is about 73 per cent water. Fat is not deposited in any quantity as yet.

PHASE IV—THE FAT GAIN PHASE

1. CLINICAL. The patient has now been discharged home, and after adding an amount of nitrogen to his body commensurate with that previously lost, he enters into the fourth phase of convalescence, which may last many weeks or months. It is characterized by a return of full bodily weight and function. During the fat gain phase, the patient usually returns to work. If the work imposes a high caloric requirement, this may considerably delay the fat-gain phase. During the adrenergic–corticoid phase, the corticoid withdrawal phase and most of the spontaneous anabolic phase, the patient has shown little sexual interest or activity, and if a female, there is cessation of the menses during this time. However, during the fat gain phase, the reproductive function, formerly held in abeyance, now returns.

The most outstanding clinical phenomena are, therefore, a gain of weight and return of sexual activity. A commonly observed variant, especially after operations on the gastro-intestinal tract, such as subtotal gastrectomy, consists of a failure to gain weight. This is due to disordered gastro-intestinal function and should not be confused with the normal convalescent pattern which involves restoration to normal weight, and which occurs where gastrointestinal function is normal. Just as the commencement of good dietary intake is permissive in the onset of phase III, so here the maintenance of an adequate caloric intake, in excess of daily work requirements, is also permissive. Fat gain "wants to begin" when lean tissue gain is complete. It cannot begin without adequate diet.

2. THE WOUND. The wound flattens, broadens, gradually turns white and local activity appears to cease.

3. METABOLIC.

A. *Nitrogen, Potassium and Sodium.* There is zero balance of these three elements, signifying respectively that body protein, intracellular electrolyte and extracellular electrolyte are unchanged.

B. *Calories.* Caloric intake must be maintained in order to produce fat gain. If the patient returns to heavy physical labor, the caloric intake must be further increased to permit storage of fat, as well as providing caloric energy for daily tasks. If the patient returns to work too soon and works too hard, resulting in excessive caloric need or inadequate time for eating, he may not show a normal fat-gain phase.

C. *Eosinophile Count and Steroid Excretion.* The eosinophile count has been normal and continues so. The steroid excretion in the urine gradually now returns to normal. It should be emphasized that during the spontaneous anabolic phase, the so-called androgenic or anabolic steroid end-product, namely 17-ketosteroids, are low in the urine. During the fat-gain phase, the patient returns sexually to normal and the urinary excretion of these steroid hormones return to normal also.

D. *Total Body Water.* The characteristic finding of this phase (which first permitted its identification) is the fact that total body water remains unchanged while weight is gained. This phenomenon of continued weight gain without change in total body water is difficult to interpret without hypothecating that fat is the issue being added to the body.

The completion of the fat-gain phase is signaled by the return of body weight to normal and at this time, metabolic convalescence appears to be complete.

III. ILLUSTRATIVE CASE

Biochemistry

The foregoing has been a clinical and metabolic account of four phases which appear to us as distinct sequences in normal convalescence. The brief presentation of an illustrative case will serve now to indicate the actual magnitude of the changes in body composition which occur in these phases of convalescence, with special reference to the starting (normal) body composition and the arithmetic calculation of changes. This case is a synthesis, based on our studies, of what we would expect to observe in a man 45 years of age, 68 kg. in weight, who has an asymptomatic carcinoma of the gastro-intestinal tract which has not yet caused loss of weight or appetite, and who then has an extensive visceral ablation and anastomosis. Under these preoperative circumstances, metabolism is normal and the mere presence of cancer does not put a stamp of depletion on the case until clinical depletion has in point of fact begun. This, then, is the case of a middle-aged, metabolically normal male faced with the necessity of extensive visceral surgery in the abdomen, about scale 6 or 7 (Figure 1).

Based on norms from our laboratory and elsewhere we start with an organism as follows:

Weight	68.0 kg.
Total Body Water	61.5% of body weight, 41.8 liters
Total Body Fat	15.7% of body weight, 10.7 kg.
Total Body Proteins	17.2% of body weight, 11.7 kg.
Total Body Nitrogen	1.9 kg.
Total Exchangeable* Potassium	45.7 mEq./kg. 3110 mEq.
Total Exchangeable Sodium	42.2 mEq./kg. 2870 mEq.
Total Intracellular K	3050 mEq.
Total Extracellular K	60 mEq.
Total "Intracellular" Na (Inc. Bone)	870 mEq.
Total Extracellular Na	2000 mEq.
Extracellular fluid:	20% of body weight, 13.6 liters

* In the case of potassium this is essentially synonymous with "Total Body Potassium." In the case of sodium, much of the bone reservoir is not measured, but the "Total Exchangeable Sodium" is the "Total Available Sodium."

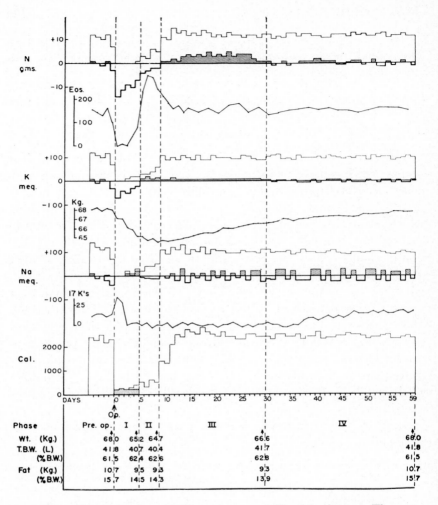

Fig. 1.—Metabolic chart of illustrative case outlined in the text. The normal response of a normal person to a scale 6–7 trauma.

Metabolic balances of nitrogen, potassium and sodium are shown, together with eosinophile counts, body weight, 17-ketosteroid excretion (mg. per 24 hours) and caloric intake. The charting convention is that described elsewhere, with the exception that negative balance is charted in white, below the zero line and enclosed in black line, rather than shaded black. As a result, the white area subtended below the intake always represents excretion whether positive or negative balance results.

Below the metabolic chart are shown weights, total body water (as liters and as per cent of body weight) and fat (as kilograms and per cent of body weight). These are the data upon which the body composition changes are based.

The vertical broken lines indicate the transition periods between the four phases referred to.

During the preoperative phase, the net metabolic balances of nitrogen, potassium and sodium are zero, on the intakes shown, which are the intakes of an individual who is a light eater and takes only a moderate amount of salt on his food. The sorts of food involved and routes of excretion are standard information, not detailed again here. The eosinophile count, body weight, steroid excretion and caloric intake are shown as normal values. The 24 hours immediately prior to operation shows the reduction in intake, slight balance changes and small eosinophile drop mentioned previously. See Figure 1 for details throughout.

The methods discussed here, of metabolic balance, total electrolyte and total water measurement are all cumbersome, time-consuming and "tricky." Short-cuts are not available; none of the methods permit easy delegation to technical personnel without close supervision by experienced professional persons. Constant check of accuracy, reproducibility and normal values is of vital importance. Although these laboratory methods have taught us much about surgical patients, they should not be confused with clinical laboratory procedures readily susceptible to mass production or used at the bedside.

PHASE 1. ADRENERGIC-CORTICOID PHASE

Day of Operation and First Four Postoperative Days. Our patient is now operated upon under pentothal-ether anesthesia. His operation might consist of a total gastrectomy and removal of the omentum (as an example of trauma in the scale 6 or 7 range). The duration of operation is four hours. The operative blood loss is 1000 cc. and this is immediately and accurately replaced with fresh whole blood. For this reason, it does not enter further into our metabolic calculations. If the blood loss had been under- or over-replaced, or if the blood were not fresh, it of course would alter body water distribution, potassium and pigment metabolism and the plasma and red cell volumes.[12]

The effect on the biological indices under consideration is shown graphically on the chart (Figure 1). These changes may be described

[12] Serial measurements of blood volume (by various techniques) in postoperative surgical patients frequently demonstrate an unexpected reduction in volume immediately after operation. This would offer interesting clinical and interpretative problems were it not for the fact that the volume then rapidly increases to normal in many instances without further transfusion. Whether this bears witness to important physiologic mechanisms not now understood, or merely to method troubles will need much more elucidation.

with reference to body composition as follows. The basis of these calculations has been described elsewhere.

1. The nitrogen loss is 51 Gm. in the five days of the adrenergic-
corticoid phase. This accounts for approximately 1530 Gm. of wet
lean tissue. This wet lean tissue contains 1.1 liters of water and 414
Gm. of lean tissue solids, mostly protein.

2. The loss of water is confined in our illustrative example to the
1.1 liters involved in the lean tissue which has been destroyed. There
is no extracellular dehydration. However, the potassium:nitrogen ratio
of the losses in the adrenergic-corticoid phase is comparatively high,
being 4.12 mEq. of potassium lost per Gm. of nitrogen. This is a characteristic finding. If we assume that each gram of nitrogen in muscle
is associated with 2.7 mEq. of K, then we can say that of the total K
lost, 137.5 mEq. formerly resided with the nitrogen which was lost.
This means that there has been an "extra potassium loss" of 72.5
mEq. This represents potassium which has moved out of the cell over
and above that predicted on the basis of cell matrix changes. As will
be noted below, this may be correlated with some intracellular sodium
shift.

3. On the basis of present information, the loss of 72.5 mEq. of potassium from muscle over and above cell matrix would represent the
loss of about 500 cc. of cell water. The changes in body composition
hypothecated here do not disclose the loss of this water from the body.
This has been our finding on several occasions. This suggests that as
potassium moves out of the cell in excess of nitrogen, the potassium
is excreted in the urine, but that the associated cell water is held in
the body during the phase of water and sodium retention. This may
increase slightly the extracellular fluid and may account, at least in
small part, for the increase in extracellular fluid observed after any
trauma.

4. Or, this water may remain in the cell, held there by sodium
which has moved in from the extracellular fluid or—a remote possibility—from bone. In our illustrative case, the plasma sodium concentration drops from 143 to 135 mEq. per liter; his extracellular phase is
about 14 liters, 112 mEq. has, therefore, apparently migrated into the
cell. The total K lost from cells during this phase has been 210 mEq.,
72.5 mEq. of which are "in excess of nitrogen." These interrelationships are about normal for this magnitude of trauma, but we do not

have the evidence at the present time to indicate clearly the net change—if any—in cell hydration. If large water infusions are given, a further drop in plasma sodium concentration may be observed, presumably a dilution effect.

In our illustrative example no sodium is given intravenously for two days; there is no excretion. The result is no flux with the environment (as indicated by a single line on the chart). On the second, third and fourth postoperative days, small sodium intakes commence with early oral fluids; 20 mEq. is retained, indicating less than 150 cc. of extra-cellular fluid (later diuresed in phase II). The amounts are so small that they do not enter the calculation. If large sodium infusions are given, the loading and the subsequent diuresis may be spectacular, and profoundly alter body composition.

5. The change in body water consists in a minor drop of only 1.1 liters (the water in 1.53 kg. of lean tissue lost) in the face of a weight loss of 2.78 kg. We can, therefore, calculate the fat loss and we find that this loss has been 1.25 kg. during the five days immediately post-operative. This fat loss can be calculated in either of two ways, either by nitrogen balance (using a coefficient of 30 for lean wet tissue), or by the Pace formula whereby

$$\% \text{ Fat } = 100 - \frac{\% \text{ Water}}{0.73}$$

Both methods of calculation rely on normal lean tissue hydration for their validity.

In this example, the two methods of fat loss calculation check perfectly (as the reader may corroborate) because the situation described does not involve any net alteration in total water content of lean tissue. There has been a small water loss from cells, but that water has been retained in the extracellular phase so that the total water content of lean tissue is not altered, even though the balance between intra- and extracellular phase is. It is important to point out that this perfect check of the two methods of calculation is not characteristic when major trauma is involved, although the discrepancy is usually small. As pointed out elsewhere post-traumatic situations often introduce a discrepancy between these two methods, traceable to alterations in the lean tissue nitrogen coefficient, at present poorly understood. In acute situations, therefore, a method of fat loss calculation involving simultaneous measurements of nitrogen balance, total body water, body weight and extracellular phase is the most reliable, although rarely attainable.[13]

This fat loss of 1.25 kg. in five days (0.25 kg. per day) is quite characteristic of trauma of this magnitude and is equivalent (on the basis of 9 calories per Gm.) to the production of 2250 calories per day from endogenous sources. This is a rate about five times that observed in semi-starvation.

If we assume that the lean tissue solids (414 Gm.) burned in the early postoperative phase are the source of the 51 Gm. of nitrogen excreted, and that these solids are largely protein, we find that this has resulted in the production of a maximum of 1645 calories (330 calories per day) by the combustion of protein. This nitrogen loss rate is only slightly in excess of that observed in the first five days of total starvation. Under circumstances of trauma of scale 7 or higher, we may observe nitrogen loss rates far in excess of this. (This example was chosen to illustrate a reasonable norm.)

6. Although these changes of the adrenergic-corticoid phase are of considerable significance, they represent only fractional changes in body composition (losses) as follows:

Of total lean tissue, 2.68%
Of total fat, 11.7%
Of total water, 2.68%
Of total potassium, 6.7%

It is noteworthy that the relative utilization of body constituents has proceeded farthest in the direction of fat utilization. A higher percentage of fat has been lost in this early phase than any other constituent. In none have we found that a greater percentage of water or lean tissue was lost than fat, in the immediate post-trauma period. The utilization of half or even three quarters of the body's fat has little permanent damaging effect on visceral function and it is reasonable

---

[13] Direct dilution methods for body fat such as those now under study by J. M. Steele and others will make a great contribution to surgical metabolism by providing an additional check on these observations; the specific gravity methods of Behnke and Pace are most informative, but not at present applicable to surgical patients.

to assume that this rapid fat oxidation does not "cost" the body anything. The loss of lean tissue is debatable as to cost. It would be our feeling that the magnitude of lean tissue (muscle tissue) loss here does not seriously cripple the patient or alter visceral function, although it may well be associated with the muscular weakness observed in the early period.

The source of this nitrogen loss is of interest. It must come from some large reservoir of protein in the body, since a total of 1530 Gm. of wet lean tissue was lost in the first five days in our illustrative example. This is only a moderate figure, and in many instances one will observe much larger losses. It is inconceivable that this much could come merely from small amounts of blood left in the peritoneal cavity, or some such adventitious source. Since there is no nitrogen intake during this time, the familiar discussion as to whether this is "catabolic" or "antianabolic" is no longer appropriate. It definitely represents nitrogen coming from some source in the body. The body has no large reserve pool of small molecular weight nitrogen compounds. It is our conviction that this nitrogen which is excreted largely as urea comes from the proteins of skeletal muscle which form the largest single mass of protein in the body, and which show clinical changes in strength and measurable changes in size in response to trauma.

PHASE II. CORTICOID WITHDRAWAL PHASE

Postoperative Days 5 to 8 Inclusive. The typical effects of this phase on the biologic indices under consideration are shown on the chart of our illustrative case. The effect of these changes on body composition are as follows:

1. The loss of nitrogen is only 11 Gm. in the four days of this period; representing only 330 Gm. of wet lean tissue, typical of the sharp reduction in loss rate observed in the second phase, but yet lacking a positive balance.

2. Potassium is gained during the phase of markedly decreased urinary potassium excretion and increasing intake, there being a gain of 52.5 mEq. Most of the "excess potassium" lost in phase I (about 70 per cent of it) now returns to the cell, and during this time, sodium diuresis occurs with the characteristic restoration of plasma sodium to normal. This sodium diuresis manifests itself largely as an increasing

excretion rate as intake increases; since there has been little sodium loading in this case (only about 20 mEq.), there is now little net loss during the diuresis phase.

3. The body water change is the loss of 240 cc., being the amount in the 330 Gm. of lean tissue destroyed.

4. Fat loss is therefore 200 Gm. for the four-day period, a loss of 50 Gm. a day (450 calories) and much nearer the starvation norm.

5. The weight loss is 0.53 kg., equivalent to the lean tissue loss (330 Gm.) plus the fat loss (200 Gm.).

6. Intake characteristically commences during this time and it is a common observation that water and electrolyte intake begin well before nitrogen and caloric intake. This is due, of course, to the water and electrolyte content of soft solids and juices taken easily before solid food is given.

The fraction of total body composition represented by these changes is very small, as will be apparent by study of these magnitudes in comparison with those of phase I.

PHASE III. THE SPONTANEOUS ANABOLIC PHASE

Days 9 to 30 Inclusive. Intake now rapidly increases to normal; during this phase the patient typically goes home. It must be re-emphasized that this all-important period of resuming strength and vigor cannot occur without resumption of diet. In our illustrative case, diet rapidly increases to 11 Gm. of nitrogen and 2400 calories, a reasonable mean of our observed data. The effect of this phase on our biologic indices is shown in the chart, and the effect on body composition is as follows:

1. The nitrogen gain is 62 Gm., equivalent to all that previously lost. In our illustrative patient, this is added at the average rate of 3 Gm. per day, so the process takes three weeks. We have seen nitrogen gained faster, but it is rare. This represents 1860 Gm. of wet lean tissue, the amount previously lost in phases I and II.

2. The potassium gain is 137.5 mEq. at a ratio of 2.7 mEq. per Gm. of nitrogen. This is a positive balance of only 7 mEq. per day. Balance methods must be very accurate (and rarely are) to demonstrate a consistent +7 mEq. balance with a daily flux of over 100 mEq. Yet during this period as a whole, a gain is recorded which restores cell matrix and electrolyte proportionally.

3. The sodium balance is zero, or very slightly positive, to cover the small extracellular phase of this tissue growth.

4. Weight is gained equal to the lean tissue synthesized (1.86 kg.).

5. The body water change is a gain of 1.36 liters, that expected from the nitrogen gain. There is, therefore, no change in absolute fat content, but a small fall in relative fat content from 14.3 per cent to 13.9 per cent.

6. The duration of the four phases is variable, as has been repeatedly emphasized. The duration of the last two phases is dependent not only upon inherent metabolic adjustments, but also upon diet and activity factors under the control of the patient and the surgeon, the gastro-intestinal function available and physical activity required.

7. Changes in steroid excretion consist of a gradual rise to normal; the eosinophile count remains normal.

PHASE IV. THE FAT GAIN PHASE

Days 30 to 60 Inclusive. The patient is now at work and must maintain a diet providing calories in excess of daily work requirements to show the characteristic weight changes of this phase. The effect of this phase on the various biologic indices under consideration is shown in the chart, and the effect on body composition is as follows:

1. With respect to nitrogen, potassium and sodium there are no significant changes. The minor variations shown in the chart are typical of daily measurement of balance; there is no consistent net change.

2. Weight gains slowly and steadily at an average rate of about 50 Gm. a day; the total here is 1.4 kg.

3. Body water shows no significant change, leaving us with the interpretation that the weight gain is fat. We had previously considered this late gain as whole tissue, and this it may be in patients who have come to operation in a depleted state; but in the normal, this late gain is fat, as indicated by consistent weight gain without change in total body water.

4. The eosinophile count remains normal; steroid excretion becomes normal, if it has not done so previously.

The close of this phase is characterized by return of weight to normal, and return of bodily vigor and strength to normal in every respect. Metabolic convalescence is complete.

The above concludes our presentation of the biochemistry of a single illustrative case. At the expense of repetition we must re-emphasize that variations are great and this illustrative case serves only to indicate the type of changes seen, and their approximate magnitudes.

IV. THE POSITIVE FORCES OF CONVALESCENCE

Endocrinology

The four phases of convalescence just described are appearances based on clinical and metabolic facts observed in surgical patients. Turning now to a discussion of the endocrine forces which produce these changes, we have a wide range of previous endocrine research to work from, but only a minimum of data from surgical patients. Some of the endocrinologic interpretation of convalescence is soundly based. As will become abundantly clear, other features of this endocrinology are quite unknown at the present time.

Preoperative. In a normal resting adult, the net endocrine forces are, in many instances, the result of a delicate balance between opposing hormones of trophic and target glands. In general, the hormones of the target gland tend to inhibit the trophic gland which, in most cases, is the pituitary. The pituitary, on the other hand, stimulates the target gland. Thus nature has set up a reciprocal relationship or "closed circle" governing mechanism which may undergo cyclic activity if the regulation is slow in responding, or in other instances may strike an even rate of activity. In the female, the reciprocal relationship between the pituitary and the gonads finds its expression in the normal menstrual cycle. About thirty days are required for the system to run one cycle. Whether or not there is any similar cyclic activity in the male is unknown. Adrenal function, thyroid function, parathyroid function and the function of the pancreatic islets similarly result from an interplay between two balanced forces which in these latter instances, maintain a more even rate of function than the female reproductive cycle.

An injury, an acute illness or an operation apparently distorts these normally balanced forces. There is set in motion a train of endocrine changes which results initially in rapid tissue catabolism and the inhibition of growth and reproduction. This endocrine sequence runs its course over a period of days or weeks, at the end of which time body composition is gradually restored to normal by forces which are re-constructive in nature.

Phase I. The Adrenergic-Corticoid Phase. Clinical appearances suggest that an outpouring of adrenal medullary substances—epinephrine and related compounds—is the first endocrine event occasioned by real or anticipated injury. Psychological factors unquestionably enter into the genesis of these occurrences since they may appear in the absence of a wound. But the wound, as a break in continuity of the organism, appears to determine certain details of duration and intensity of this initial response. Shortly after this initial change, the body undergoes an adjustment which suggests that there has been an increased secretion of anterior pituitary ACTH, with a resultant secretion by the adrenal cortex of steroid hormones.

The central nervous system is clearly important in this initial adjustment, both as evidenced by the importance of psychological factors, and by the fact that the response to injury is altered in the presence of certain types of central nervous system lesions. This matter, and the detailed neurophysiology of these central nervous system areas, are now under investigation in several laboratories in this country and abroad.

It would be inappropriate here to review the status of this work save to point out that any central nervous system areas which receive nerve impulses from the periphery and transmit endocrine impulses to the pituitary are of exceptional interest, since they represent the meeting point of the two great regulatory systems in the body, the nervous system and the endocrine system. Such centers seem to have as one of their most important functions, the subjugation of other bodily functions to survival after injury. This entire field of work is under review by Hume.

Changes in endocrine secretory rate are also under scrutiny in an effort to differentiate true secretory changes from illusory alterations in endocrine balance which might result not from actual secretory changes but from alterations in tissue reactivity, visceral inactivation or excretion. There is evidence from the adrenalectomized rat that many of the "corticoid" phenomena which follow trauma will occur without alteration in the replacement dosage of hormone. This raises the possibility that trauma does not alter the output of hormone but that the injury or the wound somehow alters the reaction of the tissues in the periphery to a constant level of hormones. In addition, decisive evidence for an increased secretion of epinephrine after injury is lacking, although circumstantial evidence dating back to Cannon is abundant. It is important to observe that changes in steroid excretion in the urine might be produced by alterations in liver function or by alterations in kidney function quite aside from alterations in the rate of activity in the hypothalamic-pituitary-adrenal axis. And finally, it is important again to emphasize that the eosinophile count in the blood may drop when epinephrine is administered, even though the adrenal glands are absent.

Whatever the findings may ultimately indicate in regard to these important endocrine mechanisms, the metabolic appearances of the first phase of convalescence resemble those produced by the injection of epinephrine and adrenal corticoids (or ACTH) into otherwise normal individuals. It appears to us that the weight of evidence at this time, based on human studies, favors the concept that there is an actual increase in the secretory activity of the pituitary and the adrenal cortex after injury and that subsequently these factors are subject to diminution or withdrawal.

It is important to emphasize that neither the administration of ACTH nor of epinephrine, even when combined with immobilization and starvation, exactly reproduce *all* the detailed metabolic features of the first phase of convalescence. Yet the effects of these hormones in normal man closely enough approximate the first ‚phase to justify terming it the "adrenergic-corticoid" phase. It must be re-emphasized that the early minutes or hours of this phase are dominated by epinephrine, with its characteristic effects on the circulatory system and carbohydrate metabolism, but as this wanes, the corticoid picture is unmasked and persists much longer.[14] The adrenergic appearance is much more marked in unanesthetized wounding than in elective surgery.

The increased rate of fat utilization demonstrated by combining body water measurements with studies of the extracellular phase and

---

[14] The posterior pituitary anti-diuretic hormone responds in a very sensitive way to dehydration. It may also respond to trauma without dehydration as a feature of the normal surgical endocrinology. (Le Quesne, P. L., and A. A. G. Lewis: Postoperative Water and Salt Retention. Lancet I, 153, 1953.) To settle this point further studies are needed of weight, water and salt metabolism in normal surgical patients not given large water and salt loads.

nitrogen metabolism appears to be an integral part of phase I. The endocrine forces producing this rate are not well understood. It is an important fact that ACTH administration may produce an increased rate of fat oxidation.[15]

The inhibition of sex function which occurs immediately following trauma suggests that stimulation of the pituitary-adrenal axis is associated with a marked falling off in activity of the pituitary-gonadal axis.

Individuals without wounds who are given ACTH do not feel "sick and weak"; they may have subjective sensations which are quite the reverse. Whether this apparent symptomatic inconsistency is due to the difference in response occasioned by the tissue damage itself, or whether the adrenal secretes a somewhat differently balanced output of steroids in response to a wound (as compared with ACTH) is not clear.

Discussion of the endocrinology of the first phase must include some provision for the variations in duration and intensity observed with varying degrees of trauma. The duration and intensity of phase I (as evidenced for example, by the duration of high urinary nitrogen excretion rate on zero intake) seem to set the tone for the whole of convalescence, the duration of the other phases being related. This raises the question of the wound itself as an "endocrine organ," circulating substances from it maintaining or intensifying the response. This idea is appealing, particularly as it relates to dissociation between corticoid-like (compound E-F) activity and desoxy-like (salt retaining) activity. In a burn, for instance, marked sodium diuresis occurs while the corticoid phase is still in progress, as evidenced by low eosinophiles and high nitrogen excretion rate. Although burn metabolism is as a whole an abnormal variant of convalescence, this would suggest that the wound can alter the endocrine sequences. On the other hand, the clinically minor response elicited by a wound in the anesthetized extremity of a paraplegic suggests that the neural path-

[15] Jenkins and Thorn have recently carried out studies of persons given cortisone (and compound F) demonstrating a rapid gluconeogenesis which outstrips the production of small nitrogenous compounds as measured by urine nitrogen. This is to be interpreted as an increased rate of fat utilization resulting from steroid therapy. Other evidence (Levin, L. and R. K. Farber: Recent Progress in Hormone Research, Vol. VII, pp. 399–423. Academic Press, New York, 1952) suggests that while cortisone is permissive in depot fat mobilization, other factors may initiate the change.

way centrally is more important than the blood stream in relating the wound to the response. This subject is under intensive clinical study at the present time and more solid interpretation will be forthcoming.

Phase II—The Corticoid Withdrawal Phase. As the end of phase I draws near, there is lessening evidence of corticoid stimulation; nitrogen excretion lessens and the eosinophiles start to rise and "overshoot." The duration of salt-retaining activity is variable, but diuresis usually occurs after the eosinophile backswing.

We find an extremely close clinical and metabolic correlation between the events of phase II and the picture of corticoid withdrawal. When a normal person is given ACTH for several days and it is then suddenly withdrawn, four things happen almost simultaneously. First, there is a rise in the eosinophile count to above normal; secondly, there is a decreased urine nitrogen excretion; thirdly, there is a marked decrease in urinary potassium excretion which may be associated with strongly positive balance; and finally, there is a tendency to sodium diuresis, the extent of which depends on the previous load. In certain instances, urinary steroid excretion is quite low, significantly lower than normal.

All these things characterize the corticoid withdrawal phase of convalescence. It is a phase of readjustment between the pressor-energy forces of the adrenergic-corticoid stimulation of phase I and the muscular growth phenomena of phase III. More important for the wound, it is a phase when the fibroplasia-inhibitors of the compound E-F group are withdrawn and fibrosis occurs rapidly, giving the wound the increase in tensile strength so characteristic of this period.[16]

The importance of the wound itself as an endocrine organic is suggested by some of the interesting variations seen in the corticoid withdrawal phase. The early sodium diuresis in burns has already been mentioned as antedating the reduction in nitrogen excretion. In certain other surgical cases, one observes a close correlation between nitrogen excretion reduction, eosinophile backswing, potassium loading and

---

[16] Although re-wounding at this time elicits a minor metabolic response and hence a minimal "lag" phase, this is a period of rapid fibrous union and hastened resumption of tensile strength. This fact may be helpful in the timing of secondary closure or delayed primary suture of surgical incisions or traumatic wounds. Whatever the endocrine interpretation, it is most advantageous to seize upon this favorable period for delayed closure. This has been repeatedly emphasized by Doctor Churchill in his works on military surgery and in his theater policies of World War II.

urinary hormone excretion, only to find that sodium diuresis is delayed for ten days or two weeks. Delayed resolution of local inflammation and edema may here constitute an example of the wound governing details of total metabolism.

Are the adrenal cortical hormones sharply withdrawn in phase II? Or are we witnessing a sudden alteration in peripheral tissue reactivity, or a sudden inactivation by the wound, either of which give a false metabolic picture of a withdrawal? This question, of overriding importance in the endocrinology of convalescence, will require much more work for a definitive answer. But just as in phase I, our interpretation of the data now available is that of an actual change in secretion rate.

Phase III—The Spontaneous Anabolic Phase. The metabolic picture of phase III is one of the addition of nitrogen and cell electrolyte to the body at a steady rate, accompanied by a low excretion in the urine of 17-ketosteroids and by zero balance of the other indices under consideration. As has been pointed out elsewhere, this is the characteristic picture of a growing child who, prior to puberty, does not add fat to his body very rapidly but is growing lean tissues such as muscle and skeleton. At puberty other factors enter, such as the deposition of fat in the female and extra skeletal muscle in the male, and the development of other secondary sex characteristics.

During this third phase, the patient gains strength, vigor and ambition in direct proportion to his diet and the addition of nitrogen to his body. It is of great interest that body weight and water increases during this period are wholly accountable by nitrogen accumulation.

The endocrine force producing this anabolism might be gonadal, or in the nature of a growth hormone. We favor the latter view. If one administers to a normal animal an anabolic steroid compound such as testosterone, a strongly positive nitrogen balance is produced. However, this is associated with a marked increase in size of the secondary sex organs. This is most readily demonstrated in the rat where the increase in the weight of the prostate is spectacular in the animal given testosterone. One must recall that development of skeletal muscle in the male is in part a secondary sex character and that increased muscle mass in the male is a feature of puberty.

In sharp contrast to the normal, however, the surgical patient in the third phase of convalescence is growing new muscle at a steady rate, and this rate cannot be further increased by testosterone. Furthermore, this nitrogen anabolism of phase III is associated with a low excretion in the urine of 17-ketosteroids. The third phase of convalescence takes place with great rapidity in a young growing child where there is comparatively little gonadal function. As previously mentioned, the role of diet is permissive in this phase and, like normal growth, phase III cannot occur without diet. This is in contrast to the overgrowth of secondary sex characteristics on testosterone, which will occur even in starvation.

For these reasons, then, we do not feel that the spontaneous nitrogen anabolic phase of convalescence is related to the nitrogen-anabolic effects of hormones of gonadal or adrenal origin. It appears, instead, to be a growth phenomenon. Further research work should indicate whether it resembles the picture produced in a normal person by the administration of pituitary growth hormones or a non-androgenic, anabolic steroid.

Phase IV—The Fat Gain Phase. Finally, the patient restores to his body all the fat previously lost. During this period the patient appears to be quite normal. Sexual activity again begins. In the female, this takes the form of the menses and in the male it takes the form of increased libido, providing caloric supply is adequate. In the absence of adequate diet, neither menstruation nor libido are returned.

The fourth phase of convalescence, like the third, cannot proceed normally without diet. Dietary calories, nitrogen, essential amino acids and vitamins are necessary for spontaneous anabolism and the redeposition of fat.

The endocrine forces producing this fat gain are not known at the present time. It is of interest to recall that in the female at puberty a differential increase in body fat is one of the most spectacular occurrences. It is conceivable that this phase is dominated by estrogen-like substances, producing deposition of body fat. Were it apparent that the third phase of convalescence resembled the anabolism produced by the male sex hormone, we might hypothecate that the third phase of convalescence is a male-type phase with increase in body muscle and that the fourth phase is a female-type phase, characterized by an increase in body fat. For reasons mentioned above, we do not feel that this is the case and we prefer to interpret them as respectively a growth phase and a fat-gain phase, leaving endocrine mechanisms to future work.

V. MEANING TO THE PATIENT

Teleology

The term "homeostasis" was coined by W. B. Cannon to mean the total biological result of the many forces acting to maintain the internal environment in a normal balance despite acute external alterations. He uses the phrase: ". . . The various physiological arrangements which serve to restore the normal state when it has been disturbed." The convalescent process is the continuation of homeostatic forces summoned by the acute injury on to complete wound healing, regrowth of lost tissues and return to activity and reproduction. The word "homeostasis" connotes a teleologic interpretation of natural events; the four phases of convalescence carry a similar connotation which will be examined briefly in this section.

Phase I—The Adrenergic-Corticoid Phase. The injured organism needs quick energy from carbohydrate for the immediate struggle; it must vasoconstrict to save blood pressure and blood flow[17] for vital organs and clot to reduce bleeding in the periphery; it must increase cardiac output to cover muscular exertion for combat or escape, and it must dilate bronchioles to improve oxygenation. These purposes are served by the adrenal medullary aspects of the initial response and will not be described further; they are the very phases of adjustment covered by Cannon's classic work.

It is not generally realized how quickly this initial adjustment is followed by a corticoid phase, nor how thoroughly (even though by other mechanisms) the corticoid phase serves two of the adrenal medullary purposes: blood pressure maintenance and endogenous energy production. Where the sympatho-adrenal response may be short-lived (1 to 12 hours), the corticoid phase is more prolonged (3 to 5 days) and carries forward similar but additional purposes.

On the score of energy, the adrenal medullary activity makes short

[17] Splenic constriction represents an interesting phase of this response and one which interested Cannon greatly. The contribution of red cells is small. There may be other species in which splenic contraction makes a significant contribution to blood volume.

shrift of body carbohydrate (400 Gm.) which is quickly burned. Fat oxidation carries on with the same objective for several days at a high rate (200 to 400 Gm./day or 1800 to 3600 calories); whether this apparently simple purpose is also served by adrenal corticoids is at present unknown, although it is probable. Degradation and oxidation of protein also proceeds rapidly in this phase, its outward manifestation being rapid nitrogen excretion in the absence of intake. Although gluconeogenesis from protein provides energy, it is our conviction that the destruction of lean tissue has as its purpose the provision of raw materials for wound healing (of which lean tissue is the only endogenous source) rather than heat energy, of which it is a very expensive and inefficient source when compared to fat.

The maintenance of extracellular water in support of plasma volume and blood pressure is served by the corticoid mechanisms for conserving water, chloride and sodium. The sodium area of the body is the extracellular phase and this is the area of body water which the plasma volume calls upon for support when it is reduced by hemorrhage. The maintenance of body sodium with an adequate store of water is essential to the refilling of plasma volume after hemorrhage. It is important to emphasize that under natural conditions or in the absence of transfusion, this mechanism is the only one available for restoration of blood volume. Here a pressor mechanism characteristically steroid in nature and biochemical in mechanism carries on where the adrenal medullary mechanism (vasoconstriction, tachycardia) left off. Whether the steroids have a direct vascular pressor effect other than on water and sodium metabolism remains to be proven.

These two pressure-maintaining mechanisms (medullary and corticoid) act initially in concert; but long-continued medullary effects may be in themselves harmful as suggested by Remington's work and by the disastrous clinical picture of late vasoconstricted-tachycardic-hypotension. By contrast, pressor mechanisms of a steroid nature may carry on for days without damage to the organism, so long as the surgeon does not over-administer fluid and salt. The medullary forces are indeed designed for the acute emergency and once it is over, the sooner they are abolished the better. The corticoid pressor mechanism is designed to carry on for a longer (but still limited) period without damaging side effects. Only when unduly prolonged (past seven to nine days) do we begin to see harmful side effects.

Also of importance in meeting hemorrhage are the mechanisms which relate to the clotting mechanism. There are data in the literature on the normal alterations in the clotting mechanism which follow injury. These data indicate that changes in the clotting mechanism are a part of the normal response to injury; whether the mechanism is adrenal medullary, adrenal cortical or hepatic (or all three) remains unsettled despite 30 years of work since Cannon's first studies.

On the score of wound healing mechanisms in phase I, it is our conviction that the metabolic mobilization of nitrogen, potassium and the other intracellular electrolytes has as its primary purpose the provision of raw materials for the healing of the wound. These materials must be mobilized in the organism which is wounded, which cannot seek food and is therefore starving. Not only must caloric energy be supplied to the starving post-trauma organism, but also the intracellular material present in food and essential to the synthesis of new protoplasm. These substances are made available from body tissues.

We are indebted to J. S. L. Browne of Montreal, for this concept of "loosening" body nitrogen to make it available for wound healing following stress. The concept appears to us a fruitful one and the evidence, that the intracellular changes of the corticoid phase have as their purpose the provision of substances for the formation of new tissue in the wound, outweighs the opposite contention that this catabolism is a deleterious effect. It is of great interest that the healthy person who heals his wound the best after a single trauma and who "does well" clinically shows this catabolism most vigorously,[18] and the depleted person who is much more apt to fail in healing (wound dehiscence, non-union of fractures) does not show a vigorous catabolism.

It may appear remarkable that the first set of endocrine responses following an injury involve an increased secretion of substances such as the cortisone-like hormones which inhibit fibrous tissue proliferation and which might be interpreted as interfering with wound union. Our interpretation is that the pressor-energy mechanisms have a higher biological priority than wound tensile strength in the early period

---

[18] There is evidence to suggest that bone trauma elicits a much more vigorous metabolic response than one would predict solely on the extent of the injury were only soft tissues involved. Recent work in our laboratories further corroborates this. Again the question arises of the wound as an endocrine organ, its detailed anatomic and biochemical characteristics altering the details of the metabolic response.

after wounding. The corticoid phase accomplishes these emergency objectives while at the same time loosening intracellular substances which are destined to make possible the subsequent rapid resumption of tensile strength which occurs when the corticoids are withdrawn and fibrosis occurs. Viewed in this light, the corticoid phase is truly the "lag period" of wound tensile strength, but a most intensive period for supply of intracellular material in the extracellular phase. The "lag" applies only to tensile strength; metabolic activity is intense.

One may inquire why so much tissue—1860 Gm. in our illustrative case—is catabolized to heal a little wound. Nature is prolific in many regards; the salmon lays many million eggs to produce a few young fish. There is an analogy here in the mobilization of intracellular substance for wound healing. In a simple abdominal laparotomy, the transverse healing of the incised wound and of any intraperitoneal manipulations involved probably does not entail the formation of much more than 20 to 50 Gm. of tissue at the very maximum. In all likelihood, the actual weight of new tissue formed is even smaller than this. But this must occur in the absence of diet. Nature makes available in the extracellular phase a continuous excess of all the substances needed to form this new tissue. The body dissolves 1.8 kg. of muscle tissue elsewhere in the body to form this crucial 20 Gm. of new tissue in the wound. For a huge wound of war, a femoral fracture or a burn, an even greater mobilization occurs. The supply of amino acids, polypeptides and intracellular electrolytes is continuously increased and made available to the wound. Since many of these substances are toxic in the extracellular phase if their concentration is increased, there is a resultant continuous increase in their excretion in the urine. As intracellular electrolyte leaves the normal cells, it is in part replaced by extracellular salts, producing the "shift" previously referred to.

In phase I the reproductive process (menses, libido) and the digestive assimilative process (peristalsis, appetite) are completely subjugated to the pressor-energy-catabolism triad of metabolic priorities. Growth likewise ceases for the duration of the emergency if injury occurs in a child.

We cannot leave the endocrinology of the first phase without reference and acknowledgment to Selye's "alarm reaction." Selye's experiments dealt with long-continued stress of a continuous nature producing "shock, counter-shock and exhaustion."[19] Many of the metabolic changes he describes in the early phase are seen in the adrenergic-corticoid phase of human convalescence; but the surgeon deals with finite trauma which ceases in due course and is not followed by counter-shock and exhaustion but instead by wound healing, convalescence and complete recovery.

Phase II—The Corticoid Withdrawal Phase. Following the completion of the adrenergic-corticoid phase, the organism is left with the slowing-down of those homeostatic mechanisms which maintain circulatory efficiency, energy production and the mobilization of cellular material for the wound. As mentioned above, the endocrinology of the first phase places circulation, energy and endogenous production of cell materials at the top priority; digestion, growth and reproduction have ceased. But as this phase ends, the crisis has been met and is passed, and priorities gradually change.

Phase II is the first step in an orderly progress by which circulatory strain, endogenous energy production and catabolism gradually recede as biological objectives to allow wound healing, digestion, growth and reproduction to resume. Phase II is a transition from emergency mechanisms to trophic mechanisms. Its metabolic events are nicely explained by corticoid withdrawal; its teleology seems to be that of stopping one adjustment which is incompatible with a second set of mechanisms, so that the second set may start and wound fibrosis occur. Amongst other things, the body makes ready for diet; phase III cannot begin without exogenous energy. Yet, all the characteristic metabolic changes of phase II can occur without intake, indicating that—whether or not it will start—anabolism is "ready to begin."

For the wound, phase II is far more than an interval between corticoid and growth phases. As the cortisone-like factors are withdrawn, fibrosis begins with a rush, and during a two or three-day period, the gross character of the wound changes dramatically. Reopened at three days, a wound "falls apart." At six days, it has to be cut. That this can—and frequently does—occur in the absence of diet is a tribute to the effectiveness of cellular mobilization in the corticoid phase, and to

---

[19] Selye's term "shock" refers to a metabolic state and makes no reference to traumatic or oligemic shock as seen by the surgeon.

the rapidity of fibrosis and collagen deposition once the corticoids are withdrawn.

Phase III—Spontaneous Anabolic Phase. As diet begins, supplying the exogenous nitrogen and calories now for the first time essential for the continuation of convalescence, the rebuilding of body composition starts and muscular strength is slowly resumed. The teleologic significance of such a step needs no further comment. Wound changes are still occurring, consisting of collagen deposition, firming up of the cicatrix and resumption of tensile strength. These wound changes are not associated with an increased cellularity, but rather with increased intercellular substance. The muscular changes appear to occur before fat is gained or full sexual (menstrual) function returns. The wound and muscle occupy top priority in this phase of regrowth.

Phase IV—The Fat Gain Phase. The wound now drops to lowest priority, activity in it ceases, the cicatrix gradually turns white and softens, and it remains the same—save for a tendency to linear contraction—for the duration of life.[20] Muscular strength has been restored and all that remains to be done is to rebuild the storehouse of energy called upon at the first—body fat. Such seems to be the teleologic purpose of this phase. Sexual activity returns to normal; survival having been tended, reproduction can resume.

Prior to this time, should the patient suffer a second injury, he will show a "depletion response"—a miniature version of normal traumatic metabolism. Now, during the fat gain phase, he is "loaded" again, and if the trigger is pulled, a full metabolic discharge will occur.

VI. DISCUSSION

This paper has described a theory of convalescence, based on the facts available. This theory encompasses four phases of convalescence, their effect on body composition, their endocrinology and their meaning to the injured organism as a whole and to the wound in particular.

As further facts become available, it will be possible to fill in many details now left uncertain as to biochemistry and endocrinology. A

---

[20] If by now the wound is not healed—a late burn, a fracture non-union—it scarcely can be made to heal save by another major operation which may have as its main effect the re-mobilization of the catabolic forces of the adrenergic-corticoid phase. The apparent beneficial effect of ACTH in treating and grafting the very late unhealed burn may be traceable to the "dummy operation" effect of ACTH in raising the wound again to a higher priority in the bodily economy.

clearer picture of time relationships will emerge, and their correlation with different grades or types of trauma will become more certain. Interrelationships between the needs of the organism and the needs of the wound will be clarified.

Any teleologic interpretation of natural phenomena is at best an outsider's view of those processes which Starling first referred to as the "wisdom of the body." This theory is no exception. But teleologic speculation often suggests fruitful avenues of investigation, and therein lies its chief importance.

Despite such shortcomings, this concept of convalescence provides a firm basis for care in normal convalescence. Beyond this daily care of the normal patient lies the large group of abnormal convalescent metabolic states seen by the surgeon. These include starvation, depletion, multiple trauma, renal or heart failure, infection, excessive injury, gastro-intestinal dysfunction, endocrinopathy, liver disease and many others. These abnormalities in convalescence can be treated most effectively when the departure from the normal pattern of recovery is clearly understood.

VII. SUMMARY AND CONCLUSIONS

1. Four phases of convalescence are described; their biochemistry, endocrinology and teleology are briefly discussed.

2. These four phases are as follows:

    I—The Adrenergic-Corticoid Phase.
    II—The Corticoid Withdrawal Phase.
    III—The Spontaneous Anabolic Phase.
    IV—The Fat Gain Phase.

3. These phases are viewed as an orderly sequence in which emergency mechanisms (circulation, energy) are first replaced by wound healing, then by digestion, regrowth of other tissues and reproduction, as the top priorities for the organism.

4. The duration of each phase depends on the extent and duration of the trauma; for extensive anastomotic gastro-intestinal surgery, the four phases last about five, four, twenty and forty days respectively.

5. The endocrinology is as yet poorly understood; the importance of conceiving convalescence as the net resultant of interlocking and sequential biologic forces is stressed. These forces bear not only on

the wound as a break in continuity of the organism, but also on survival of the organism in the acute emergency, mobilization of substances to heal the wound during the inevitable period of transient
starvation, and then a reconstruction of the body to accomplish growth
and reproduction on the one hand, or, if necessary, a new adjustment
to injury on the other. The normal human body is geared to nego-
tiate the first two phases, through and including the healing of the
wound to high tensile strength, without diet; the final two "reconstructive" phases require exogenous diet in adequate amounts, for
completion.

6. An understanding of the normal pattern of recovery is the basis
for the care of the normal surgical patient and the treatment of the
abnormal.

4. Wound Healing and Infection

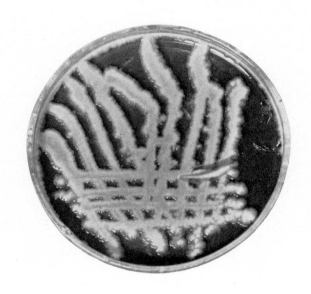

PREFATORY COMMENTS

THE CARE OF THE WOUND

From time immemorial caustic agents of various types have been poured on wounds. Scalding oil was considered the panacea until Paré cried out in protest. Even at the present time some surgeons have a fetish for using antiseptics and medicaments which they feel might promote wound healing. It has been emphasized by Dr. Samuel Harvey, late Professor of Surgery at Yale University School of Medicine, that it is difficult if not impossible to accelerate the normal rate of healing. On the other hand, it is quite easy to retard wound healing by the wanton use of irritating and necrotizing agents. Often the patient's attempt to repair his injury is frustrated by the overzealous application of noxious irritants. Moyer presented the problem squarely when he stated "Let he who would commit an act upon a burned surface or put a substance upon it first apply that treatment to his conjunctiva or an experimental scald imposed upon himself. It is likely that nowhere else in the field of surgery has the dictum 'prima non nocere' been more assiduously ignored than in the primary care of the burn-wound."

Lister is usually credited with the introduction of the antiseptic method. There is no doubt that he made a great contribution to surgery but, at the risk of blasphemy, we contend that his precepts have not stood the test of time. Though he created interest in antiseptics his method placed emphasis on the atmosphere around the wound and encouraged the application of irritants to the wound. He detracted from the importance of the proper care of the wound itself and started a fruitless search for a universal antiseptic solution. On the other hand, Dr. Reid has emphasized the principles that have

155

stood the test of time, viz., gentle cleansing of wounds, meticulous handling of tissues and accurate hemostasis. He emphasized the fact that the art of surgery is gentleness.

ANTIBIOTICS

One of the classic examples of serendipity in medicine is the discovery of the antimicrobial properties of penicillin. Revelatory accidents occur frequently, but only when they are observed by an individual with a prepared mind do they become great discoveries. Fleming's ability to recognize the potentialities of this antibiotic was the result of astute observations made during his experiments. In accepting the Nobel prize for his discovery, he stated with typical humility: "My only merit is that I did not neglect the observation and that I pursued the subject as a bacteriologist."

Unfortunately the excessive use of penicillin and other antibiotics created many difficulties. First of all, resistant organisms became prevalent. Whether these organisms were resistant at the time of their implantation or developed resistance in the host by mutation after prolonged treatment with the antibiotic is of little practical significance. As a matter of fact, it is probable that both modes of action occur. At any rate, the wide use of antibiotics has helped rear many strains of bacteria which were formerly sensitive but are now resistant to the agent. With the introduction of each new antibiotic, the incidence of sensitivity of the organisms to that agent is high but it is soon followed by a period of increasing resistance and the development of a hardier race of bacteria. We have seen this phenomenon of resistance well documented in the case of the *Staphylococcus aureus* which soon acquired resistance to penicillin and later to erythromycin. Chloramphenicol was used most sparingly for several years because of reports of aplastic anemia in a few patients. When the restrictions to its use were lifted, the drug seemed to be more efficacious than it had been prior to its restriction. Time may have erased many of the previously chloramphenicol-resistant organisms and substituted for them a new progeny of sensitive bacteria. If this point could be proven convincingly, it might be advisable to outlaw the use of a wide-spectrum drug for a year or two and to introduce it again at a later date. Finland of Boston has stated: "The routine use of antibiotics prophylactically in large numbers of patients in hospitals is probably the major cause for the rapid increase in the incidence and pathogenic significance of antibiotic-resistant staphylococci. In any event, the prophylactic use of antimicrobial agents, particularly for long periods and in large numbers of persons, may actually increase the probability that infections when they do occur will be due to organisms resistant to just those antibiotics used in the prophylaxis."

In addition to the problem of invoking resistance, many of these agents are capable of producing manifestations of hypersensitivity. In the case of penicillin, the severity of these reactions is enhanced by the use of repository forms. Because of the transient appearance of L. E. cells during penicillin reactions it has been suggested that some cases of collagen disease may be attributed to the use of antibiotics. Gastrointestinal disturbances occur in many patients treated with antibiotics. There is an increasing number of reports concerning resistant staphylococci, capable of producing a severe pseudomembranous enterocolitis. Moreover, superinfection with resistant bacteria may develop after the elimination of the sensitive organisms. All of these pitfalls associated with chemotherapy should be fully appreciated by the surgeon. It is our contention that once he becomes cognizant of the dangers inherent in these agents, his indications for their prophylactic use will be curtailed sharply. McKittrick in 1955, in his analysis of 175 patients undergoing abdominal surgery at the Massachusetts General Hospital, came to the following conclusion: "This study failed to demonstrate benefits which are necessary to compensate for the discomforts, expense, and possible dangers associated with the prophylactic use of antibiotics following most elective operations on the gastrointestinal and biliary tracts." Many of us are aware of the fact that prior to the antibiotic era the incidence of infection as a surgical complication was extremely low in competent hands. As early as 1893 Halsted stated: "Our hernia wounds illustrate admirably the danger of constricting tissues. We never resort to drainage of any kind for fresh wounds. And with the exception now and then of a hernia wound (*not more than 1–2 cases a year*) *none of our fresh wounds suppurate.* [*Ed. Note:* Italics ours.] Inasmuch as we rarely if ever have occasion to constrict tissue in other fresh wounds, it is almost certain that the occasional stitch abscess in a hernia wound is due to tissue constriction plus, of course, the infection. To provide for a good circulation in every particle of tissue in and immediately about a wound is as much a part of our technique as are the ordinary anti-septic precautions."

For the surgeon, the greatest objection to the injudicious use of antibiotics lies in its insidious abrogation of the time-tested principles of meticulous surgery. McKittrick compares the surgeon's dependence on antibiotics to the wearing of a bib. He makes the analogy to eating lobster in a restaurant which features bibs for patrons. Invariably, these bibs are badly stained at the end of the meal. These same diners seldom come away with stained shirts when the bib is not available and more care is used in eating. The refinements in technique, which were so important in bringing about this present golden age in surgery, are being de-emphasized. The tendency to rely upon antibiotics to cover up breaches in technique should not be condoned.

In our denunciation of the abuses of antibiotics, we must not lose sight of the advantages. Weinstein compared these chemotherapeutic agents to a two-sided coin when he stated: "To limit the inspection of the 'chemotherapeutic coin' to the unattractive side alone is just as misleading and unrevealing of the truth as to view only the face which gleams with the picture of the benefits to be derived. In order to determine the true value of the entire coin, it becomes imperative, therefore, to examine both sides carefully and to reach a conclusion only after each has been evaluated in terms of the other and in proper relation to the whole. So, only through long experience and unbiased, critical evaluating of the good and the bad in antibiotic therapy can an intelligent understanding of its real benefits and limitations be reached. I will have failed miserably indeed if what I have said leaves the impression that the drugs which have been discussed are only harmful, or that their dangers outweigh the benefits to be derived from their proper use. To act on such an impression would mean the loss of countless lives and the permitting of untold suffering and pain.

"The fact that harmful effects may follow the use of antibiotic sub-stances must never discourage the physician from the use of any of them in any situation in which they are definitely indicated. It should, however, make him very careful in their use when they are required, and very cautious and hesitant about employing them in instances in which indications for their application are either entirely lacking or, at most, only slightly suggestive. To do otherwise is to run the risk, at times, of converting a simple, benign and self-limited disease into one which may be serious or even fatal. The physician must always be mindful of the fact that the use of any powerful therapeutic agent is always accompanied by a calculated risk. The antibiotics are no different; to condemn them on the grounds of their potential dangers is no less unrealistic and unwise than to accept them as universally applicable, completely beneficial and entirely harmless."

It is unlikely that Paul Ehrlich's dream of a single agent to eradicate all infection (*therapia magna sterilisans*) will ever be realized. As with many other weapons in surgery, this sword has a double edge.

MONT ROGERS REID (*1889–1943*)

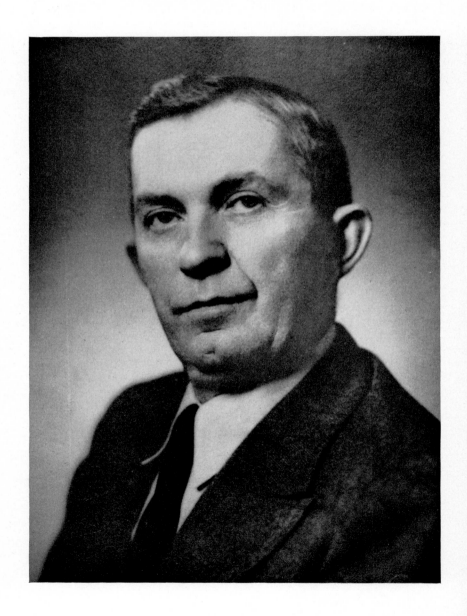

Mont Rogers Reid was born on April 7, 1889, at Oriskany, Virginia. His medical education was received at The Johns Hopkins Medical School where he was graduated in 1912. There he continued his surgical training as one of the most gifted pupils of William Stewart Halsted. In 1922 he went to Cincinnati University as Associate Professor of Surgery, and in 1931 was appointed Christian R. Holmes Professor of Surgery, Head of the Department of Surgery at the College of Medicine, and Director of the Surgical Services of the Cincinnati General and affiliated hospitals. In this position, he attained national fame as a surgeon, investigator and teacher.

Dr. Reid's additions to the science and art of surgery were many and varied. Among surgeons he was perhaps most widely known for his research and clinical experience in vascular surgery. He also contributed notably in other fields, especially in the study of the care and healing of wounds, the surgery of the thyroid gland, bile duct, appendix, and sympathetic nervous system. These achievements brought him memberships in the leading medical and surgical societies of the country, many prizes and awards, and appointment as a member of the National Advisory Cancer Council.

He died on May 11, 1943.

SOME CONSIDERATIONS
OF THE PROBLEMS
OF WOUND HEALING

BY MONT R. REID, M.D.

The subject of this evening's lecture is irritation" (wound healing), "which, being the foundation of surgical science, you must carefully study, and clearly understand, before you can expect to know the principles of your profession, or be qualified to practice it creditably to yourselves, or with advantage to those who may place themselves under your care."—ASTLEY COOPER.

"The proper treatment of wounds is to be regarded as the most important requirement for the surgeon."—BILLROTH.

I offer these two quotations in lieu of any apology for the subject of this occasion's address. Should there need be any other I should only make mention of the prevalent feeling that wound healing is a subject to be mastered by the student in a course of pathology and later to serve as a filler in the first part of modern textbooks of surgery. At the onset I would make a plea for discarding this perfunctory attitude toward our problem and for re-establishing, as of old, the idea that a thorough knowledge of the principles of wound healing and its daily, thoughtful application is of the most fundamental importance in

From the *New England Journal of Medicine,* 215:753, 1936. Reprinted by permission.

Figures 5, 6 and 7 have been omitted.

the practice of surgery. The importance of our subject is in no manner dimmed by the fact that anesthesia and modern methods of controlling hemorrhage have immeasurably widened and multiplied a thousand-fold the incidence of wounds. Nor is there any justification for the attitude that the discovery of bacteria and the subsequent development of countless aseptic and antiseptic procedures have to the slightest degree lessened the necessity of understanding the fundamental principles of wound healing. To me the reverse attitude seems to be the obvious one.

Wound healing is wound healing under whatever circumstances it may occur and the reparative processes are essentially the same, except in degree, regardless of whether the wound heals by first, second, third or any other intention; and whether it be considered infected or clean. Nobody could deny the importance of the presence or absence of bacteria in wounds but I hold it to be equally true that, in the problem of wound healing, their presence in a wound should be regarded as an incident or complication which cannot be intelligently evaluated or treated without a thorough knowledge of the process of wound healing and of what living tissue itself, in this process, can do with such a complication. Viewed in this light it is questionable if bacteria assume a role of greater importance in wound healing than do necrosis, débris and devitalized tissue, or granulation tissue, or fibrin or other factors which must be taken into consideration. Some day we may yet find Paré worshipped by the surgeons on an equal basis with Pasteur.

Throughout our surgical literature we read that the brilliant progress of surgery has been due to anesthesia, the control of hemorrhage and the control of infection. At the risk of accusation of heresy and ingratitude I would suggest that we change "the control of infection" to read "a knowledge of wound healing" which, naturally embracing a consideration of infection, will, I believe, lead to a more intelligent practice of our art as well as to a greater perfection of it.

Wound healing is a daily problem in the life of nearly every doctor. Yet it would be interesting to know how few wounds are treated on the basis of study and thought to determine what form of treatment they need. My own experience with students, interns and doctors in the management of wounds is constantly disappointing. They seem always to be asking for a routine of therapy which, it is clear to me, should be evidently impossible of adoption by anyone who understands even the merest fundamentals of the processes of wound healing. For instance, I am repeatedly asked when skin sutures should be removed and my answer is when the wound is sufficiently healed. Or, how should open wounds be treated and my reply is to look at them and study them and then do what you think the wound demands. For a long time it has seemed to me that routines of wound treatment and thoughtfulness or ignorance of wound healing go hand in hand. And this statement is just as true in the management of deliberately planned wounds as it is in the case of traumatic, ulcerated and infected wounds.

To discuss any of the problems of wound healing in this paper it is, of course, necessary to assume that the reader has a knowledge of the well-established principles or processes of wound healing. Among these must be mentioned the prevention or elimination of necrotic tissue and débris in wounds. Paré's original observations with respect to the importance of this consideration may well be compared with those of Lister in connection with the use of carbolic spray to prevent infection. Yet, only the most casual observation of operative technics reveals that the subsequent refinements of aseptic or antiseptic procedures have far surpassed those which should have followed the original observations of Paré. Pasteur's work told the world what was causing the infection of wounds and unloosed, beginning with Lister and his carbolic acid, a veritable flood of bactericidal agents which show no signs of abating even today. Paré astounded himself and the surgical profession of his time when he learned that the sloughing incident to the burning of wounds with boiling oil or the actual cautery had a very deleterious effect upon the healing of wounds. He learned that the gentlest cleansing of the wounds with the commonest innocuous substances at his disposal at that time, such as water and soap, gave the best wound healing. Today, with our knowledge of the delicacy of growing living cells and of their lethal susceptibility to alcohol, ether, iodine, mercurochrome, merthiolate, carbolic acid, bichloride of mercury, and countless other substances, people go blithely on pouring them into open, fresh wounds to kill living cells and to complicate the process of wound healing and to promote the chances of infection. So far as fresh traumatic wounds are concerned we would today be far better off with a total ignorance of all chemical bactericidal agents and if we only utilized our knowledge of bacteria and of wound healing by gentle mechanical cleansing of the surrounding skin and open wound of all dirt, foreign bodies, dead or devitalized tissue and by flooding the invisible bacteria away by means of sterile salt solution. Paré was, in the light of modern knowledge, densely ignorant but he acted with amazing sanity; today, with a colossal knowledge of the properties of both bacteria and living cells, many wounds are being treated with a lack of sound judgment. This fundamental principle of wound healing which Paré taught the surgical profession over four hundred years ago is constantly being disregarded. In order to worship at the shrine of Paré we must be rid of our bondage to advertising pharmaceutical concerns which delude our profession into the belief that the one essential aid to wound healing is the killing of germs with agents which they do not tell us are also killers of countless invisible delicate living cells. To date, you can accept it as a fact that all germicidal agents are also capable of killing growing cells or of damaging the medium in which they must grow.

REST

For many centuries, and especially since the writing of Baron Larry [sic] upon this subject, rest of the wound has been recognized as one of the essential aids to wound healing. Let me quote from Billroth: "Hitherto I have not mentioned that the absolute rest of an injured part is always necessary; it may seem singular that I should mention it at all, you may think this should be considered a matter of course. I lay particular stress on it, because injurious substances are taken from the wound into the blood: hence every muscular movement, and every consequent congestion of the wound, in short, everything that drives the blood and lymph more strongly into the vicinity of the wound, may eventually prove injurious. Of late, I rarely see contused wounds do so well as compound fractures of the extremities, where plaster dressings are at once applied; hence we have a strong hint to compel absolute rest of an extremity with a large contused wound without fracture, by applying a fenestrated plaster-splint. The cases where I have done this did remarkably well; even after amputations of the hand and foot, where the patient was very restless, I have applied the plaster-splint with excellent result, and think this mode of treatment, which we shall describe more fully under compound fractures, may be more extensively used than hitherto." Complete recognition of a principle in the abstract is by no means followed by an intelligent application of it. There can be little doubt that for a generation or two there has been a great neglect in the use of this unquestioned aid to the healing of wounds. Of late there has been some re-emphasis of its value, especially by Orr, Koch and others, and the results have led to astonishment on the part of those who have recognized the manifest indications for the employment of the principle of rest in wound healing. And, perhaps, the spirits of Billroth and Baron Larry are rejoicing. In this instance, too, Homans is vindicated for writing that "In Surgery, however, as in every other art, fundamental matters are perennially being discovered, discredited, forgotten, rediscovered and reaffirmed."

BLOOD SUPPLY

There is also no argument in principle that a third important factor in the healing of wounds is the blood supply. But I venture the belief that there is a great lack of consideration of this fundamental factor in the routine practice of surgery in this country. Men will readily agree that there are vast differences in the healing of wounds of the aged and the young individuals, of the debilitated and the robust persons, and yet make very little allowance for these differences in the planning of incisions, the tying of ligatures and sutures. The whole problem of the harm of tension within wounds is directly linked with this matter of blood supply to them. Its consideration will dictate to the thoughtful surgeon the position in which he wishes a wound to be kept in order to secure for it the maximum blood supply. To him the crippling effects of edema on blood supply may indicate the elevation of a wound in a healthy part while a sluggish, trickling arterial supply may make him choose for the wound a position somewhat below the level of the heart. Recently an arteriosclerotic patient insisted on sitting up all night because of the relief he got from an agonizing pain he was suffering in an ulcer of his great toe. He had been thus trying to sleep for months. By simply elevating the head of his bed four inches he slept comfortably all night and for him this was well worth a trip from a distant part of the country. A practical regard for blood supply will substantiate the spacing of skin sutures so that a moist dressing, kept moist by the overlying oil silk or gutta percha will relieve tension by permitting the oozing of serum and blood during the period of swelling or edema in the wound.

Time will not permit me to cite other obvious applications which, no doubt, occur to you in connection with a consideration of this universally accepted principle of the rôle of blood supply in the healing of wounds.

HEMOSTASIS

A fourth generally accepted aid to the healing of wounds is ideal hemostasis. The qualifying word "ideal" is used deliberately instead of the more generally accepted term "complete." There is no question that a hematoma of a wound interferes by tension with blood supply, prolongs wound healing, injects the presence of a large foreign body, and immeasurably encourages the development of the clinical signs and symptoms of infection and suppuration. Yet the excessive devitalization of living tissue by unnecessary ligatures of small blood vessels and too many tight sutures also interferes with blood supply, prolongs wound healing and invites infection (fig. 1). Thus, in a measure, the utilization of the principle of hemostasis in wound healing may run counter to Ambroise Paré's principle of the value of eliminating from wounds all necrosis. In the World War, experiences with the secondary closure of wounds taught us a great deal about the role that ligatures and buried sutures may play in the healing of wounds. The greatest successes resulted whenever it was not necessary to bury any ligatures or sutures. Plastic surgeons have perhaps the keenest appreciation of this great principle of surgery. They will spend literally hours in controlling bleeding by means of gentle pressure and warm saline compresses when surgeons less appreciative of the value of Paré's contribution would hastily resort to ligatures. They know that devitalized tissues and infections are the greatest wreckers of the success of their work. The same principles are equally applicable to all forms of surgery. This fourth principle in the healing of wounds, namely, hemostasis, injects forcibly, for the first time in this paper, the necessity for the great element of judgment if one would attempt to weigh and evaluate in the practice of surgery the contradictions inherent in the application of the fundamental principles of wound healing. Reared in a school of complete hemostasis, and cherishing this

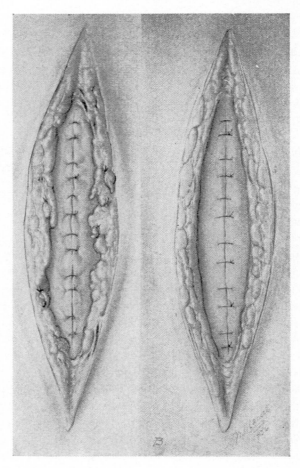

Fig. 1.—The improper and proper methods of closing a wound. With an equal amount of contamination wound *A* [*left*], which has been traumatized and the sutures tied too tightly, runs a much greater chance of suppuration than does wound *B* [*right*], in which the tissues have been properly approximated and no devitalized tissue left in the wound.

principle perhaps above all others, I would nevertheless like to acknowledge the debt of an apology to both Paré and Larry. A due regard for the harmful effects of necrotic tissue and the beneficial hemostatic effects of complete rest of a wound would probably have saved me the necessity of tying countless numbers of knots.

INFECTION

A fifth great consideration in the healing of wounds is the prevention and treatment of infected wounds. Nobody can deny that efforts along this line should and do take the rank of first importance in the problems of wound healing. Modern surgery owes its very life to our knowledge of bacteria and the methods and means of preventing and treating their complications to the problem of wound healing. But are we not in the lethargy of perfect satisfaction with an unprecedented and almost miraculous spurt in our art of surgery which is yet far from its goal? Are we not in the doldrums of further progress by our slavery-like submission to the dictates of the manufacturers of germicides? Surely the use of every one with which I am familiar involves some sacrifice of other fundamental principles of wound healing. Is there no way of determining the price to be paid for their use and of deciding whether it is too great to be justified? In the matter of asepsis of the skin perhaps a recent reply to a salesman of a patented antiseptic solution may be permissible. He asked me what germicide I used for the skin and I said that I did not care so long as the skin was first made macroscopically clean by the use of soap and water, alcohol, and ether and the germicide was free of germs and would not burn the skin. Except for the sin of using skin antiseptics in lieu of careful mechanical cleansing of the skin of all dirt, the modern preparation of the skin seems not often to violate the other fundamental principles of wound healing. When, however, it comes to using bactericidal agents in open fresh wounds one is confronted with the fact that if they are capable of killing micro-organisms they are also capable of killing or damaging the delicate living cells which in turn become excellent food for the growth of germs.

In general it may be stated that the conditions which are ideal for the destruction of bacteria are in no sense ideal for the growth of living cells. Likewise, some of the conditions which are ideal for the growth of living cells may be very conducive to the growth of bacteria. The very medium in which living cells must grow is usually quite attractive food for bacteria. And both bacteria and cells have about the same optimum temperature for reproduction. Thus it frequently happens that one's efforts to promote the healing of wounds may help the growth of bacteria and the reverse is also true. In the course of the healing of an infected granulating wound it is usually desirable to be switching back and forth from tissue reproducing measures to bactericidal treatment in order to get the best result. When the wound is relatively sterile the adoption of a policy of rest, optimum temperature and noninterference may result in a rapid healing, until the multiplication of organisms becomes so numerous that the plasma or medium for the growth of cells is all devoured by them. Then healing comes to a halt and attempts at further sterilization are in order.

"The sterilization of freshly made wounds is, like the sterilization of the skin, a relative and not an absolute matter." (Homans.) Thus

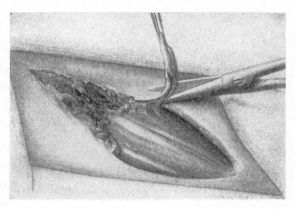

Fig. 2.—Debridement of a fresh traumatic wound. Note how the devitalized tissue is being removed by sharp dissection.

logically as well as practically the use of tissue damaging chemicals in an attempt at sterilization of fresh wounds is not often justified, for the resultant necrosis encourages too much the growth of the organisms not killed. Débridement of dead or devitalized tissue and of foreign materials plus a careful flooding away of the bacteria with sterile water or normal salt solution will usually leave the tissues in such a healthy state that they can cope with the few organisms present without exhibiting the evidences of clinical infection (fig. 2). The harm which has resulted from pouring strong antiseptics into open wounds cannot possibly be estimated. It is impossible to estimate the harm and suffering which have come from the use of iodine for this purpose. For the less powerful antiseptics an appeased conscience which has led to the ignoring of some of the fundamental principles of simple cleansing has often compensated for the lessened damage to the living cells. To quote again from Billroth: "For the first treatment of the part poisoned by cadaveric matter, I advise you to let cold water run on the wound for a long time, and not check the bleeding, if there be any. In many cases the injurious matter will be washed out, and there will be no further infection. Cauterization immediately after contact with the poison, from a considerable experience on myself and on my students in the course of operations, I consider unadvisable." It may be argued that he did not have at his disposal the modernly refined antiseptics and this may be met by saying that he was not aware of the delicacy of living cells or of the power of them to destroy bacteria. He was not even familiar with the rôle of bacteria in wounds and yet he made true observations which are constantly being ignored today.

Not long ago a friend of mine brought his boy hurriedly to my home because of a laceration of the end of his thumb. If the boy had not held his wound under running water the father would not have been so worried; he would have put some iodine on it and wrapped it up. As it was he was very afraid of an infection from the water. You can imagine his surprise when, after cleansing the skin about the wound with benzine and then cutting away some dead fragments of skin, I gave the boy a stool by the sink and told him to run warm water on the wound while the father and I discussed fishing. After the lapse of ten or fifteen minutes a large amount of vaseline was placed on the wound and secured in place by a soft dressing incorporating a splint to immobilize the thumb. The hand was placed in a sling and the father was instructed not to bring him for an inspection of the wound for a week unless he should show an elevation of temperature or complain of pain. No antiseptics were used in the open wound. There was practically no pain and no fever. At the end of a week the wound was healed. The father, like thousands of other people of our generation, had been imbued since birth with the necessity of using iodine or some antiseptic to kill the germs in such a wound. He had never seen a wound like that heal without getting red and painful. He didn't know why I had used a splint or why the hand was put in a sling or why the fragments of dead tissue were cut away. To him the one essential on such an occasion had always been to kill the germs at whatever cost in pain, suffering and infection. He could only shake his head and say, "I do not understand."

This father's attitude reflects, I believe, the viewpoint of the average layman today with regard to the handling of trivial wounds and probably that of the vast majority of the doctors of our time with respect to all wounds.

I have dwelt at some length upon this fifth consideration in the healing of wounds because it is my belief that the modern antisepsis of fresh wounds does not justify the wholesale violation of some of the other fundamental principles of wound healing, notably those dealing with the harmful effects of necrosis and débris and the beneficial effects of rest. In this whole important business of the control of infection in fresh wounds, there is a crying need for a sane modification of our viewpoint so as to make it fit more harmoniously with other established principles of wound healing rather than permit it to usurp them.

GRANULATION TISSUE

An understanding of the problems of wound healing presupposes an appreciation of the importance of granulation tissue. Its formation is essential to the healing of every wound. Besides, in the absence of an epithelial or endothelial protection, it becomes the body's best defense against invasion of bacteria. Nearly seventy-five years ago Billroth reported the following experiments to his students:

"If you inject a drachm of putrid fluid into the subcutaneous cellular tissues of a dog, the result will be inflammation, fever and septicemia. If you make a large granulating surface on a dog, and dress it daily with charpie soaked in putrid fluid, it will have no decided effect. On the borders of the inflammatory new formation the lymphatic vessels are closed; on the granulating surface there are no open lymphatic vessels, hence no reabsorption takes place." Hence, the protection of granulation tissue from traumatization and insults of any nature becomes of paramount importance in the consideration of wound healing. On its exposed surface there are always bacteria and I am sure that those of you who have had any considerable experience with wounds can recall fatal cases of septicemia resulting from the making of granulation tissue bleed as well as numerous examples of local exacerbation of the infection. Its appearance usually reflects accurately the severity of the surface infection, as well as the adequacy of its blood supply. In the absence of surface infection, granulation tissue always assumes its healthiest possible appearance. Juicy, pale and swollen granulations probably represent their best efforts to combat infection. The obvious indication is to help rid them of the infection and not to rid the body of their protection. Once relatively free of infection whether by their own efforts or with the aid of Dakin's solution, some other mild germicide or moist pressure dressings, they will spontaneously return to what is regarded as their normal, red, granular appearance. It seems to me that it is fair to assume that granulations are always doing the best they can under any given circumstances and that there is no justification for speaking of healthy and unhealthy granulation tissue. It would appear that they are most pleased when least disturbed.

TISSUE GROWTH

While I have made hasty mention of the five or six factors which most surgeons agree are of fundamental importance in understanding the behavior of wounds and in the intelligent treatment of them, I believe that the more modern work of Carrel, Lewis and many others with tissue culture, justifies the addition of another important factor which should be necessary and helpful, namely, some understanding of the actual process involved in the growth of living cells in a wound. For, after all, it is the multiplication and growth of cells which cause the healing of a wound, save for what is accomplished by the process of contraction.

In a large sense nearly all of the principles of wound healing which I have been discussing have a rationale in the beneficial effect they have on the growth of living cells. Dead or devitalized tissue diverts the energies of growing cells from the problem of repair to one of elimination of foreign materials. Rest of wounds promotes the growth of living cells just as it does in the case of the medium for tissue growth in vitro. Nourishment for the growth of cells comes from the blood stream and hence the more perfect the blood supply, the more ideal will be the medium in which the cells must grow. In addition to the poisonous effects of their toxins upon the living cells and body mechanism as a whole, bacteria also devour the medium for the growth of cells in wounds just as they do the medium for the growth of cells in vitro. Hemorrhage, as well as the surgeon's necrosis, gives to the cells the burden of removing additional foreign bodies. A casual observation of the behavior of superficial wounds in the winter and summer, illustrates the effect of temperature upon the growth of cells in wounds just as its effect is well known upon the growth of cells in vitro.

If you will imagine a straight clean wound accurately approximated, the medium for the growth of cells which repair that wound will lie in a small crevice between the cut edges (fig. 3A). If you

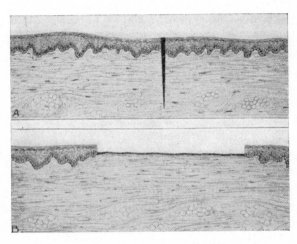

Fig. 3.—Schematic illustration of a closed fresh wound and an open wound. In either instance the healing processes are essentially the same. The fibrin serves as the medium into which granulation tissue and epithelium must grow.

will then imagine that wound spread open like the leaves of a book, the medium will lie on a surface with one side exposed instead of being compressed into a thin line between two opposing surfaces of living tissue (fig. 3B). In either instance the process of repair is essentially the same except in the amount of the growth of epithelium. In both instances this medium is absolutely essential to the growth and multiplication of cells. The epithelial cells do not push themselves out over the surface nor do the elements of tissue which form granulation tissue divide and jut out into space. They grow into and devour this coagulum of fibrin which is constantly forming on raw surfaces and granulation tissue. If, as we have repeatedly shown, a fresh wound is so energetically dakinized that no fibrin or media can accumulate, then there will be no formation of granulation tissue or growth of epithelium (fig. 4). When possible, nature's ideal way of preserving this medium for the growth of living cells is the formation of a sterile scab. To her I suspect that this means healing by first intention regardless of whether the edges of wounds are closely approximated or widely separated. Infection, traumatization, dressings which

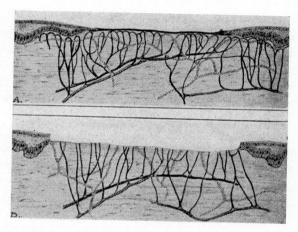

Fig. 4.—*A.* A granulating wound. The vessels and the lymphatics are closed. When there is no traumatization there is no absorption and the underlying tissues are best protected.

B. An open wound without fibrin showing the open vessels and lymphatics. Absorption takes place rapidly from such a surface.

pull it away, interference with the blood which supplies it, and the unwise use of chemicals and bactericidal agents which may destroy it are the principal handicaps to the preservation of this medium. In the experiment just cited, if the wound be covered with vaselinized gauze and left undisturbed for twenty-four hours the base will become covered with healthy granulations and there will be obvious growth in epithelium. Perhaps in a few days, infection may likewise destroy the medium and halt the processes of healing. Striking an optimum balance, in such a wound, between methods to promote the growth of tissue and those to help control the infection can be no haphazard routine. It must be based on careful observation.

Would it not be well to regard every wound as a new growth in which, paradoxically, our every effort should be to promote its growth, knowing that some as yet not understood, biologic principle will terminate the process when healing is complete? With this conception constantly before us it seems to me that we would be more likely to evaluate properly our efforts to assist and, moreover, what is probably more important, develop an alertness to change them to meet the ever-changing demands of a healing wound.[1]

With this general discussion of the fundamental principles which should be considered in the treatment of wounds it may be permissible for me to describe for you the attitude adopted in our clinic toward the treatment of certain types of wounds. This seems especially advisable since, as I have indicated, the utilization of some of these principles is often not compatible with the employment of others.

SURGICAL WOUNDS

In the minds of most people there are two types of wounds—clean, and contaminated or infected—, and the division between them is as sharp as between night and day. Little thought is given to the fact that every open wound, surgical or accidental, receives bacterial organisms and that the term *infection* is applied only in those instances in which the processes of wound healing exhibit obvious difficulties, in varying degrees, in combating this contamination. Little do we appreciate the natural protective forces inherent in wound healing. For every obvious difficulty with infection the processes of wound healing probably spare us the worry a hundred times by taking care of similar bacterial contaminations.

It is reasonable to assume that with the modern methods of sterilizing supplies and instruments, with the universal wearing of masks and gloves, and the effective preparation of the skin there is not a wide variation in the actual bacterial contamination of surgical wounds. In the vast majority of instances clinical infection is directly traceable to the burden of added insults heaped upon the tissues of the wound by the operator and his assistants. Viewed in this light there was never a

---

[1] Throughout this discussion of wound healing I have deliberately omitted any mention of restoration of function of the wounded parts. From the pure standpoint of the principles of wound healing it does not merit serious consideration, but from the viewpoint of the results of healed wounds it may become a matter of some importance.

truer statement than that of Homans in which he says that, "The patients' best defense against infection lies in the perfection of the operator's technique."

In the performance of identical operations and with presumably the same bacterial contamination, one surgeon may get an infected wound while the other will get primary healing. Some surgeons can excise a badly infected breast or close a severely contaminated laparotomy wound and virtually get healing by first intention while others will invariably get infected wounds.

The answer is in how well the soil has been prepared for the growth of the bacteria by the production of necrosis, traumatization of tissues and interference with blood supply. Definite efforts to avoid this invitation to the growth of bacteria are made in our clinic. Whenever possible blood vessels are tied before division and the end projecting beyond the ligature is removed. As few clamps as possible are used and whenever they are, a definite effort is made to grasp only the bleeding vessels. Vessels which in the judgment of the operator will not bleed upon removal of the clamps are not tied. When mass ligation is unavoidable, transfixion ligatures are employed and tied only tight enough to stop the bleeding and leave the included tissue viable. All obviously nonviable tissue, whether caused by ligatures, clamps or trauma, is excised if possible. Sharp dissection with the knife in the belief that it is less damaging to living tissue is the almost invariable rule. The use of clamps on the peritoneum and other tissues for purposes of traction demands an extraordinary excuse. The use of retractors and especially the self-retaining ones is reduced to a minimum. The placing of sutures in fat or muscle is almost never done because of the delicacy of these structures as well as the almost invariable uselessness of such sutures. Sutures are tied with extreme care lest their tightness or subsequent tightening due to edema will interfere with circulation (fig. 1). Some surgeons will tie with great force the sutures buried in the infinitely more delicate tissues and then close the skin loosely. If there is any justification for this I cannot understand it. Before closing a wound it should be free of bleeding, of air and of blood clots. In the case of local anesthetics the patient is made to cough or strain to see if any untied vessels will begin to bleed. Pressure with gauze for a few moments on the freshly cut surfaces of a wound may reduce by 50 to 75 per cent the number of clamps which otherwise might have been used. Finally the wound, when closed, should present tissues, as nearly as possible, as healthy in appearance as when the incision was first made. Drainage of clean wounds is never employed. In wounds where there is known to be serious bacterial contamination or considerable oozing of blood, deliberate provision is made for gaping, between the skin sutures. In the case of such abdominal wounds, no sutures are placed in the line of the incision but, instead, the wound is closed with through-and-through silver wire sutures placed far removed from the edges of the wound. Most dressings are applied and kept moist for a considerable time by means of a rubber protective so that tension of the wound may be relieved by seepage during the period of edema or slight hemorrhage (fig. 5) [*Ed. Note:* Figure omitted]. The wound is placed in the position of optimum general circulation and completely immobilized when thought necessary and especially during the period of recovery from anesthesia. Unless indicated by pain or evidence of infection or hemorrhage, the wound is left undisturbed until it is thought it may be desirable to remove some of the stitches.

It is obvious that these are only a few of the safeguards against the development of infected wounds due to errors of operative technique. It is not necessary to mention any others, for, when an operating surgeon works with a mind acutely conscious of wound healing, he will unconsciously adopt all of them; if he does not, what I have already said becomes well-nigh useless and the patients will go on paying the price in pain, disablement and even death.

It must be added that in many, many instances the very efforts of a surgeon to prevent the infection of surgical wounds constitute the direct cause of the infection. His very efforts at destruction of germs have made the living tissues incapable of coping with a contamination which otherwise they might have handled with ease.

Finally a good aid to the healing of surgical wounds is to make every unexpected infection or failure of an even hoped-for primary union a matter for serious investigation. This policy in any clinic is always beneficial to the problems of the healing of surgical wounds.

Traumatic Wounds. We are paying for the advancement of industry and for our economic development an enormous price in wounds, disability and lives. Nearly seventy-five years ago Billroth said, "You may imagine, not only how much sweat, but how much blood clings to the many evidences of modern culture." When one reads such a statement the usual reaction is a smile if one thinks of Billroth's remarks in comparison with the problems of our time. The differences in the magnitude of the problems of his time and of ours may be just cause for a smile, but there is serious doubt if genuine chagrin should not be the result if we should consider the progress which has been made in handling these problems. Viewed in this light the surgeons of today are face to face with a distinct challenge lest our efforts in the treatment of traumatic wounds be subject to censure by the surgeons of the not distant future.

To meet this challenge we have endeavored to develop in our clinic methods of treatment of traumatic wounds which we believe are based upon the accepted principles of wound healing of our time. Our application of these fundamental principles of wound healing in this very large field of surgery may, of course, be wrong but our conscience is free in that we may not be accused of acting without thought or under the influence of domination by the bactericidal therapeutists.

In the case of all traumatic wounds, bleeding of any consequence is first controlled preferably by elevation of the part and pressure or when absolutely necessary the clamping of individual vessels. The wound and surrounding skin are then flushed rather vigorously with a large quantity of sterile normal salt solution. The skin about the wound is shaved, washed with soap and water, alcohol, ether and possibly painted with some of the accepted skin antiseptics. None of the alcohol, ether or antiseptic is permitted to enter the fresh wound. Next sterile draping is done as though for a clean surgical operation. If any clamps were placed to control hemorrhage they are held up by an assistant during the washing and skin preparation and are now removed by him and replaced, when necessary, by fresh sterile clamps by the operator. If the operation is to be done under local anesthesia the skin infiltration is made well away from the edges of the wound. With this preparation the wound, and skin edges, are debrided by sharp dissection of all debris, dead, crushed, devitalized or dirt-stained tissues. Frequently it is necessary to use soap and water on the fresh wound in order to remove greasy dirt. The fewest possible ligatures are placed in the wound. After this another very careful and thorough irrigation of the wound with hydrogen peroxide followed by sterile normal salt solution, is done. The wound is then ready for surgi-

cal repair and dressing. Only when absolutely essential are buried
sutures used. Skin sutures are tied loosely and widely spaced so that
there will be free seepage from the wound into the moist dressing.
Usually it is far better to use no skin sutures which may in any way
imperil the blood supply to either side of the skin edges. An avulsed
flap of skin is far more useful alive and unsutured than dead from
the anemia of the tension of the sutures which place it beautifully
back into perfect position. To tack a flap of skin loosely back one-half
inch or more from the opposing edge is, I think, the hardest thing in
the world for a young surgeon to do. About six months ago a young
girl of fourteen years received in an automobile accident an extensive
laceration and contusion of the left thigh. A large triangular flap, of
skin and muscle was turned upward from just above the knee. The
transverse tear extended from the lateral side of the thigh across the
top to the mesial aspect where it met a vertical laceration which extended upward for more than six inches. The muscles were torn and
loosened up as far as the greater trochanter, exposing the bone from
which a considerable area of periosteum had been removed. The tissues were badly stained and there were many stones of varying sizes
throughout the extent of the wound. After a painstaking irrigation and
débridement such as described above, requiring more than an hour,
the triangular flap of skin and subcutaneous tissue was gently laid
back and sutured with three sutures which failed by one and a half
inches to approximate the skin edges. A moist dressing was applied
and the leg was encased in a large plaster spica which included the
abdomen and foot. Although this patient was unconscious from a
concussion of the brain and incontinent for three days during which
the dressings became soaked with urine, the first dressing was not
made for ten days. Healing was by first intention. The function of
the leg is unimpaired even though much of the quadriceps and lateral
leg muscles was cut away. No buried sutures were placed in the wound.
It is amazing with how little scarring even large open wounds will
heal if there has been little or no loss of skin.

In many instances, when no attempt at closure is made, the wound,
after the preparation described, is filled with vaseline, dressed and immobilized for many days without even inspection unless pain or fever
may indicate an infection which the tissues may need some help to
handle.

INFECTED WOUNDS

In the problems of an infection or an infected wound it is obvious that time will not permit me to be specific even if it were possible to deal specifically with the countless problems which arise. This subject must of necessity be dealt with in general terms.

Our only hope of aiding in the solution of these problems must be based, first, on an intensified effort to disseminate to students and doctors a thorough knowledge of the fundamental principles of wound healing as we understand them and, secondly, in an endeavor to make every act in behalf of an infected wound conform to a judgment which should be arrived at only in the light of one's best knowledge of these principles. If infected wounds were so handled there could be no criticism of thoughtlessness, of addiction to a routine or of slavery to one principle of wound healing when the application of others might be more indicated by the condition of the wound. Such an approach to these problems would at least have the virtue of wounds being treated according to the abilities of those handling them, which I fear is very far from the facts at the present time.

One thing very essential to the intelligent handling of infected wounds is a correction of the more or less prevalent feeling that such wounds are either treated or not treated depending upon whether they are operated upon and subjected to antiseptic therapy. The care of infected wounds is not by any means solely a problem of drainage and germicidal therapy. Many kinds of wound infection are often best treated by a stressing of some principle of wound healing other than that of active control of the infection. An unwillingness to cut into acute infections such as lymphangitis, furunculosis, cellulitis, where there is no suppuration may easily be justified by an avoiding of traumatization and necrosis, a refusal to open up new avenues for a spread of the infection and by a desire to observe the fundamental principle of rest. The use of moist warm dressings to prevent edema, the forcing of fluids, transfusions and various kinds of intravenous therapy, all find a rationale in an effort to improve the blood supply.

A course of procedure based on such reasoning is just as much a part of the problem of treating infected wounds as is incision and antiseptic therapy. That some infected wounds such as osteomyelitis, certain types of joint infections as well as other kinds of infections may do best under a stressing of the principle of absolute rest and, as a corollary, nontraumatization has been amply proved. In general, when antiseptic fluids cannot be made to reach a part of an infected wound, it is always a question whether the traumatization incident to their use justifies the harm which may result from a disregard of the value of rest.

Prior to actual suppuration it is difficult for me to justify any incisional measures in the treatment of infected wounds. It has always seemed to me that the price to be paid in the nature of traumatization, necrosis, and the opening up of new avenues for the spread of the infection, is not warranted by the good which may result from the release of tension or the establishment of drainage for subsequent suppuration. It is most unusual for this to be done in our clinic.

When, however, suppuration has occurred, sooner or later some form of external drainage or excision becomes necessary in order to avoid the damage of tension, accumulated toxins, and the spreading of the infection in undesirable directions. Deciding when to do this and how are obviously problems of such magnitude and variation that they cannot be considered. Even if it were possible to consider this phase of our problem, I would have to admit that it is impossible for me to put in writing my course of procedure. I can decide only after careful study of each individual instance of suppuration as it arises. I would venture the one generalization that radical procedure is not often a fault of the modern surgery of suppurating wounds. That it, however, should be done with the least amount of damage to the existing granulation tissue is obvious.

I realize the inadequacy of my treatment of the subject of infected wounds, but I do trust that I have indicated the necessity for carefully considering and weighing all the fundamental principles of wound healing before deciding upon a course of procedure in any given case of infection. This process should become second nature to one's mental behavior each and every time an infected wound is inspected.

GRANULATING WOUNDS

It now remains for me to make only a few comments on the treatment of open granulating wounds. My assumption will be that all of them are infected, for it is the rarest occasion to see such a wound of any size heal under the benign influence of a sterile scab.

It is obviously essential that anyone charged with the responsibility of treating a given granulating wound should have clearly in mind what he wishes to accomplish with it. If it is desired to perform a secondary closure, then intensive bactericidal therapy (with Dakin's solution in our clinic) until the wound is macroscopically free of necrosis and exhibits in the smears and cultures of its secretions a very minor degree of bacterial contamination seems clearly to be the course to follow. To us it also seems the wisest course to follow in preparing granulations for the reception of any kind of skin grafts. If the granulating surface is but a mere incident to some deep-seated more important pathologic process, such, for example, as osteomyelitis, it is often most illogical to treat it at the expense of rest and nontraumatization which may be clearly indicated for the more important underlying process. The granulations, if not interfered with, will nearly always provide adequate protection to the body against invasion of bacteria while adopting the principle of rest in treating the other condition. If, however, the time arrives when there will be no or very little sacrifice to deep healing, we believe that efforts to promote epithelization of the granulations by skin grafting or otherwise up to the point of sinus should be begun.

By far the most frequent problem in connection with granulating wounds is simply to get the epithelium to grow over the surface either from the edges or from islands of grafted skin (fig. 6) [Ed. Note: Figure omitted]. In the minds of most doctors, efforts to promote this process are regarded as cut-and-dried simple problems, but it is my belief that in the handling of this kind of a wound is to be found the greatest sinning against the principles of wound healing. Throughout the country there must be in practice literally thousands of different ways of treating such wounds and in probably over 80 per cent of the instances the granulating wounds are healing in spite of, or under the handicap of, what is being done for them. Reduced to its simplest terms the main problem is to get the granulating surface covered with the best possible medium for the growth of epithelial cells. As I have said before nature's ideal way is the formation of a sterile scab but this very rarely occurs over a large granulating surface. Thus practically all granulating wounds should be so handled that this medium will form to the best advantage even in the presence of infection, for without any medium, the epithelial cells cannot grow.

Dakinization or antiseptic therapy may be so thorough and energetic as to make a granulating surface practically sterile and of a most healthy, red, firm appearance and yet no epithelization will occur because the medium for the growth of cells is also dissolved away (fig. 7) [*Ed. Note:* Figure omitted]. Or, granulations may be so infected with bacteria which practically destroy all this medium that the growth of epithelial cells will come almost to a standstill. Again, coarse gauze placed next to the surface may at each dressing remove practically all of this medium which becomes enmeshed in it, as well as cause bleeding which opens up avenues for the spread of infection (fig. 8). Dependent edematous parts with granulating surfaces may so interfere with circulation as to hinder the formation of this fibrinous medium as well as cause the exudation of serum which carries it away. In connection with such ulcers Billroth has this to say: "It is remarkable how rapidly the common ulcer of the leg begins to improve in appearance as soon as the patient has taken a warm bath, simply applied a wet compress to the ulcer, and remained in bed quietly for twenty-four hours." Time and again I have seen amazing results when the responsibility for the care of a chronic ulcer which has been dressed daily for months in a clinic has been thrown back upon the patient with advice such as that quoted from Billroth. The thick, dried, contracting dirt and sebaceous material on the skin about the ulcer disappears, the circulation improves, granulations take on a healthy appearance, fibrin forms on their surface, and epithelization takes on a new impetus. The only warning has been that under no circumstances should the granulation tissue be made to bleed. The good results are undoubtedly due to the improvement of the circulation which, in turn, improves the supply of medium for the growth of epithelial cells.

If a doctor would, therefore, treat a granulating wound intelligently, he must keep constantly in mind the process by which it must eventually heal; he must be willing to change his procedures to meet the demands of the wound. When antiseptic therapy has been pushed so far that it is stealing away the medium for the growth of cells, he must be willing to let up on its use and, vice versa, when bacteria are devouring all of it he must be willing to reemphasize the use of antiseptics. Efforts should be made to get to the wound the best possible blood supply. Dressings which stick to the wound, and then pull away

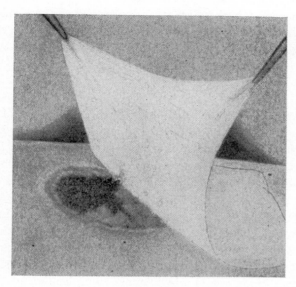

FIG. 8A.—Drawing showing effect of removal of dry gauze from a granulating wound. Note the bleeding and the removal with the gauze of the delicate fibrin covering the wound.

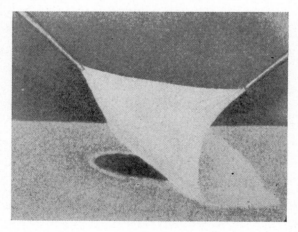

FIG. 8B.—Drawing showing the condition of a wound which has been treated by the application of vaselinized old linen. The delicate fibrin layer is not removed by this dressing.

the fibrinous medium, should never be employed (fig. 8). When, as occasionally happens, a nice layer of healthy fibrin is seen covering a granulating surface, every effort should be made to preserve it instead of, as I have frequently seen, to remove it (fig. 8).

SUMMARY

This paper is a plea for re-emphasis of the importance of the study and application of the fundamental principles of wound healing. It is the author's belief that the amazing progress of surgery during the past generation and a half has made our profession and the public satisfied with results which fall far short of those possible to obtain. In a large measure this progress has been the result of a knowledge of germs and of efforts to control their harmful effects in wounds. However, wound healing is not alone a problem of germ destruction. Throughout this paper it has been repeatedly stressed that the price of aseptic and antiseptic procedures frequently means the sacrifice, at a loss, of other fundamental principles of wound healing.

Among these other principles which are discussed are the gross and invisible necrosis of living cells, rest, hemostasis, blood supply, the protective value of granulation tissue and an adaptation of the knowledge gained from tissue culture to the processes of a healing wound.

Only when it becomes our constant aim to evaluate all these considerations of the problems of wound healing, both in the art of making wounds as well as in the treatment of them, will there result the greatest benefit to those whose misfortune it is to bear them.

SIR ALEXANDER FLEMING (1881–1955)

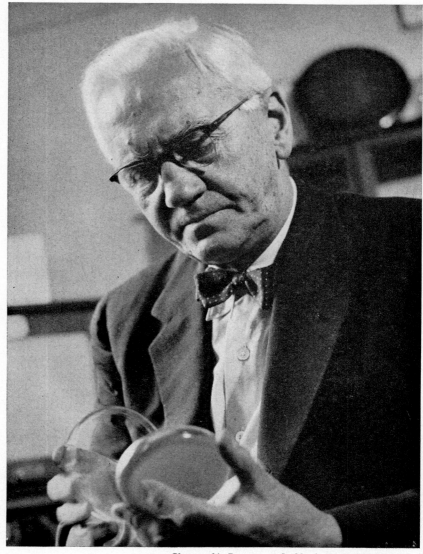

Alexander Fleming was born on August 6, 1881, in Ayrshire, Scotland, and received his early schooling at Kilmarnock Academy. He studied medicine at St. Mary's in London and won almost every prize and scholarship available. He became Professor of Bacteriology at St. Mary's Medical School in 1928 and in 1948 became Professor of Bacteriology at London University. His association with Sir Almoth Wright gave him a fine experimental background. During World War I he devoted himself to the problems of sepsis and developed an antiseptic proteolytic substance, lysozyme. In 1945 he received the Nobel prize for his work on penicillin.

Much fantasy and legend exists regarding Fleming's discovery of penicillin. His own description gives us much insight into his character. While working on a purely academic bacteriological problem with staphylococci, "I hit on penicillin. The very first stage in the discovery of penicillin was due to a stroke of good fortune. As soon as you open a culture plate, things drop from the air. One of those bits of trouble happened to be penicillin. A mould spore, coming from I don't know where, dropped on the plate. That didn't excite me, I had often seen such contamination before. But what I had never seen before was staphylococci undergoing lysis around the contaminating colony. Obviously something extraordinary was happening.

"With the background that I had, this was far more interesting to me than staphylococcal research, so I switched promptly. I am now glad that for years my interest had been directed to antiseptics and that some years before I had found in a somewhat similar manner another naturally occurring antiseptic, lysozyme. But for that previous experience it is likely that I would have thrown the plate away as many bacteriologists must have done before. . . . Instead of casting out the contaminated culture with appropriate language, I made some investigations." The laboratory in which he discovered penicillin has ben described as "dingy and dun

colored." His own reply to slightly astonished Americans when he went to their country and was shown their "sterilized sanctums," shining and spotless, was: "Wonderful, but penicillin could never have been discovered in a lab like this one!" Of course, no spores could live in that uncontaminated air!

He was referred to as a quietly-spoken man with a sharp sense of humor, passionately attached to his work yet interested also in art, in sport and in the life in the open air.

In his Linacre Lecture in 1946, "Chemotherapy Yesterday, Today and Tomorrow," Sir Alexander concluded with a quotation from Mervyn Gordon which typifies the little-known men in the laboratory who unselfishly provide us with our tools.

"No research is ever quite complete. It is the glory of a good bit of work that it opens the way for something still better, and thus rapidly leads to its own eclipse. The object of research is the advancement, not of the investigator, but of knowledge."

ON THE ANTIBACTERIAL ACTION OF CULTURES OF A PENICILLIUM, WITH SPECIAL REFERENCE TO THEIR USE IN THE ISOLATION OF B. INFLUENZAE

BY ALEXANDER FLEMING, F.R.C.S.
*From the Laboratories of the Inoculation Department,
St. Mary's Hospital, London*

While working with staphylococcus variants a number of culture-plates were set on the laboratory bench and examined from time to time. In the examinations these plates were necessarily exposed to the air and they became contamined with various microorganisms. It was noticed that around a large colony of a contaminating mould the staphylococcus colonies became transparent and were obviously undergoing lysis (see fig. 1) [*Ed. Note:* Figure omitted].

Subcultures of this mould were made and experiments conducted with a view to ascertaining something of the properties of the bacteriolytic substance which had evidently been formed in the mould culture and which had diffused into the surrounding medium. It was found that broth in which the mould had been grown at room temperature for one or two weeks had acquired marked inhibitory, bactericidal and bacteriolytic properties to many of the more common pathogenic bacteria.

From the *British Journal of Experimental Pathology*, *10*:226, 1929.
Figures 1 and 2 and Table III have been omitted.

CHARACTERS OF THE MOULD

The colony appears as a white fluffy mass which rapidly increases in size and after a few days sporulates, the centre becoming dark green and later in old cultures darkens to almost black. In four or five days a bright yellow colour is produced which diffuses into the medium. In certain conditions a reddish colour can be observed in the growth.

In broth the mould grows on the surface as a white fluffy growth changing in a few days to a dark green felted mass. The broth becomes bright yellow and this yellow pigment is not extracted by CHCl₃. The reaction of the broth becomes markedly alkaline, the pH varying from 8.5 to 9. Acid is produced in three or four days in glucose and saccharose broth. There is no acid production in 7 days in lactose, mannite or dulcite broth.

Growth is slow at 37° C. and is most rapid about 20° C. No growth is observed under anaerobic conditions.

In its morphology this organism is a penicillium and in all its characters it most closely resembles *P. rubrum*. Biourge (1923) states that he has never found *P. rubrum* in nature and that it is an "animal de laboratoire." This penicillium is not uncommon in the air of the laboratory.

IS THE ANTIBACTERIAL BODY ELABORATED IN CULTURE BY ALL MOULDS?

A number of other moulds were grown in broth at room temperature and the culture fluids were tested for antibacterial substances at various intervals up to one month. The species examined were: *Eidamia viridiscens, Botrytis cineria, Aspergillus fumigatus, Sporotrichum, Cladosporium, Penicillium,* 8 strains. Of these it was found that only one strain of penicillium produced any inhibitory substance, and that one had exactly the same cultural characters as the original one from the contaminated plate.

It is clear, therefore, that the production of this antibacterial substance is not common to all moulds or to all types of penicillium.

In the rest of this article allusion will constantly be made to experiments with filtrates of a broth culture of this mould, so for convenience and to avoid the repetition of the rather cumbersome phrase "Mould broth filtrate," the name "penicillin" will be used. This will denote the filtrate of a broth culture of the particular penicillium with which we are concerned.

METHODS OF EXAMINING CULTURES FOR ANTI-BACTERIAL SUBSTANCE

The simplest method of examining for inhibitory power is to cut a furrow in an agar plate (or a plate of other suitable culture material), and fill this in with a mixture of equal parts of agar and the broth in which the mould has grown. When this has solidified, cultures of various microbes can be streaked at right angles from the furrow to the edge of the plate. The inhibitory substance diffuses very rapidly in the agar, so that in the few hours before the microbes show visible growth it has spread out for a centimetre or more in sufficient concentration to inhibit growth of a sensitive microbe. On further incubation it will be seen that the proximal portion of the culture for perhaps one centimetre becomes transparent, and on examination of this portion of the culture it is found that practically all the microbes are dissolved, indicating that the antibacterial substance has continued to diffuse into the agar in sufficient concentration to induce dissolution of the bacteria. This simple method therefore suffices to demonstrate the bacterio-inhibitory and bacteriolytic properties of the mould culture, and also by the extent of the area of inhibition gives some measure of the sensitiveness of the particular microbe tested. Fig. 2 [*Ed. Note:* Figure omitted) shows the degree of inhibition obtained with various microbes tested in this way.

The inhibitory power can be accurately titrated by making serial dilutions of penicillin in fresh nutrient broth, and then implanting all the tubes with the same volume of a bacterial suspension and incubating them. The inhibition can then readily be seen by noting the opacity of the broth.

For the estimation of the antibacterial power of a mould culture it is unnecessary to filter as the mould grows only slowly at 37° C., and in 24 hours, when the results are read, no growth of mould is perceptible. Staphylococcus is a very suitable microbe on which to test the broth as it is hardy, lives well in culture, grows rapidly, and is very sensitive to penicillin.

The bactericidal power can be tested in the same way except that at intervals measured quantities are explanted so that the number of surviving microbes can be estimated.

PROPERTIES OF THE ANTIBACTERIAL SUBSTANCE

EFFECT OF HEAT. Heating for 1 hour at 56° or 80° C. has no effect on the antibacterial power of penicillin. Boiling for a few minutes hardly affects it (see Table II). Boiling for 1 hour reduces it to less than one quarter its previous strength if the fluid is alkaline, but if it is neutral or very slightly acid then the reduction is much less. Autoclaving for 20 minutes at 115° C. practically destroys it.

EFFECT OF FILTRATION. Passage through a Seitz filter does not diminish the antibacterial power. This is the best method of obtaining sterile active mould broth.

SOLUBILITY. It is freely soluble in water and weak saline solution. My colleague, Mr. Ridley, has found that if penicillin is evaporated at a low temperature to a sticky mass the active principle can be completely extracted by absolute alcohol. It is insoluble in ether or chloroform.

RATE OF DEVELOPMENT OF INHIBITORY SUBSTANCE IN CULTURE. A 500 c. c. Erlenmeyer flask containing 200 c. c. of broth was planted with mould spores and incubated at room temperature (10° to 20° C.). The inhibitory power of the broth to staphylococcus was tested at intervals.

After 5 days complete inhibition in 1 in   20 dilution.
  ” 6 ” ”   ”   ” 1 in 40 ”
  ” 7 ” ”   ”   ” 1 in 200 ”
  ” 8 ” ”   ”   ” 1 in 500 ”

Grown at 20° C., the development of the active principle is more rapid and a good sample will completely inhibit staphylococci in a

TABLE I. EFFECT OF KEEPING AT ROOM TEMPERATURE ON THE
ANTI-STAPHYLOCOCCAL POWER OF PENICILLIN

Growth of staphylococcus in dilutions of penicillin as under

	$\frac{1}{20}$	$\frac{1}{40}$	$\frac{1}{60}$	$\frac{1}{80}$	$\frac{1}{100}$	$\frac{1}{200}$	$\frac{1}{300}$	$\frac{1}{400}$	$\frac{1}{600}$	$\frac{1}{800}$	$\frac{1}{1000}$	Control
At time of filtration	−	−	−	−	−	−	−	−	−	±	++	++
After 4 days	−	−	−	−	−	−	−	−	−	±	++	++
" 7 "	−	−	−	−	−	−	−	±	+	+	++	++
" 9 "	−	−	−	−	−	−	±	+	+	++	++	++
" 13 "	−	−	−	−	−	+	+	+	+	+	++	++
" 15 "	−	±	+	+	+	+	+	+	+	+	++	++

TABLE II. Inhibitory Power of Penicillin (Heated and Unheated)
on Various Microbes (Agar Plate Method)
Extent of inhibition in mm. from penicillin embedded in agar,
serum agar, or blood agar plates

Type of microbe	Unheated	Boiled for 1 minute
Experiment 1:		
Staphylococcus pyogenes	23	21
Streptococcus "	17	17
" viridans (mouth)	17	15
Diphtheroid bacillus	27	22
Sarcina	10	10
Micrococcus lysodeikticus	6	7
" from air (1)	20	16
" " " (2)	4	9
B. anthracis	0	0
B. typhosus	0	0
Enterococcus	0	0
Experiment 2:		
Staphylococcus pyogenes	24	
Streptococcus "	30	
" viridans (mouth)	25	
Pneumococcus	30	
Diphtheroid bacillus	35	
B. pyocyaneus	0	
B. pneumoniae (Friedlander)	0	
B. coli	0	
B. paratyphosus A	0	
Experiment 3:		
Staphylococcus pyogenes	16	
Gonococcus	16	
Meningococcus	17	
Experiment 4:		
Streptococcus pyogenes	17	
" epidermidis	18	
Streptococcus pyogenes	15	
" viridans (faeces)	5	
B. diphtheriae (2 strains)	14	
Diphtheroid bacillus	10	
Gram-negative coccus from the mouth (1)	12	
" " " " " " (2)	0	
B. coli	0	
B. influenzae (Pfeiffer) 6 strains	0	

1 in 500 or 1 in 800 dilution in 6 or 7 days. As the culture ages the antibacterial power falls and may in 14 days at 20° C. have almost disappeared.

The antibacterial power of penicillin falls when it is kept at room temperature. The rate of this fall can be seen from Table I.

If the reaction of penicillin is altered from its original pH of 9 to a pH of 6.8 it is much more stable.

The small drops of bright yellow fluid which collect on the surface of the mould may have a high antibacterial titre. One specimen of such fluid completely inhibited the growth of staphylococci in a dilution of 1 in 20,000 while the broth in which the mould was growing, tested at the same time, inhibited staphylococcal growth in 1 in 800.

If the mould is grown on solid medium and the felted mass picked off and extracted in normal salt solution for 24 hours it is found that the extract has bacteriolytic properties.

If this extract is mixed with a thick suspension of staphylococcus suspension and incubated for 2 hours at 45° C. it will be found that the opacity of the suspension has markedly diminished and after 24 hours the previously opaque suspension will have become almost clear.

INFLUENCE OF THE MEDIUM ON THE ANTIBACTERIAL TITRE OF THE MOULD CULTURE. So far as has been ascertained nutrient broth is the most suitable medium for the production of penicillin. The addition of glucose or saccharose, which are fermented by the mould with the production of acid, delays or prevents the appearance of the antibacterial substance. Dilution of the broth with water delays the formation of the antibacterial substance and diminishes the concentration which is ultimately reached.

INHIBITORY POWER OF PENICILLIN ON THE GROWTH OF BACTERIA

Tables II and III [*Ed. Note:* Table III omitted] show the extent to which various microbes, pathogenic and non-pathogenic, are inhibited by penicillin. The first table shows the inhibition by the agar plate method and the second shows the inhibitory power when diluted in nutrient broth.

Certain interesting facts emerge from these tables. It is clear that penicillin contains bacterio-inhibitory substance which is very active towards some microbes while not affecting others. The members of the coli-typhoid group are unaffected as are other intestinal bacilli such as *B. pyocyaneus, B. proteus* and *V. cholerae.* Other bacteria which are insensitive to penicillin are the enterococcus, some of the Gram-negative cocci of the mouth, Friedlander's pneumobacillus, and *B. influenzae* (Pfeiffer), while the action on *B. dysenteriae* (Flexner), and *B pseudo-tuberculosis rodentium* is almost negligible. The anthrax bacillus is completely inhibited in a 1 to 10 dilution but in this case the inhibitory influence is trifling when compared with the effect on the pyogenic cocci.

It is on the pyogenic cocci and on bacilli of the diphtheria group that the action is most manifest.

Staphylococci are very sensitive, and the inhibitory effect is practically the same on all strains, whatever the colour or type of the staphylococcus.

Streptococcus pyogenes is also very sensitive. There were small differences in the titre with different strains, but it may be said generally that it is slightly more sensitive than staphylococcus.

Pneumococci are equally sensitive with *Streptococcus pyogenes*.

The green streptococci vary very considerably, a few strains being almost unaffected while others are as sensitive as *S. pyogenes*. Gonococci, meningococci, and some of the Gram-negative cocci found in nasal catarrhal conditions are about as sensitive as are staphylococci. Many of the Gram-negative cocci found in the mouth and throat are, however, quite insensitive.

B. diphtheriae is less affected than staphylococcus but is yet completely inhibited by a 1% dilution of a fair sample of penicillin.

It may be noted here that penicillin, which is strongly inhibitory to many bacteria, does not inhibit the growth of the original penicillium which was used in its preparation.

THE RATE OF KILLING OF STAPHYLOCOCCI BY PENICILLIN

Some bactericidal agents like the hypochlorites are extremely rapid in their action, others like flavine or novarsenobillon are slow. Experiments were made to find into which category penicillin fell.

To 1 c.c. volumes of dilutions in broth of penicillin were added 10 c.m.m. volumes of a 1 in 1000 dilution of a staphylococcus broth culture. The tubes were then incubated at 37° C. and at intervals 10 c.m.m. volumes were removed and plated with the following result:

	Control	$\frac{1}{80}$	$\frac{1}{40}$	$\frac{1}{20}$	$\frac{1}{10}$
		Number of colonies developing after sojourn in penicillin in concentrations as under:			
Before	27	27	27	27	27
After 2 hours	116	73	51	48	23
After 4½ "		13	1	2	5
" 8 "		0	0	0	0
" 12 "		0	0	0	0

It appears, therefore, that penicillin belongs to the group of slow acting antiseptics and the staphylococci are only completely killed after an interval of over 4½ hours even in a concentration 30 or 40 times stronger than is necessary to inhibit completely the culture in broth. In the weaker concentrations it will be seen that at first there is growth of the staphylococci and only after some hours are the cocci killed off. The same thing can be seen if a series of dilutions of penicillin in broth are heavily infected with staphylococcus and incubated. If the cultures are examined after four hours it may be seen that growth has taken place apparently equally in all the tubes but when examined after being incubated overnight, the tubes containing penicillin in concentrations greater than 1 in 300 or 1 in 400 are perfectly clear while the control tube shows a heavy growth. This is a clear illustration of the bacteriolytic action of penicillin.

TOXICITY OF PENICILLIN

The toxicity to animals of powerfully antibacterial mould broth filtrates appears to be very low. Twenty c.c. injected intravenously into a rabbit were not more toxic than the same quantity of broth. Half a c.c. injected intraperitoneally into a mouse weighing about 20 gm. induced no toxic symptoms. Constant irrigation of large infected surfaces in man was not accompanied by any toxic symptoms, while irrigation of the human conjunctiva every hour for a day had no irritant effect.

In vitro penicillin which completely inhibits the growth of staphylococci in a dilution of 1 to 600 does not interfere with leucocytic function to a greater extent than does ordinary broth.

USE OF PENICILLIN TO DEMONSTRATE OTHER BACTERIAL INHIBITIONS

When materials like saliva or sputum are plated it is not uncommon to see, where the implant is thick, an almost pure culture of streptococci and pneumococci, and where the implant is thinner and the streptococcal colonies are more widely separated, other colonies appear, especially those of Gram-negative cocci. These Gram-negative cocci are inhibited by the streptococci (probably by the peroxide they produce in their growth) and it is only when the mass effect of the streptococci is reduced that they appear in the culture.

Penicillin may be used to give a striking demonstration of this inhibition of bacteria by streptococci and pneumococci. Sputum is spread over one half of it. After incubation it may be seen that on the half untreated with penicillin there is a confluent growth of streptococci and pneumococci and nothing else, while on the penicillin-treated half many Gram-negative cocci appear which were inhibited by the streptococci and pneumococci and can only flourish when these are themselves inhibited by the penicillin.

If some active penicillin is embedded in a streak across an agar plate planted with saliva an interesting growth sometimes results. On the portion most distal from the penicillin there are many streptococci, but these are obscured by coarsely growing cocci, so that the resultant growth is a copious confluent rough mass. These coarse growing cocci are extremely penicillin sensitive and stop growing about 25 mm. from the embedded penicillin. Then there is a zone of about 1 cm wide of pure streptococci, then they are inhibited by the penicillin and as soon as that happens Gram-negative cocci appear and grow right up to the embedded penicillin. The three zones of growing produced in this way are very striking.

[*Ed. Note:* The experiments on the effect of penicillin on *B. influenzae* have been omitted.]

DISCUSSION

It has been demonstrated that a species of penicillium produces in culture a very powerful antibacterial substance which affects different bacteria in different degrees. Speaking generally it may be said that the least sensitive bacteria are the Gram-negative bacilli, and the most susceptible are the pyogenic cocci. Inhibitory substances have been described in old cultures of many organisms; generally the inhibition is more or less specific to the microbe which has been used for the culture, and the inhibitory substances are seldom strong enough to withstand even slight dilution with fresh nutrient material. Penicillin is not inhibitory to the penicillium used in its preparation.

Emmerich and other workers have shown that old cultures of *B. pyocyaneus* acquire a marked bacteriolytic power. The bacteriolytic agent, pyocyanase, possesses properties similar to penicillin in that its heat resistance is the same and it exists in the filtrate of a fluid culture. It resembles penicillin also in that it acts only on certain microbes. It differs however in being relatively extremely weak in its action and in acting on quite different types of bacteria. The bacilli of anthrax, diphtheria, cholera and typhoid are those most sensitive to pyocyanase, while the pyogenic cocci are unaffected, but the percentages of *pyocyaneus* filtrate necessary for the inhibition of these organisms was 40, 33, 40 and 60 respectively (Bocchia, 1909). This degree of inhibition is hardly comparable with 0.2% or less of penicillin which is necessary to completely inhibit the pyogenic cocci or the 1% necessary for *B. diphtheriae*.

Penicillin in regard to infections with sensitive microbes, appears to have some advantages over the well-known chemical antiseptics. A good sample will completely inhibit staphylococci, *Streptococcus pyogenes* and pneumococcus in a dilution of 1 to 800. It is therefore a more powerful inhibitory agent than is carbolic acid and it can be applied to an infected surface undiluted as it is non-irritant and nontoxic. If applied, therefore, on a dressing, it will still be effective even when diluted 800 times which is more than can be said of the chemical antiseptics in use. Experiments in connection with its value in the treatment of pyogenic infections are in progress.

In addition to its possible use in the treatment of bacterial infections penicillin is certainly useful to the bacteriologist for its power of inhibiting unwanted microbes in bacterial cultures so that penicillin insensitive bacteria can readily be isolated. A notable instance of this is the very easy isolation of Pfeiffer's bacillus of influenza when penicillin is used.

In conclusion my thanks are due to my colleagues, Mr. Ridley and Mr. Craddock, for their help in carrying out some of the experiments described in this paper, and to our mycologist, Mr. la Touche, for his suggestions as to the identity of the penicillium.

SUMMARY

1. A certain type of penicillium produces in culture a powerful antibacterial substance. The antibacterial power of the culture reaches its maximum in about 7 days at 20° C. and after 10 days diminishes until it has almost disappeared in 4 weeks.

2. The best medium found for the production of the antibacterial substance has been ordinary nutrient broth.

3. The active agent is readily filterable and the name "penicillin" has been given to filtrates of broth cultures of the mould.

4. Penicillin loses most of its power after 10 to 14 days at room temperature but can be preserved longer by neutralization.

5. The active agent is not destroyed by boiling for a few minutes but in alkaline solution boiling for 1 hour markedly reduces the power. Autoclaving for 20 minutes at 115° C. practically destroys it. It is soluble in alcohol but insoluble in ether or chloroform.

6. The action is very marked on the pyogenic cocci and the diphtheria group of bacilli. Many bacteria are quite insensitive, e.g. the coli-typhoid group, the influenza-bacillus group, and the enterococcus.

7. Penicillin is non-toxic to animals in enormous doses and is non-irritant. It does not interfere with leucocytic function to a greater degree than does ordinary broth.

8. It is suggested that it may be an efficient antiseptic for application to, or injection into, areas infected with penicillin-sensitive microbes.

9. The use of penicillin on culture plates renders obvious many bacterial inhibitions which are not very evident in ordinary cultures.

10. Its value as an aid to the isolation of *B. influenzae* has been demonstrated.

5. Surgery of the Head and Neck

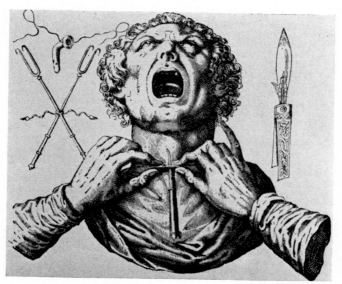

PREFATORY COMMENTS

The pioneers in head and neck surgery were faced with the problems of infection, hemorrhage, shock and flooding of the tracheobronchial tree with secretions. They displayed an undue degree of timidity because of their realization that more vital structures per unit of area passed through the neck than through any other region of the body. Their enthusiasm was further dampened by the unsightly cosmetic result and by the persistence of the disease.

In 1838 Regnoli had performed intraoral operations through a neck incision. Little progress was made throughout the nineteenth century. The basis for our present-day methods was provided by George Crile, who in 1906 reported 132 cases of cancer of the head and neck treated by radical excision. It is interesting that only one month before, in the same journal, Dr. Crile had described his method for direct blood transfusion by anastomosis of the donor's and recipient's vessels.

The development of radiotherapy in the nineteen thirties and the esthetic appeal of this medium to the patient and to the physician caused interest in the radical extirpation of head and neck cancer to wane. In the past twenty years, the value of en bloc dissection has become evident and many large series of cases attest to the value of the procedures advanced by Crile.

Goitre has been referred to in historical writings for more than 3500 years. One of the earliest attempts to extirpate a goitre was that of Albucasis in Bagdad about A.D. 1000. During the next 800 years sporadic attempts at goitre removal were made by many venturesome surgeons, e.g., Celsus, Paulus Aegineta, Giovanni di Vigo and Desault.

205

In 1920 William S. Halsted published an exhaustive 166-page study entitled *The Operative Story of Goitre* in which he reviewed 375 sources of information. The history was so involved that it was necessary to categorize the developments from each of nine countries in separate tables.

Obviously it is difficult to single out one man who made the greatest contribution. We feel, however, that to Theodor Kocher belongs this honor, for it was by placing emphasis on meticulous technique that he was able to make thyroid surgery safe. In 1898, Kocher reported 600 thyroidectomies with only one death and this could be attributed to the use of chloroform. For this accomplishment and his contributions to the physiological functions of the thyroid gland he received the Nobel prize. Before his death in 1917 more than 5000 thyroidectomies had been performed in his clinic.

We have elected to reproduce excerpts from Halsted's monograph which describe the obstacles that beset the pioneer in the field of thyroid surgery and the evolution of a safe surgical approach.

THEODOR KOCHER (1841–1917)

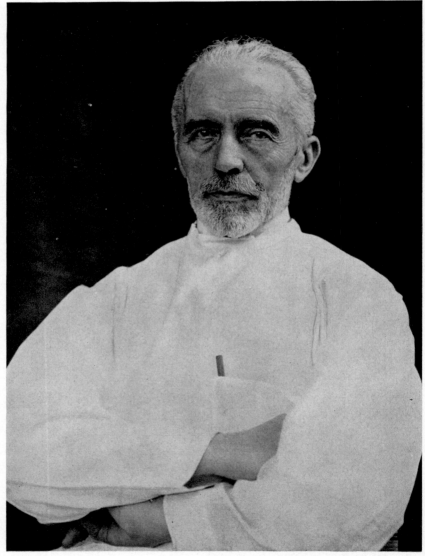

Theodor Kocher was born in Berne, Switzerland, on August 25, 1841. He was a pupil of Langenbeck and Billroth, and spent his entire medical career in Berne where he became Professor of Surgery at the University in 1872. He wrote valuable treatises on hernia, osteomyelitis, artificial anus and antisepsis. The Kocher maneuver for reduction of dislocated shoulders is still in use. He received the Nobel prize in 1909 "for his work on the physiology, pathology and surgery of the thyroid gland." He first excised the thyroid gland in 1872 and was known for meticulous technique resulting in a 4½ per cent mortality for more than 2000 thyroidectomies that he had performed personally. The incontestable proof of his ability rests in the fact that almost every patient upon whom he performed a total thyroidectomy developed myxedema, but only a single one developed tetany. Other contemporaries had many cases of tetany following attempted total thyroidectomy, but few of myxedema. Kocher did considerable experimental surgery and worked on a material to accelerate coagulation in internal hemorrhage. He is considered one of the ablest technical surgeons of all time and provided the example that Halsted attempted to follow.

He died on July 27, 1917 following an operation for an intestinal ailment.

EXCERPTS FROM
THE OPERATIVE STORY
OF GOITRE

BY WILLIAM S. HALSTED

The extirpation of the thyroid gland for goitre typifies, perhaps better than any operation, the supreme triumph of the surgeon's art. A feat which today can be accomplished by any really competent operator without danger of mishap and which was conceived more than one thousand years ago might appear an unlikely competitor for a place in surgery so exalted.

There are operations today more delicate and, perhaps, more difficult, but they have followed naturally and easily in the paths made clear for them. But is there any operative problem propounded so long ago and attacked by so many which has cost so much thought and endeavor and so many lives before its ultimate solution was achieved? And further, is there any problem in surgery having required for its solution such intrepid throbbing and prolonged striving of the world's greatest surgeons which has yielded results so bountiful and so adequate?

For thousands of years, probably, goitre has been a familiar malady. An unsightly and frequently fatal disease, it was accepted as an inoperable affliction or dispensation of Providence in communities where it prevailed, and paraded the streets exciting the curiosity of the popu-

From the Johns Hopkins Hospital Report, *xix:*71, 1920. Reprinted by permission.

lace in towns where it was unusual. The sufferers sought relief from suffocation, difficulty in swallowing, failure of the heart and from a distressing disfigurement. Thus this conspicuous tumor of the neck was a perpetual challenge to the physician, and to the surgeon a stigma as well.

My interest in the thyroid gland may be traced to the time, 40 years ago, when Wölfler was writing his classic monograph on *Die Entwickelung und Bau des Kropfes*. Anton Wölfler, first assistant of Billroth and later professor of surgery in Prague, occasionally came to the laboratory in which I was working in Vienna in 1879 and 1880 to study my sections of the salmon, with reference to the development and structure of the thyroid gland in the fish. I do not recall, however, having seen an operation for goitre in the clinic of Billroth, which I attended quite regularly.

From 1880 to 1886, the period of my surgical activities in New York, I neither saw nor heard of an operation for goitre, except that in one instance I assisted Dr. Henry B. Sands to extirpate a small tumor from the right lobe of the thyroid gland.

[*Ed. Note:* Historically, many early references are made to operations for goitre. However it is difficult to ascertain whether the thyroid gland itself or other neck glands were being extirpated. According to Halsted, the first established operation took place in 1595: "In the year 1595 an empiric attempted to remove a goitre in the case of a ten year old girl. She died under the operation, and the surgeon was imprisoned." (*Fabric. Hildanus* vol. ii, p. 399)]

[*Ed. Note:* Sporadic attempts to operate on the thyroid were made throughout the first half of the nineteenth century. Independent simultaneous advances were made in several countries but the results were so discouraging that the procedure was often abandoned after a few cases. This attitude is well exemplified in the following quotation from Samuel D. Gross, an honest and reputable surgeon who commanded the respect of his colleagues.]

SAMUEL, D. GROSS, *A System of Surgery.* Philadelphia, 1866, 4th ed., vol. ii, p. 394.

"When the tumor resists our curative efforts, and endangers suffocation, it has been proposed to afford relief by extirpation; but the question arises, is such a procedure proper or justifiable? In a word, can the thyroid gland, when in a state of enlargement, be removed with a reasonable hope of saving the patient? Experience emphatically answers, no. This conclusion is not invalidated by the fact that the operation has, in a few instances, been successfully performed. By no means. It only proves that an undertaking may occasionally be accomplished under circumstances apparently the most desperate. What has once been effected may be effected again. But no sensible man will, on slight considerations, attempt to extirpate a goitrous thyroid gland. If a surgeon should be so adventurous or foolhardy as to undertake the enterprise, I shall not envy him his feelings while engaged in the performance of it, or after he has completed it, should he be so fortunate as to do this. Every step he takes will be environed with difficulty, every stroke of his knife will be followed by a torrent of blood, and lucky will it be for him if his victim live long enough to enable him to finish his horrid butchery. Should the patient survive the immediate effects of the operation, if thus it may be called, death will be almost certain to overtake him from secondary haemorrhage, or from inflammation of the cervical vessels, esophagus and respiratory organs. When the tumor is large, the wound is of frightful extent, involving all the most important and delicate structures of the neck, and rendering it altogether improbable, from the constant motion of the windpipe and esophagus, that much of it will unite by first intention. Thus, whether we view this operation in relation to the difficulties which must necessarily attend its execution, or with reference to the severity of the subsequent inflammation, it is equally deserving of rebuke and condemnation. No honest and sensible surgeon, it seems to me, would ever engage in it."

[*Ed. Note:* Such was one man's opinion. We return now to Halsted's description of Kocher's operation of 1874 and subsequent modifications reported in 1883.]

THEODOR KOCHER. *Zur Pathologie und Therapie des Kropfes.* D. Zeitschr. f. Chir., Leipzig, 1874, Bd. iv, p. 417.

Hardly a year has passed since Kocher was called to the chair of surgery at the University of Bern in which one or more papers on goitre have not appeared from his pen.

Among Kocher's significant contributions to the subject are: (1) Discovery of the fact that total extirpation of the thyroid gland is followed by body changes, to which he gave the name cachexia thyreo- or strumipriva; (2) the studies with his life-long friend Langhans of malignant tumors of the thyroid gland; (3) the perfecting of the operation of thyroidectomy; (4) the stimulus which he gave to the operative treatment of Graves' disease and to the study of the milder forms of hyperthyroidism; (5) the recognition of engrafted forms of Graves' disease; (6) the demonstration of the value of the ligature of the arteries as a preliminary step to lobectomy, in the highly toxic cases; and (7) the danger of the indiscriminate administration of iodine to patients with goitre.

In 1872, Theodor Kocher, at the youthful age of 31, succeeded Lücke as director of the surgical clinic in Bern, his native town. Stimulated, presumably, as I have said, by Lücke's success in the operative treatment of goitre and by the great number of patients suffering from this disease who must have applied for relief at the surgical clinic of Bern, Kocher in the first two years of his incumbency, was able to credit himself with 13 extirpation operations upon the thyroid gland. Among these were two total excisions and two évidement or "Ausschälung" operations; the remainder were, seemingly, enucleations of circumscribed tumors. Two of his patients died—the first and the last, and from infection. In both of the cases of total excision recovery took place. Billroth, at this time, had apparently, discontinued operating for goitre, being convinced that the danger, chiefly from sepsis, was too great. He had performed only one total excision; this patient died within 48 hours, probably from haemorrhage—plus, perhaps, infection. Kocher writes:

"The chief danger in extirpation is the profuse bleeding which occurs from the numerous arteries, but much more from the enormously developed venous plexus about the glandula thyroidea. To attempt to lessen the haemorrhage by ligating the four arteriae thyroideae, as has been proposed of late, seems theoretically very rational, but such a procedure is almost identical with extirpation of the goitre itself."

In six cases the indication for operation was dyspnoea. In five of these the tumor was of the "goitre plongeant" variety. The incision employed was either along the edge of the sternomastoid muscle (for laterally situated tumors) or in the midline.

"It is absolutely essential for the most successful carrying out of the operation that the operator should not permit himself to be frightened off by any difficulty from dissecting down to the goitre tissue proper; he must not leave the thinnest connective tissue capsule undivided. *It would be better to cut into the goitre itself, to make sure, rather than in the deliverance of the tumor behind, to find oneself floundering in the lateral tissues of the neck."*

Kocher's operation in 1883: To a vertical incision of skin from manubrium to cricoid cartilage was added an oblique incision outwards and upwards from the cricoid cartilage to the anterior border of the sternomastoid muscle (Kocher's Winkelschnitt). The chief object of this incision was to give the operator free access to the lower pole "where the largest veins develop," and to the trachea in the region of the gland's attachment. The oblique portion of the incision, which divided the platysma as well as the skin, crossed the subcutaneous veins and thus made possible, at the outset, the double ligation of the anterior and oblique jugular veins and, if necessary, of the external jugular also. The sternohyoid, sternothyroid and omohyoid muscles were then divided in line with the oblique cut of the skin.

"Contrary to Billroth and to our own earlier method, we no longer split the capsule of the goitre at this stage of the operation. Our further procedure is determined by the intention to isolate and ligate each of the larger arteries and veins before dividing it and especially by the desire to have completely freed the tumor before undertaking to separate its pedicle from the trachea.

"At the outset we proceed to ligate the superior artery and vein. By following the vessels on the anterior surface and mesial edge of the tumor to the extreme tip of the upper pole, one easily and surely is guided to the main trunks which form the stem-like continuation upwards and outwards of the upper pole. These vessels are then ligated and divided, having been isolated with the aid of a specially designed 'Kropfsonde,' provided with three grooves. Proceeding from the upper pole downwards along the outer edge one encounters the transverse vena thyroidea superior accessoria, in case it is present, and divides

it after double ligation. Then, tracing along the mesial edge of the
upper horn, one treats in the same manner the vena thyroidea communicans superior, which courses over the trachea along the upper
edge of the isthmus. Thus the upper pole is free, and now one turns
to the lower pole. If feasible, the finger is made to encircle the lower
pole which is then drawn upwards. In the case of strongly compressing
strumas causing considerable dyspnoea it is often necessary for the
sake of better narcosis to deliver the struma promptly, especially in
cases of struma descendens.

"From the inner edge downwards there stretches the vena thyroidea ima, often a very large vessel, which must be ligated and divided. Outwards and downwards from the lower pole stretches the
ordinarily smaller, but occasionally equally large, vena thyroidea inferior, and further to the side and upwards the transverse vena thyroidea inferior accessoria. Both of these must be doubly ligated. At the
lower edge of the isthmus when there is a double vena thyroidea ima
one may find a vein connecting the two; this may be called the vena
thyroidea communicans inferior. Except for a few small irregular little
veins, the tumor, at this stage, is held only by its pedicle; namely, by
the isthmus which binds it to the upper rings of the trachea. The goitre
is then rolled inwards and taken into the hand, and now the moment
has arrived when one must keep close to the surface of the gland. The
capsule (*the external capsule—not the capsula propria, which must
remain intact*) being split and the tumor thus further released, the
trunk of the inferior thyroid artery must be isolated and tied far away
from the tumor, as near as possible to the carotid. The isolation must
be done with the greatest care, and one must assure oneself that the
recurrent nerve is not being caught in the ligature. Keeping close to
the gland, one works without haste along its posterior surface towards
the trachea, and, relying on pressure to occlude the peripheral lumina,
catches each spurting vessel as finely as possible. The isthmus being
reached, it is gradually divided as, one after the other, each vessel is
secured.

"By following this method the recurrent nerve can often be beautifully dissected out; but injury to it can with certainty be avoided
without this direct exposure. Since we have adhered strictly to this
procedure, the hoarseness, formerly so frequently observed after operation, has now become exceptional."

I have quoted from Kocher's description of his operation at such
length that the reader, contrasting his method of 1874 with that of
1883, might note the progress made by him in nine years.

Whereas, formerly, he had urged the operator not to be frightened
off by any difficulty from dissecting down to the goitre tissue proper,
and hence to extirpate it from within its intrinsic capsule, he now
dissects along the plane external to the external capsule (two planes
removed), and only after he has ligated both thyroid arteries and delivered the tumor does he split the external capsule. He now accomplishes with ease the clean dissection of the "pedicle" (isthmus)
from the trachea, tying each vessel as it spurts, an act which, in 1874,
he thought insuperably difficult. Paralysis of the recurrent nerve,
which very often was then observed, is now an accident of rare occurrence. The larger blood vessels are being isolated before tying, and
ligation en masse of the pedicle, in toto or in parts, is in disfavor.

The value of the artery clamps is not likely to be overestimated.
They determine methods and effect results impossible without them.
They tranquilize the operator. In a wound that is perfectly dry, and
in tissues never permitted to become even stained by blood, the operator, unperturbed, may work for hours without fatigue. The confidence gradually acquired from masterfulness in controlling haemorrhage gives to the surgeon the calm which is so essential for clear thinking and orderly procedure at the operating table.

In this classic paper Kocher makes a contribution to physiology even
greater than to surgery. Eighteen patients of 34 with total excision returned for examination. Of these only two were free from the symptoms which we now know to be due to loss of the thyroid gland. He
describes at length and discusses quite exhaustively the possible causes
of the mental and other physical changes characteristic of hypothy-
roidism, notes the striking resemblance to cretinism, and for the syndrome purposes the name cachexia strumipriva.

[*Ed. Note:* The ensuing quotations from Halsted reveal the remarkable degree of safety brought to thyroid surgery in the brief span of
one generation.]

In April, 1895, at the annual meeting in Berlin of the Deutsche
Gesellschaft für Chirurgie, Kocher announced that he had operated
upon more than 1000 cases of goitre. Twelve years before, on the
occasion of the presentation of his famous paper on *Cachexia thy-*

reopriva, he gave the results of operation in his first 100 cases. He had then established the fact that not one of his cases of total excision had escaped the cachexia. Since 1883, therefore, in only one instance had he removed the entire gland; in his exceptional case, and only in this one, the cachexia had developed. Tetany, regarded as the acute form of the cachexia, manifested itself transitorily in a number of instances, but only once (operation for carcinoma) in severe form. In the 900 cases operated upon in the 12 years the mortality was a little over 1 per cent, exclusive of the malignant and Basedow cases.

A new series of 600 operations was reported by Kocher in 1898. In this series for the first time his assistants, Roux, Tavel, Lanz, de Quervain, Schwyer, Fischer, Albert Kocher and others, were permitted to operate upon some (150) of the patients. For more than two years he had employed cocaine anaesthesia and states that the danger in complicated cases was greatly lessened thereby. Now, too, he recommends the collar incision.

"The first distinctive feature of our method, consists in this, that we make, as a rule, a so-called collar incision, namely, a transverse bow-shaped cut with its convexity below, which leaves a much more beautiful scar than any other. This we have demonstrated sufficiently often before gatherings of physicians. Occasionally we make an angle cut (*Winkelschnitt*) which together with the collar incision we have described in detail in our book (*Operationslehre*). . . . Further, we do not, as we have so frequently seen, make a transverse division of the muscles; we go between them and free only above and partly the attachments of the muscles which stretch from the sternum to the larynx, of the sternohyoid and sternothyroid, in order to insure for them an intact nerve supply. . . . As a third essential act of our method we regard the luxation of the goitre, a procedure already described by us. When the connective-tissue capsule has been split with precision down to the gland and, when necessary, the accessory veins described by us have been ligated, the circumference of the goitre is freed so that it can be rolled over to the tracheal side. This luxation being accomplished, the act of ligating the main vessels is made easier. This again we regard as one of the special features of our operation, that we make it a point to ligate these vessels before shelling out the goitre. . . . This difficulty of determining beforehand the side on

which to make the excision brings us to the question of total excision
in the cases, for example, in which the surgeon ascertains too late that,
having removed the larger lobe, it is the other lobe which is making
the pressure on the trachea. It would seem useless to waste further
words on this subject, after having in 1883 brought proof that each
total excision in man leads to a greater or less danger of cachexia
thyreopriva and since subsequent experiments and clinical observations have confirmed my statements. But we note from recent letters
and publications that this question still agitates certain minds. Thus
Munk in Berlin insists that the consequences of total excision are attributable to accidental traumatisms in course of the operation. And
Bottini in a work on the surgery of the neck declares that he has not
seen harm result from total excision of the gland. It is superfluous for
us to state that since the spring of 1883 we have made no total excision
without compelling conditions. . . . In this case both thyroid halves
were removed because on both sides a high degree of pressure was exercised upon the trachea. In addition to circumstances such as this we
find necessity for removing both halves when, in absence of a thin
isthmus, the two lobes are welded together in a mass over the trachea.
In such cases an attempt to divide the firm colloid masses may be accompanied with haemorrhage so severe that *ex indicatione vitali* one
might better remove the whole tumor. With the exception of these two
possibilities only the malignant nature of a struma can justify the total
excision."

Of the 600 new cases reported by Kocher in this paper of 1898, 556
were colloid strumas. Chloroform was the cause of the only fatality
in this series. The patient had a greatly enlarged thymus gland. The
mortality was only $18/100$ of 1 per cent.

At the 30th Congress der Deutschen Gesellschaft für Chirurgie,
April, 1901, Kocher reported a second thousand operations for goitre.

GEORGE WASHINGTON CRILE (1864–1943)

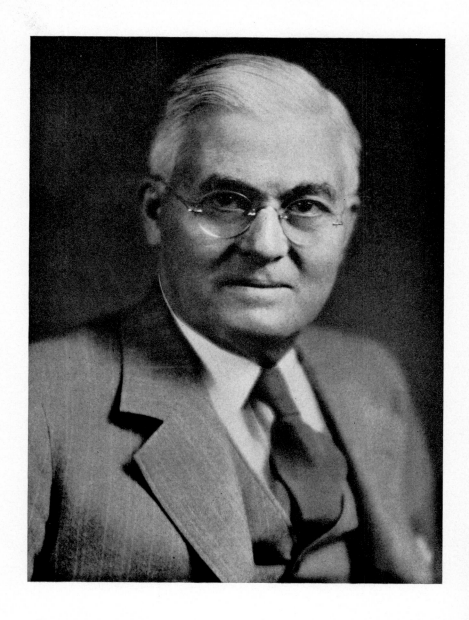

George Washington Crile was born in Chili, Ohio, on November 11, 1864. He matriculated at Ohio Northern University and in 1887 he was graduated from the University of Wooster Medical Department, Cleveland (now Western Reserve University). He then studied in Vienna, London and Paris. He ultimately became Professor of Surgery at Western Reserve from 1911 to 1924. He was also director of research and co-founder of the Cleveland Clinic. His awards and memberships in scientific societies numbered more than thirty. He was active in the military service and received many honors.

Dr. Crile was a prolific contributor to scientific literature. Early in his career his work on shock received widespread recognition. He was one of the first, if not the first, to give a direct blood transfusion. His work on surgery of the neck is reproduced in this volume. His theories on anoci-association led to many developments in reducing surgical shock. His writings embraced philosophy and an appraisal of the phenomena of life.

Dr. Crile's forceful, individualistic personality fascinated the men who came under the spell of his charm. Franklin H. Martin describes him well on the occasion of his accepting an invitation to talk on shock: "He was a young man under thirty years of age, handsome as a prince, with an enthusiasm that fairly took our breath, and with a convincing manner that captivated us, old and young."

EXCISION OF CANCER OF THE HEAD AND NECK

With Special Reference to the Plan of Dissection Based on One Hundred and Thirty-Two Operations[1]

BY GEORGE CRILE, M.D.

Cleveland, Ohio

Though signal advances have been made recently in many surgical problems, the treatment of cancer of the head and neck has, it would seem, neither received the attention nor kept the pace of progress in other fields. These unhappy cases are too often regarded as specters at the clinic. The operative treatment is hampered by tradition and conventionality, and the tragic ending of so large a proportion of these cases has held back lay and even professional confidence.

In this paper it is intended to present an outline sketch of the conclusions regarding the surgical treatment of cancer of the head and neck in the curable stage. The etiology, the diagnosis and the pathology will not be considered. It is generally admitted that cancer is primarily a local disease. Each case, then, is presumably at some period curable by complete excision.

The immediate extension from the primary focus is principally by lymphatic permeation and metastasis in the regional lymphatic glands.

[1] Read in the Section on Surgery and Anatomy of the American Medical Association, at the Fifty-seventh Annual Session, June, 1906.

From the *Journal of The American Medical Association*, Dec. 1, 1906. Reprinted by permission.

Secondary foci in distant organs and tissues are probably due to cancer emboli. A careful study of 4,500 cases, exclusive of the thyroid gland, traced to their original report in literature, made for me by Dr. Hitchings, showed that in less than 1 per cent have secondary cancer foci

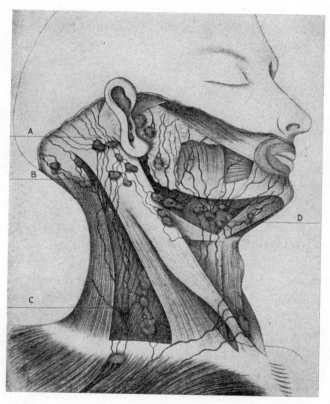

Fig. 1.—(From Gray, Poirier, Cuneo and Toldt.) The distribution of the superficial lymphatics. *A.* Posterior auricular glands. *B.* Occipital gland. *C.* Superficial cervical gland. *D.* Submaxillary gland.

been found in distant organs and tissues. That is to say, in cancer of the head and neck, death almost always occurs by local and regional development of the disease. The collar of lymphatics of the neck forms an extraordinary barrier through which cancer rarely penetrates (Figs.

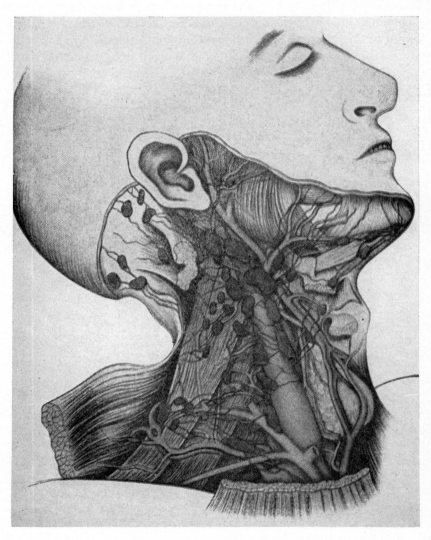

Fig. 2.—(Modified from Gray and Cuneo.) The intimate relationship between the venous and the lymphatic systems and the difficulty of entirely excising the lymphatic system and leaving the venous intact. Also how easily both may be excised together.

1 and 2). Every portion of this barrier is surgically accessible. Paired organs or distinctly one-sided foci usually metastasize regularly, while unpaired organs, as the tongue, or the mesial tissue, such as the nose and the middle of the lip, metastasize irregularly (Fig. 3).

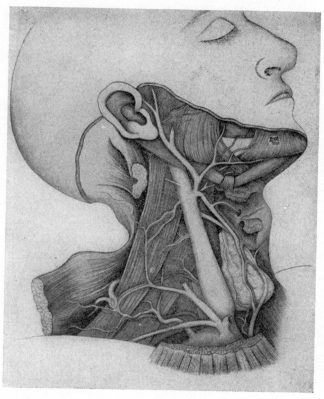

FIG. 3.—(Gray.) Emphasizing the venous tree, easy to excise *in toto* but difficult to dissect individually from lymphatics.

After the lymphatic stream has been blocked, as by carcinomatous invasion, it may flow in any direction and every sort of irregularity in the further metastases may follow, but always somewhere within the accessible lymphatic collar. After all, how much more favorable such distribution is than that of certain other organs, as, for instance, the

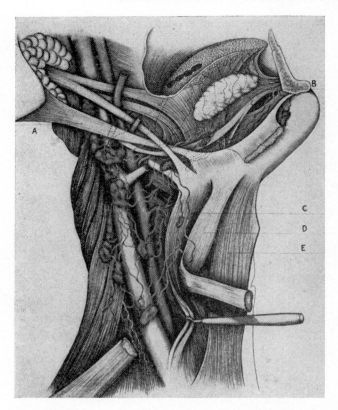

Fig. 4.—(From Poirier and Cuneo.) In cancer of the tongue the metastases extend well down as this cut illustrates. Sometimes the first point of metastasis is in the gland lying between the internal jugular and the omohyoid. *A*. Posterior belly of digastric. *B*. Submaxillary gland. *C*. Thyrohyoid. *D*. Omohyoid. *E*. Sternohyoid.

breast with its thoracic and abdominal metastases, the stomach and intestines with their inaccessible retroperitoneal metastases?

What, then, is the best method of surgical attack? An incomplete operation disseminates and stimulates the growth, shortens life and diminishes comfort. Local excision of the primary focus only is as unsurgical as excision of a breast, leaving the regional glands. Excision of individual lymphatic glands, as one would excise a tuberculous gland, not only does not afford permanent cure, but is usually followed by greater dissemination and more rapid growth. Judged by analogy and experience, the logical technic is that of a "block" dissection of the regional lymphatic system as well as the primary focus on exactly the same lines as the Halsted operation for cancer of the breast. Such a dissection is indicated whether the glands are or are not palpable. Palpable glands may be inflammatory and impalpable glands may be carcinomatous. A strict rule of excision should, therefore, be followed (Figs. 4 and 5).

In the last 63 cases we have divided them into two classes: (a) those in which the lymphatics were obviously enlarged, (b) those in

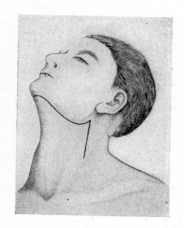

Fig. 5.—An incision which exposes the regional lymphatics which are excised in cases of lateral cancer of the lip without palpable metastases. After metastases have occurred, excision of the entire lymphatic bearing tissue of the side of the neck should be done.

which they were not enlarged. The enlarged lymphatics were presumed to be carcinomatous (this was, of course, not always correct). In this group the lymphatic-bearing tissue was widely (the entire lymphatic-bearing tissue of that side) excised, because when once the lymph stream is choked by metastasis further dissemination may travel in any direction. When there are no palpable glands the lymphatic drainage area only is excised.

Next in importance to the block regional and local excision is that of a strict avoidance of all handling of carcinomatous tissue so long as the lymphatic channel remains intact, thereby avoiding further dissemination of the growth. Retraction should be entirely on sound tissue and blunt dissection should be the exception.

If the foregoing be mainly true, what, then, are the salient features of the plan and technic, and what are the principal dangers to be avoided? We shall not here consider the preliminary preparation of the patient nor the after-care, but shall address ourselves to the immediate operative problem as to how to secure the highest immediate recovery rate and the most probable permanent cure. What, then, are the immediate dangers attending such operations? Infection, local and broncho-pulmonary, stands first, then hemorrhage, shock and exhaustion.

INFECTION

In the present status of surgery, infection may be dismissed without discussion in all clean dissections of the neck in which the wound does not communicate with the mouth, the air passages or the esophagus. The greatest infection risk exists when an extensive dissection wound of the neck communicates with the mouth or air passages, as in cancer of the tongue or of the larynx. In the latter instance experience has emphatically taught us that the primary wound in the neck should not be made at the same time that the larynx is excised. A preliminary tracheotomy is doubly indicated, as, aside from the short circuiting of respiration and fixing the trachea, it produces a wall of protective granulations across the top of the dangerous mediastinal area. After the establishment of this barrier, together with the superficial treatment of the stump of the trachea, but little risk of broncho-pulmonary infection remains.

In the case of the tongue the operation is best made in two stages. It is now well known that the immediate and perhaps the most important factor in the causation of broncho-pulmonary infection in operations within the mouth is the inspiration of blood at the time of the operation. This may be absolutely prevented by the adoption of a simple method which I have heretofore described in the *Annals of Surgery*. The method consists of passing closely fitting rubber tubes through the nares into the pharynx, opposite the epiglottis, then close gauze packing of the pharynx, after drawing the tongue well forward. With the exception of operations requiring the removal of the entire base of the tongue, complete control of blood inhalation is thereby accomplished. Incidentally, this separates the surgeon and the anesthetizer, permitting each to do his work unhampered by the other. Mucus that otherwise might collect in the throat is absorbed at once by the gauze packing. The prevention of vomiting is almost wholly under the control of an even anesthesia. The many other features of the prevention of infection will not here be considered.

HEMORRHAGE

The control of hemorrhage is important on its own account and almost equally on account of the maintenance of a dry field, affording opportunity for a clean and precise dissection. The arterial hemorrhage is best controlled by temporary closure of the common or external carotid artery. Permanent closure of the common carotid, on account of the high percentage of cerebral softening in the cancer period of life, should be avoided. Permanent closure of the external carotid, while it is not attended by this risk, carries with it approximately a 2 per cent mortality rate from the washing away of the thrombus of the ligatured stump, causing cerebral embolism. At all events, it is unnecessary. In 61 cases I have temporarily closed the common or the external carotid without immediate or remote complications. Proper closure of this vessel should be attended with little more risk of thrombosis or embolism than closure by tourniquet or by pressure applied on the skin. This part of the technic must be done with absolute gentleness, the lumen merely closed, the walls not compressed. The troublesome venous hemorrhage may be minimized by placing the patient in the partial upright posture with a sufficient even pressure on the lower extremities and the trunk up to the costal borders to prevent gravitation of blood. Probably the most convenient means for accomplishing this is by my rubber pneumatic suit. By this device almost any posture may be assumed without serious risk of cerebral anemia by gravity. It is interesting to note the collapse of the veins as the patient is taken from the horizontal to the head-up inclined posture. In atheromatous subjects, presenting a high blood pressure, I have seen marked hemorrhage, even pulsating hemorrhage, from the branches of the external carotid when the common was closed. This is easily demonstrated to be due to the passing of the blood of the opposite artery through the brain, causing a reverse stream through the internal carotid of the clamped side to the bifurcation of the common, then up the external carotid, causing pulsating hemorrhage from the branches of the latter. When this occurs, as soon as the external has been exposed, its lumen may be closed by a clamp, thereby ending the reverse as well as the direct stream of blood.

SHOCK AND COLLAPSE

In these extensive operations prevention of shock and collapse may be effectively accomplished. The important shock-producing factors are: the number and intensity of surgical contacts, as forcible retraction, vigorous and repeated sponging, blunt dissection, tearing, etc.; the loss of blood; mismanaged anesthesia, and the duration of the operation. The principal factors causing collapse are: interference with the trunk and certain branches and terminals of the vagus, excessive hemorrhage, air emboli and anesthetic accidents.

To minimize the foregoing, the operative field should be subjected to the very minimum trauma by the employment of ample operative space, sharp dissection, minimum retraction, by preserving the field free from blood and minimizing the sponging. The loss of blood may be reduced to a minimum by methods already suggested. A hypodermic injection of atropin is given half an hour before beginning the operation for the purpose of paralyzing the nerve endings of the vagus in the heart, thereby wholly preventing an inhibitory collapse from direct or reflex inhibition through the vagus or its branches and controlling bronchial secretion. Morphin favors quiet anesthesia and partially supplements the general anesthetic. By taking advantage of the distribution of the sensory nerves, the supply of which is rich in the skin and superficial fascia while scanty in the deeper planes of the neck, but little ether, in addition to the morphin, is required during the latter dissection. This is analogous to the ether-morphin anesthesia in certain prolonged abdominal technics, in which the less painful part of the operation is done principally under the morphin factor of the anesthetic alone. The factor of hemorrhage may now be practically eliminated, and with it air embolism.

In operations on the tongue it is well to remember that the lingual arteries may be closed by the firm pressure of the gauze packing at the base of the tongue in the technic of tubage. In neck dissections the desired standard of the technic is attained when the field is so clear that the minute tissues, such as individual lymphatic vessels, are clearly and distinctly seen, and when one would not expect to damage even the sympathetic nerve intentionally.

In estimating the possible shock, collapse or exhaustion, it is well to bear in mind that in the cancer period of life there are apt to be cardio-vascular changes of importance. A high degree of atheroma, a senile heart, or a chronic myocarditis are all important factors which should be met before the day of operation by such therapeutic measures as digitalis, nitroglycerin, etc., as may be indicated. Unless these factors are anticipated but little can be done in the midst of an operation toward their mitigation. When the wound is large, one must not forget the importance of moist saline compresses to prevent the effect of exposure to the air.

The practical application of the foregoing data may be illustrated in the technic for the excision of carcinoma of the floor of the mouth invading the lower jaw with extensive metastases in the submaxillary lymphatic glands. In this instance one would be compelled to take the double risk at one seance. Assuming all preliminary preparations to have been made, the patient is given an injection of $\frac{1}{4}$ morphin and $\frac{1}{100}$ atrophin half an hour before beginning of anesthesia. After completion of anesthesia the pharynx is cocainized to prevent reflex inhibition from manipulation; two rubber tubes closely filling the nares and having perforations at the distal end are pushed down to the level of the epiglottis, the tongue is then drawn well forward, a large piece of gauze packed firmly into the pharynx, completely filling it, the brunt of the packing being made at the sides of the tubes, preventing their compression; the patency of the tubes and easy respiration is readily verified; a T-tube is then connected up with an inhaler and the anesthetizer takes his place a foot or more from the field of operation, giving him the opportunity of continuing an even, uninterrupted anesthesia, allowing the surgeon full control of the operative field, absolutely preventing the entrance of any blood into the pulmonary tract, and permitting the operator to place the patient in any position he wishes.

The rubber suit has been placed and laced during the administration of the anesthetic, and is now sufficiently inflated to merely support the circulation of the extremities and the abdomen up to the costal arches. The patient is then placed in the inclined posture, head up, and the skin incision over the common carotid artery just above the clavicle is made (Fig. 6). The artery is exposed by an intermuscular separation of the sternomastoid, its outer sheath nicked, the vessel

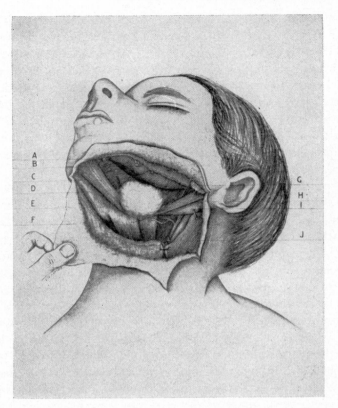

FIG. 6.—(Continuation of Fig. 5.) The regional lymphatic bearing tissue is removed by a block dissection, leaving the salivary gland in the cases in which the lymphatics are free from metastases, and excising it when any of the regional glands are involved. *A.* Submental. *B.* Facial veins and artery. *C.* Gustatory. *D.* Digastric. *E.* Submaxillary. *F.* Platysma. *G.* Parotid gland. *H.* Lingual. *I.* Digastric. *J.* Sternocleidomastoid.

exposed and temporary closure made. The complete skin incisions are then made, the skin reflected back over the entire area of the field. The sternomastoid is divided, the internal and the external jugulars are secured, tied double and divided at the base of the neck (Fig. 7). The dissection is then carried from below upward into the deep plane of the neck behind the lymphatic glands, working first at the sides, then posteriorly, carrying upward all the fascia, muscles, veins, fat and

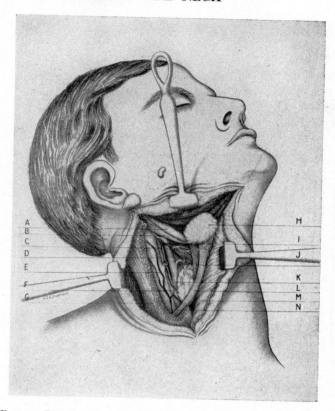

FIG. 7.—Drawing from a case of epithelioma of the face near the ear. There were no palpable glands. The local block dissection here included a portion of the sternomastoid so as to afford a better exposure of the parotid groups of glands, thereby protecting against injury of the facial nerve or the jugular. In this instance the lower part of the parotid gland was excised. The submaxillary was left. *A.* Sternohyoid. *B.* Digastric. *D.* Internal carotid. *F.* Carotid. *G.* Sternocleidomastoid. *H.* Submaxillary gland. *I.* Hypoglossal. *J.* Thyrohyoid. *K.* External carotid. *L.* Omohyoid. *M.* Platysma. *N.* Internal jugular.

connective tissue until the floor of the mouth is reached (Fig. 8). The lower jaw is then divided at a safe distance on each side of the growth. The floor of the mouth and the border of the tongue are then similarly divided, completing the block.

In very critical cases, an assistant experienced in the use and pur-

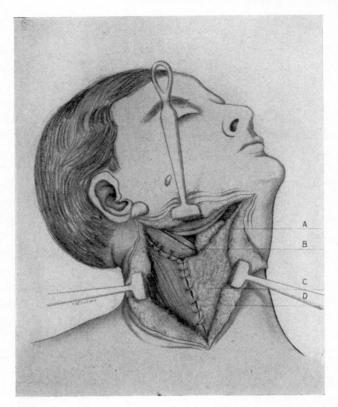

Fig. 8.—(Continuation of Fig. 7.) A method of closing the deeper plane of the neck by suturing the longitudinally split border of the sternomastoid to the platysma and the digastric. *A*. Submaxillary gland. *B*. Posterior belly of digastric. *C*. Platysma. *D*. Sternomastoid.

pose of the sphygmomanometer is placed in charge of the management of the circulation. If the pressure falls below a certain point the pneumatic pressure is increased, and after the operation the suit is gradually decompressed, but in operations in the mouth in which there may be some oozing, and in which the posture of the patient may measurably prevent inhalation of blood, by continuing the rubber suit the patient may be allowed to come out of the anesthetic in the head-up posture. The pneumatic suit may be gradually decompressed after the circulation has reached a safe physiologic status.

CLINICAL

My experience consists of 132 operations for cancer of various parts of the head and neck. A study of the literature convinces me that one could obtain the safest conclusions from his own experience, as it is impossible to get a precise knowledge of the plan, purpose and descriptions of the work of other surgeons. I have, therefore, depended largely on my own tables for my conclusions.

In the first part of this series we now appreciate as we could not then, that incomplete operations do more harm than good. Our principal errors on this point consisted in the removal of individual glands, in allowing insufficient space for the dissections, in regarding hemorrhage too lightly, in handling carcinomatous tissue, in limiting the dissection only to tissues known to be infected; in short, in not doing a complete, comprehensive operation. The early and vigorous return growth clearly proved the fallacy of our technic. Experience, too, more clearly taught us what cases should be considered inoperable. We have never seen benefit from excising a recurrent malignant tumor which had transgressed lymphatic glands and freely invaded the deeper planes of the neck. If, on the other hand, the deep planes were free and the skin involved, there still remained hope of cure.

Superficial epitheliomata in aged subjects, appearing on various parts of the skin of the face, usually about the nose, rarely metastasize. The block dissection when done in cases in which the lymphatic glands of the neck are already involved, is most radical. In all these the key to the situation is the complete excision of the internal jugular vein (Fig. 2). In one case both the internal and external jugulars of one side were excised their whole length from the bottom to the top of the neck; when, several months later, metastasis appeared on the opposite side of the neck, a similar excision of both veins was made on this side also, but only after it was discovered what the compensating route for the return circulation was. It was found that some of the superficial branches of the jugular had assumed the size of the internal jugular and were evidently the principal veins of compensation. Following the excision of the internal and external jugulars of the opposite side of the neck there was not the slightest circulatory disturbance, congestion or any hint of insufficient return circulation (Fig. 9).

Since the adoption of the plan and practice as here described, in 1898–1899, we have seen most encouraging results not only in the immediate recovery rate, but in the permanent cures. We have now apparent cures in patients in whom at the time of operation, various stages of cervical metastases were demonstrated. Among them was a case that was so large and so extensively involved the skin that the patient's physician lanced it, supposing it to be an abscess. This has passed the three-year period. Better selection of cases and improved technic have materially reduced the immediate mortality rate.

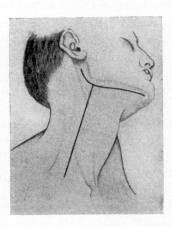

FIG. 9.—Skin incision for block excision of the gland bearing tissue of the entire side of the neck. A procedure always done when glands are involved.

It is not intended here to assume that all cancers in the various tissues of the head and neck are alike curable, but when once the lymphatics of the neck are involved the surgical problem and the risk are independent of the location of the primary lesion.

There were twenty-three operations for cancer metastases in the cervical lymphatics following operations for the excision of the primary focus alone. Some of these were in my own early cases in which

SUMMARY OF AUTHOR'S OPERATIVE CASES
NUMBER OF CASES, 132
Age

Mean age 50, youngest 28, oldest 77; 90 observations.
Cases between ages of 20 and 30 years.   1
Cases between ages of 30 and 40 years.   14
Cases between ages of 40 and 50 years.   21
Cases between ages of 50 and 60 years.   18
Cases between ages of 60 and 70 years.   29
Cases between ages of 70 and 80 years.   6
Sex and Social State
Females, 15; males, 96   Married, 40; single, 10.

LOCATION OF PRIMARY FOCUS AND IMMEDIATE RESULTS

Location	Operations	Recoveries	Deaths
Epithelioma lateral margin eye..........	6	6	0
Carcinoma of face (including maxillae)....	15	14	1
Carcinoma of lips......................	31	31	0
Carcinoma of floor of mouth.............	4	1	3
Carcinoma of soft palate................	1	1	0
Carcinoma of alveolar process...........	2	2	0
Carcinoma of pharynx..................	1	1	0
Carcinoma of tongue...................	12	10	2
Carcinoma of tonsil....................	2	2	0
Carcinoma of nose.....................	5	5	0
Carcinoma of scalp....................	2	2	0
Carcinoma of lymphatic glands..........	23	20	3
Carcinoma of parotid..................	5	5	0
Carcinoma—branchiogenic.............	4	4	0
Carcinoma of larynx...................	15	13	2
Carcinoma of thyroid..................	4	4	0
	132	121	11

(8 per cent)

OTHER DATA

Mean duration of disease prior to operation, 1 year. In the last 21 operations there has been no fatality.

Total number of cases operated.............................	132
Total number of cases traced...............................	106
Number of these known to be living.........................	47
Number of these that did not have radical block dissection...... ..	96
Number of these operated over 3 years ago...................	67
Number of these traced....................................	48
Number who have passed 3 years............................	9
Number of radical block dissections........................	36
Number of block dissections over 3 years...................	19
Number of these traced....................................	12
Number of block dissections of patients living who have passed the 3-year period..	19

0 to 1 year.............	5	6 to 7 years............	1
1 to 2 years.............	5	7 to 8 years............	0
2 to 3 years.............	0	8 to 9 years............	0
3 to 4 years.............	2	9 to 10 years............	0
4 to 5 years.............	2	10 to 11 years............	1
5 to 6 years.............	3		

Number that did not have block dissections now living.......... 28

0 to 1 year.............	6	4 to 5 years............	3
1 to 2 years............	10	5 to 6 years............	2
2 to 3 years............	3	7 to 8 years............	3
3 to 4 years............	0	16 to 17 years............	1

I was led to excise only the primary focus, either by the pleading of the patient or because the trifling primary lesion scarcely seemed to warrant excision of the regionary lymphatics (Figs. 10 and 11). The majority have been drawn from other sources. It would seem that the end results in this class of cases are the real test of the effectiveness of

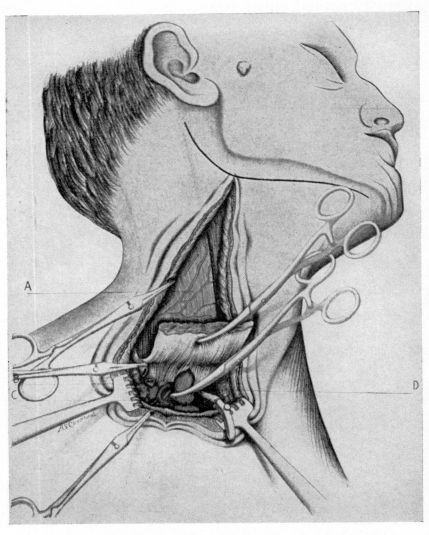

Fig. 10.—The sternomastoid is divided near the clavicle. The vein is exposed, tied in two places, and divided. The carotid is closed with the author's special clamp. The skin and the platysma are then dissected back on the entire side of the neck. The deep plane of the neck down to the region having no lymphatic gland tissue is opened from below and laterally upward, and the relation of the sternomastoid muscle and the cervical fascia is noted. The most complete exposure of the deep lymphatics is afforded by a complete excision of this muscle. This and the following cut suggest again the necessity of doing a dissection in planes parallel to the surface. *A.* Sternocleidomastoid. *B.* External jugular. *C.* Internal jugular. *D.* Common carotid.

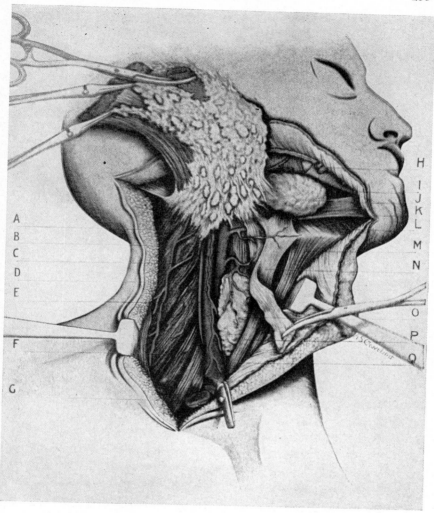

Fig. 11.—The entire mass of lymphatic-gland-bearing tissue is excised en bloc, and handled as little as possible. This dissection becomes
easy when followed in the deep plane. The entire block of tissue is
finally divided above, including the vein. A. Splenius. B. Hypoglossus
descendens. C. Spinal accessory. D. Elevator ang. scapuli. E. Pneumogastric. F. Scalenus posticus. G. Internal jugular. H. Facial vein and
artery. I. Submental. J. Submaxillary. K. Digastric. L. Mylohyoid. M.
Sternohyoid. N. Omohyoid. O. Thyroid gland. P. Thyrohyoid. Q.
Carotid.

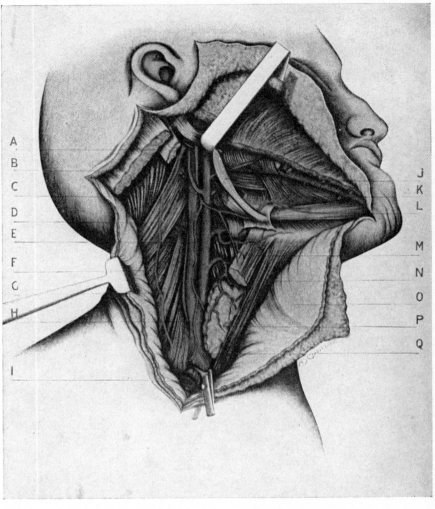

Fig. 12.—(Drawn from life.) Complete block excision of the regional lymphatic system. Note complete removal of all tissue lying between the platysma and the deep muscular plane in which no lymphatic glands lie. The artery and nerves remain. The excised block includes fascia, fat, salivary and part of the parotid glands, sternomastoid, omohyoid, part of the stylohyoid, the entire venous system, and all the lymphatic vessels and glands in this region. This is quite as comprehensive and complete as the Halsted excision of the breast. *A*. Digastric. *B*. Sternocleidomastoid. *C*. Spinal accessory. *D*. Splenius. *F*. Elevator anguli scapuli. *G*. Pneumogastric. *I*. Internal jugular. *J*. Stylohyoid. *K*. Mylohyoid. *L*. Digastric. *M*. Omohyoid. *N*. Sternohyoid. *O*. Platysma. *P*. Thyroid gland. *Q*. Carotid.

any method. The end results here are certainly equal to that of cases of axillary involvement in breast cancer. Increasing experience confirms us more and more in the belief that there has been too much conventionality in the technic. The evolution of the technic has so much minimized the operative risks that the chief consideration at present may be given to the complete excision of the last vestige of the disease along the lines of the principles underlying operations for cancer in general.

I would direct especial attention to the fact that among the 48 traced cases operated on more than three years ago, in which the radical block dissection was not made, nine are living; while among 12 traced cases among the block dissection cases operated on more than 3 years ago nine are living. The radical block dissection has, therefore, shown itself to be four times more effective than the less radical (Fig. 12).

Our general conclusions are that, since the head and neck present an exposed field, cancer here, unlike that of the stomach, the intestines, or even the breast, may be recognized at its very beginning; that every case is at some time curable by complete excision; that the field of regional metastases is exceptionally accessible; that cancer rarely penetrates the extraordinary lymphatic collar of the neck; that the growth tends to remain here localized; that by applying the same comprehensive block dissection as in the radical cure of breast cancer and by freely utilizing the modern researches of surgery the final outcome in cases of cancer of the neck and head should yield better results than that of almost any other portion of the body.

6. Surgery of the Breast

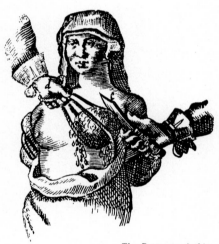

PREFATORY COMMENTS

The first true advance in the treatment of cancer of the breast came when Halsted, and soon afterwards Willy Meyer, introduced their radical operation. Since then, there have been no major changes in the surgical approach unless one considers the superradical approach as advocated by Wangensteen, Urban and others, or the more conservative approach propounded by McWhirter, as advances. These divergent views represent controversial opinions which may be negated when the final results are known. Adair's statement that "I doubt very much that the average patient with early breast cancer has any better opportunity for cure today than 60 years ago" attests to the excellence of Halsted's original operation. The sad plight of breast surgery before 1894 is revealed in Halsted's article in which he stated: "Everyone knows how dreadful the results were before cleaning out the axilla became recognized as an essential part of the operation. Most of us have heard our teachers in surgery admit that they never cured a case of cancer of the breast." In this article he reported a local recurrence of 6 per cent as compared to 58 to 85 per cent by other authors.

As an example of the many perpetuated misquotations in the literature, Halsted is credited with describing his operation in 1894. Actually his original description is buried in an article published in the *Johns Hopkins Hospital Reports* in 1891. We have elected to reprint this article which occupies only a small portion of a delightful discourse on "The Wound." In this paper he describes in detail operations for tuberculosis of the bones and joints; inguinal hernia; amputations; arthrodesis; varicose veins and many other conditions. His description of the meticulous use of sutures and ligatures, of the preparation of the hands, of the skin of the patient and of operating room techniques are classics in themselves.

245

WILLIAM STEWART HALSTED (1852–1922)

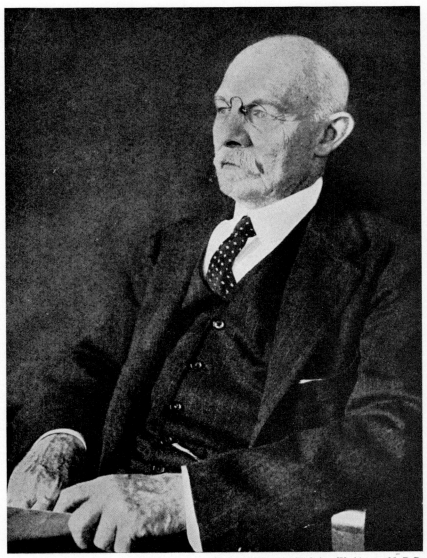

William Stewart Halsted was born in New York City on September 23, 1852. His undergraduate training took place at Yale and in 1874 he entered the College of Physicians and Surgeons at Columbia. He interned at Bellevue Hospital where he worked under Janeway, Loomis and Jacobi. In Vienna he studied under Chiari, Pollitzer, Kaposi, Zuckerkandl, Billroth, Mynert, Wölfler and Mikulicz. He returned to New York where he founded the outpatient department at Roosevelt Hospital. In 1886 he accepted a position in Dr. Welch's laboratory in Baltimore. In 1889 he became associate professor of surgery at the newly formed College of Medicine at Johns Hopkins University. In 1892 he became professor of surgery, a position he held until his death on September 7, 1922, after an operation for the removal of a common-duct stone.

Dr. Halsted founded a school in American surgery which is reminiscent of Billroth's school in Vienna. His students have made innumerable contributions to surgery. His own contributions fill two volumes and many were of such milestone importance that it was difficult not to include more of them in this volume. These include blood transfusions, the introduction of rubber gloves, the mattress intestinal suture, the subcuticular stitch, special emphasis on the blood clot in the management of dead spaces in the treatment of wounds, which has led to its more widespread use and appreciation; the introduction of conduction (so-called block) anesthesia; circular and lateral intestinal anastomosis; the bulkhead method of end-to-end intestinal suture; original operations for the radical cure of inguinal hernia, cancer of the breast, goitre; aseptic intestinal anastomosis; the partial, progressive and complete occlusion of the aorta and other large arteries by metal bands in the cure of aneurysm; the successful ligature of the left subclavian artery in its first portion for cure of a huge subclavian aneurysm; the transplantation of the parathyroid glands; replantation of entire limbs without vessel suture.

Matas has described his early impression of Halsted. "His reserve and caution in making new acquaintances, his formality, made him rather *difficult of approach and kept at a distance men who were eager to meet him." Matas then described Halsted's marked affection for his assistants, his gentleness, kindness and great concern for his patients. Matas refers to him as a modern replica of a knight of the medical profession described by Guy de Chauliac six centuries ago:*

"Bold in those things that are safe, or that he can safeguard by his own judgment and experience; fearful in those that are dangerous, avoiding all evil methods and practices, tender to the sick, honorable to the men of his profession, truthful, wise in his predictions; chaste, sober, pitiful, merciful, not covetous nor extortionate."

Many biographers have had difficulty in depicting Halsted's dual personality. The daring, spectacular operator at Bellevue who had an aggressive social personality was completely different from the slow, painstakingly methodical surgeon at Johns Hopkins who was shy, retiring and antisocial. In the early years of his investigation of cocaine, Halsted and several of his associates innocently became addicted. This affliction undoubtedly made its inroads on his personality. At the insistence of his close friends he abandoned his work for one year to attain a cure. Much speculation exists, but his closest associates, Heuer, Reid and others, were of the opinion that he overcame his addiction.

Two incidents give us some insight into his early personality. In 1881, at the age of 29, he happened to visit his sister who had just had an exsanguinating postpartum hemorrhage. He immediately drew some of his own blood into a syringe and gave her a transfusion which saved her life. One year later he was called to Albany to see his mother who was seriously ill with empyema of the gallbladder. In the presence of competent surgeons, the 30-year-old Halsted operated on his mother, drained the empyema and removed seven stones. His mother recovered. This was one of the earliest planned operations on the biliary tree in the United States. In after years, he referred to this case at a presentation, but made no reference to the fact that the patient was his mother. This impersonal approach was characteristic of his later personality.

Whatever the combination of ingredients that were necessary to develop this surgical giant, they might well be studied in detail, for there is probably no one man who has had a more profound effect upon American surgery than William Halsted.

THE TREATMENT OF WOUNDS WITH ESPECIAL REFERENCE TO THE VALUE OF THE BLOOD CLOT IN THE MANAGEMENT OF DEAD SPACE

V. Operations for Carcinoma of the Breast

BY WILLIAM S. HALSTED, M. D.

13 cases. Nos. 58, 177, 216, 326, 360, 373, 381, 385, 388, 407, 408, 454, and 489. Typical healing in all of the cases.

EXAMPLE. No. 381. Wealthy Mason, aet. 47 was admitted to the Hospital March 20, 1890.

About one year ago the patient noticed a lump no larger than a pea just external to the left nipple. The lump has gradually increased in size and is now about as large as a hen's egg. The axillary glands are large enough to be felt.

Operation. March 21, 1890. The knife was introduced at a point from 3 cm. to 5 cm. below the middle of the clavicle and drawn outwards on to and down the arm to a point a little below the insertion of the pectoralis major muscle. The knife was then reintroduced at the starting point and the tumor circumscribed by a skin incision which gave the diseased tissues at every point a wide berth—a berth of at least 5 cm. Each bleeding point as it presented itself was caught at once by an artery clamp. The tumor, the entire breast and all of the healthy tissues which had been circumscribed by the skin incision were

From the *Johns Hopkins Hospital Reports*, Volume II, 189. Reprinted by permission of the Johns Hopkins Press.

removed in one piece from within outwards, by cutting and tearing, from the ribs and from the fascia which covers the greater pectoral muscle. The triangular skin flap was dissected back to its base. The loose fascia which stretches from the lower border of the free edge of the pectoralis major muscle to the chest wall was torn through with the fingers, the major muscle was raised up from the chest wall and from the pectoralis minor muscle and cut away close to its trunk attachments and at about 5 cm. from its insertion into the humerus. The pectoralis minor muscle was divided transversely at about its middle and drawn upwards so as to completely expose the extreme apex of the axilla under the clavicle. The loose cellular tissue about the first portion of the axillary vein was dissected away with the fingers so as to clearly expose the axillary vein. Starting from this point the tissues were dissected clean from the axillary vessels and nerves, down almost to the lower limit of the skin incision on the arm. Going back again to the apex of the axilla, the axillary contents and with them all the cellular tissue and fat which covers the front and side of the exposed chest wall were dissected off clean from the ribs. The somewhat wedge-shaped contents of the axilla were thus removed in one piece from the apex to the base or floor of the axilla. The floor of the axilla had already been reflected in the triangular skin flap. The last cutting act of the operation, therefore, was to dissect the base of the wedge-shaped contents of the axilla from the reflected triangular flap of skin.

Two strong silk approximation sutures were taken from the under side of the skin at about 1.5 cm. from its cut margins. These sutures stretched across the open wound, did not touch the ribs but were suspended in the air about midway between the ribs and the level of the skin. The flap was then pressed up into the axilla to as high a point as possible and was held there by an assistant while its edges were stitched with buried skin sutures to the skin of the chest wall. The open wound was allowed to fill with blood. The approximation sutures became completely buried in the blood clot. The blood clot was protected from the dressing by strips of gutta-percha tissue. The fornix of the axilla was made as high as possible and its high position was maintained by a wedge of gauze which was held in place by a firmly applied bandage. The inner dressing was of sterilized gauze and the outer dressing of cyprus moss.

April 7. The wound is dressed. It has healed in the typical way.

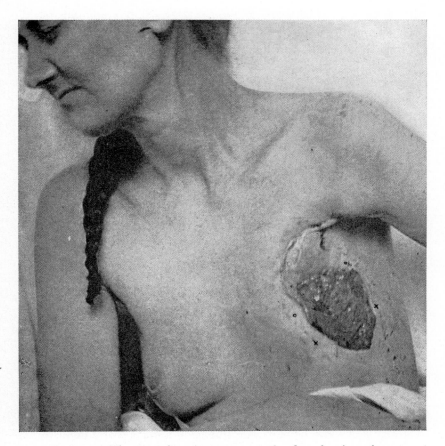

PLATE I.—The wound as it appears at the first dressing after an operation for the removal of carcinoma of the breast. The open wound is completely filled with a blood clot. The little convexities, *O, O,* and *X, X,* of the skin at the margin of the clot are caused by the approximation sutures which are buried in the clot. The white spots at the upper part of the open wound represent the decolorized parts of the blood clot. The dark spots at and near the inner edge of the open wound represent deeply pigmented areas of the blood clot. This case illustrates well the use which is made of the triangular flap to cover the defect. The apex of the flap was originally about 2.5 cm. below the centre of the clavicle. It is now almost on the line of the nipples.

The blood clot, which is already almost completely organized, fills the open wound up to the level of the skin. The approximation sutures are buried out of sight in the blood clot. The positions of the approximation sutures are indicated by little convexities of the skin at the margins of the blood clot: *vid*. Plate I, *O, O,* and *X, X.* A little above the centre of the open wound white spots may be seen in the photograph, and at the lower part of the open wound near its inner edge are some dark spots. The white spots represent the decolorized remains of the blood clot, and the dark spots represent the most deeply pigmented areas of the blood clot. The granulation tissue had reached the surface everywhere except at these light and dark spots. Sometimes at the first dressing the approximation sutures may be seen shimmering through the surface of the blood clot. They soon become entirely concealed by the granulation tissue.

About eight years ago I began not only to typically clean out the axilla in all cases of cancer of the breast but also to excise in almost every case the pectoralis major muscle, or at least a generous piece of it, and to give the tumor on all sides an exceedingly wide berth. It is impossible to determine with the naked eye whether or not the disease has extended into the pectoral muscle.

From the careful microscopical examination of many very small cancers of the breast I am convinced that the pectoralis major muscle is usually at the time of the operation involved in the new growth. Strange to say, no authority so far as I know suggests the advisability of always removing the pectoralis muscle or a portion of it in operations for the cure of cancer of the breast; and still stranger there are many surgeons of the first rank—surgeons in favor of methodically cleaning out the axilla—who instead of recommending the excision of the muscle advise the removal of the fascia only from the pectoral muscle. Konig, for example, in the fourth edition of his *Surgery* says: "When the fascia over the pectoralis muscle is diseased it (the fascia) must be removed." Surely it is absurd not to remove the muscle when its fascia is, even to the naked eye, diseased.

Kuster in describing his method says: "Now the breast and with it the fascia pectoralis is detached from below upwards." He adopts Volkmann's technique and apparently accepts his views on the importance of removing the pectoral fascia.

Volkmann in his *Beitrage zur Chirurgie* writes as follows: "I make it a rule never to do a partial amputation for cancer of the breast, but remove the entire breast even for the smallest tumors, and at the same time I take away a liberal piece of skin. The skin defect is, of course, very great when one operates in this manner, and the wound, in consequence, requires a long time for healing. Furthermore, in making the lower incision I cut right down to the pectoralis muscle and clean its fibres as I would for a class-room dissection, carrying the knife parallel with the muscular fasciculi and penetrating into their interstices. The fascia of the muscle is, accordingly, entirely removed. I was led to adopt this procedure because on microscopic examination, I repeatedly found when I had not expected it that the fascia was already carcinomatous, whereas the muscle was certainly not involved. In such cases a thick layer of apparently healthy fat separated the carcinoma from the pectoral muscle and yet the cancerous growth, in places demonstrable only with the microscope, had shot its roots along the fibrous septa down between the fat lobules and had reached and spread itself out in flat islands in the fascia. It seems to me, therefore, that the fascia serves for a time as a barrier and is able to bring to a halt the spreading growth of the carcinoma."

7. Surgery of Hernia

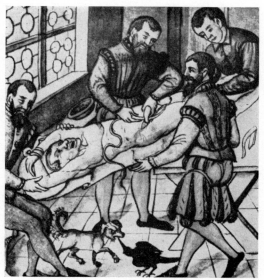

The Bettmann Archive

PREFATORY COMMENTS

For more than five thousand years hernia represented an enigma to surgeons. An overwhelming number of devices was used by an equally impressive number of surgeons. Strangulation usually meant death and operative repair of any type was often synonymous with castration. In Paré's writings, he makes reference to the gelders "which are greedy of children's testicles by reason of the great gain they receive from thence." The use of the *punctum aureum* was an interesting innovation. The contents of the sac were reduced and a gold suture was taken through the ring and the ends left outside the skin. The tissues were allowed to slough and although some cures resulted from the inflammatory reactions, recurrence of the hernia and loss of the testicle were the rule.

Bassini's report has been termed the first great advance in the treatment of hernia in more than two thousand years. He was the first to attempt to displace and preserve the cord, to reconstruct a more oblique canal and to provide an anterior and posterior wall for the inguinal canal.

Since that time many variations have come into common usage but the basic principles remain the same. Halsted, a contemporary of Bassini, devised a similar operation for the repair of inguinal hernia. At a later date, he transferred the cord to the subcutaneous space by imbricating the fascia of the external oblique under the cord.

Since Halsted's time numerous innovations have been devised by a host of surgeons including Bloodgood, McVay, Zimmerman, Gallie and others. More recently, Zimmerman has emphasized the advisability of suturing the transversalis fascia instead of the conjoined tendon

257

to Poupart's ligament. In the final analysis the basic principles of high ligation of the sac and apposition of fascia-to-fascia have stood the test of time. Finally, we have entered a surgical era when we are encouraged to employ prosthetic materials, e.g. tantalum and other meshes, to replace man's attenuated and weakened structures. These materials are being used with increasing satisfaction in patients who formerly would show a high rate of recurrence.

Bassini first presented his treatise on hernia at the Congress of Italian Surgeons in March, 1888, and again in Moscow in August, 1897. The original article is extremely long and includes 262 case reports. We have excluded the case reports and have abstracted the original text.

EDOARDO BASSINI (1844–1924)

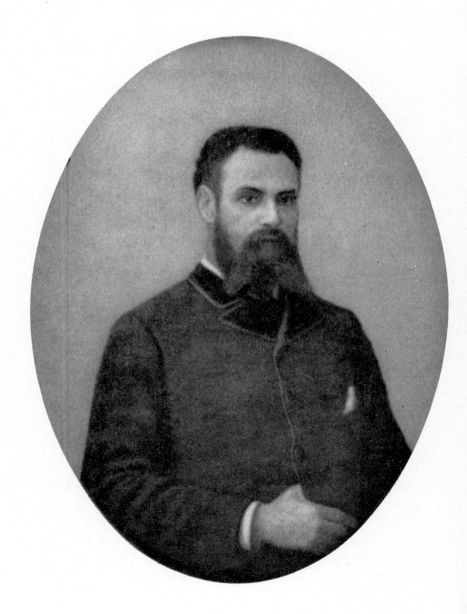

Edoardo Bassini was born in a sixteenth century castle in Pavia, Italy, on April 14, 1844. He was brought up amid the splendor of classic Italian culture and developed a strong sense of patriotism which played an important part in his life. At the age of twenty-two, Bassini received his medical diploma at the university at Pavia. He then volunteered as a foot soldier in the war against Austria and served with the 4th Alpine Chasseurs in active combat. After the armistice he returned to Pavia but the next year rejoined the army. He sustained a severe bayonet wound to the abdomen and spent an entire year under the care of Luigi Porta, Professor of Surgery at Pavia. Later, he traveled extensively and studied under von Langenbeck, Billroth and Lister. In 1877, on a return trip to London, he came under the influence of Spencer Wells. He held many teaching appointments and eventually became Professor of Surgery at the University of Padova where he remained until he was retired at the age of seventy-five.

He was a man of great simplicity and diligence. In 1904, when he was appointed Senator for his scientific and patriotic accomplishments, his students bought him a gold bistoury. When they presented it to him between operative cases, his comment was, "Thanks, thanks, but let's get back to work." On one occasion when a very wealthy patient sent him a 100,000 lire fee for a simple operation, he returned it with a one word note: "Esagerazioni!" Spangaro described him as follows: "He spoke as he felt, he wrote as he spoke, he spoke and wrote with a natural simplicity."

Bassini had a large personal museum of pathological and bacteriological specimens and wrote 32 scientific monographs. Segattini, his biographer in a publication entitled "Il Bassini" credits him with preceding Kocher with the transverse incision for thyroidectomy, with performing a cholecystoduodenostomy in 1882, and with being the first to perform a gastroenterostomy. One thing is certain, viz., his work on the radical cure of hernia has immortalized his name.

He died in 1924 at his estate at Vigasio di Verona.

CONCERNING THE TREATMENT OF INGUINAL HERNIA

BY EDOARDO BASSINI

[Ed. Note: In his introductory remarks, omitted here, the author mentions the works of Wood, Segond and Lucas Champonnière. He then points out that all methods in current use are variations of the procedures used by Wood and von Czerny.]

Wood closes the enlarged inguinal canal by inverting part of the hernial sac and closing the walls of the canal and the angles of the external ring. Czerny, however, removes the inguinal sac, buries its lower neck and closes the external canal with deep, buried sutures. Wood's method is applicable only in a reducible hernia and therefore has only limited use. The last publication by Wood (*Lectures on Hernia and its Radical Cure*, London, 1886) shows he repaired 339 reducible hernias: 17 with a hemp sling; 49 with straight pins and an intertwining suture; 273 with subcutaneous wire sutures, the latter nine times bilaterally. Reoperation was necessary in eleven instances. Of those 339 cases, if we subtract 91 unknown results and 7 deaths, there remain 189 cures and 52 recurrences. I have used this operation twice in medium-sized reducible hernias. Both recurred after one year.

Translated, with permission, from *Archiv für klinische Chirurgie*, Band 40, 1890.

262

Czerny's operation can be used in all hernias, reducible or incarcerated. Antisepsis makes this operation safe but recurrences occur if a truss is not worn. . . . Lucas Champonnière declares that the wearing of a truss after hernia operation is absolutely necessary and regards it as a factor necessary for the cure of a hernia. . . .

In both Wood's and Czerny's operations the hernial opening is closed by a scar which incorporates the aponeurosis of the external oblique muscle through which the spermatic cord travels. In Wood's operation the inverted part of the hernial sac becomes atrophic, is absorbed, and only a scar which corresponds to the opening of the hernia remains. In Czerny's method the closure is made by a scar of the external opening of the inguinal canal. But a scar which goes through the abdominal wall, and especially one in which the spermatic cord is incorporated, is not well fitted to withstand the pounding and pressure of the abdominal contents. Thus it is clear that all patients operated upon by these methods are always in danger of a recurrence if they discontinue wearing a truss.

Because of these observations I thought, early in 1883, about modifications in the operation of inguinal hernia to achieve a radical cure in such a way that the patient would not have to wear a truss afterwards.

[*Ed. Note:* Bassini then describes his first modification which he used in seven cases with poor results.]

Now I thought of how I could restore the inguinal canal in a physiological way, viz. a canal with two openings, one abdominal and one subcutaneous; with two walls, a posterior and an anterior, through the middle of which the spermatic cord travels obliquely. With the aid of a knowledge of the anatomy of the inguinal canal and with experiments on the cadaver, it was easy for me to find an operation which made possible a radical cure without the subsequent wearing of a truss. Since 1884 I have used this method exclusively and now advise it. I have operated on 262 hernias, 251 of which were reducible and 11 of which were incarcerated. Before I describe the results of this operation I think it better first to describe the operation itself. In the external, acquired inguinal hernia I proceed as follows: The patient is deeply anesthetized and rigid antiseptic technique is maintained. I incise the skin of the inguinal-scrotal region where the hernia is, expose the aponeurosis of the external oblique wide enough so that it corresponds to the inguinal canal (opening of the hernia), thus exposing the angle of the subcutaneous inguinal ring, and control all bleeding. This is the first stage of the operation. Secondly I cut the aponeurosis of the external oblique muscle starting at the outer inguinal ring and extending up to the region over the internal inguinal ring. I then separate the aponeurosis of the external oblique above and below in the form of two folds and elevate the spermatic cord and hernial sac *in toto*. Holding my index finger under these structures, I separate the neck of the hernial sac from the elements of the spermatic cord. In the acquired or congenital hernia, this isolation encounters no great difficulties with the use of blunt dissection. The isolation of the neck of the sac has to be extended into the iliac fossa, i.e., to above the neck of the hernial sac. Next I isolate the body of the sac and turn it to the outside, open the sac and note whether the contained intestines have adhesions or not, and whether the omentum is thickened. If either condition exists, I divide the adhesions and remove as much of the omentum as is necessary. After replacing the intestines, I twist the sac, put a ligature on proximally and cut 0.5 cm. distal to the ligature. Where the hernia is very large and therefore the neck and opening of the sac are very wide, I add to the simple ligature, two suture ligatures, to insure closure and to prevent slipping of the ligature. The ligated peritoneum retracts to the internal iliac fossa. With the extirpation and ligature of the sac, the second part of the operation comes to a close. In the third part I isolate the spermatic cord by gently pulling it up to the abdominal wall. If necessary, the same is done with the testicle which is pulled out of the scrotum. With sharp, wide retractors the lower part of the external oblique aponeurosis is pulled down and the upper part is pulled upwards, thereby exposing the groove which is formed by Poupart's ligament and its shelving portion. Then I separate the external edge of the rectus and the three-fold layer or "dreihaupt" which is formed by the internal oblique, the transversus and the fascia verticales Cooperi (transversalis fascia), from the aponeurosis of the external oblique and from the subserous adipose connective tissue, until the above-mentioned threefold layer can be approximated to Poupart's ligament. After this has been done I sew these two parts together for a distance of 5 to 7 cm. from the iliac crest beneath the spermatic cord, which has been moved 1 cm. toward the anterior superior iliac spine, using interrupted sutures. This terminates the third stage of the operation and the internal or abdominal opening and the posterior wall of the inguinal canal have been reconstructed.

It is advisable to use interrupted silk buttonhole sutures for the above, and to stay 2–3 cm. away from the edge of the threefold muscle-aponeurotic layer. The first two sutures starting close to the iliac crest also incorporate the outer edge of the rectus abdominis muscle. When this part of the operation is finished one can see, if one makes the patient vomit (and I did this in my first 50 cases), that the inguinal region can withstand the strongest intra-abdominal pressures; and that the threefold musculo-aponeurotic layer which has been fastened to Poupart's ligament remains immovable under rigid tension in its new position.

In the fourth part of the operation I reposition the spermatic cord and also the testicle. The external oblique aponeurosis is united with sutures until the edges are close to the spermatic cord. The skin is then sutured and dressings are applied. I use drainage only in large, old hernias where dissection and isolation of the sac are difficult. This is how the inguinal canal is reconstructed with an internal opening and a posterior wall, both constructed by the fixation of the threefold musculo-aponeurotic layer to the posterior edge of the groove made by Poupart's ligament; and an anterior wall made by the united flaps of the aponeurosis of the external oblique with a narrow external or subcutaneous opening. In external hernias, especially large ones, the inguinal canal loses its oblique direction and becomes straight or almost straight. Through this operation the canal regains its normal direction and the spermatic cord passes obliquely through the thickness of the abdominal wall. The deep suture lines do not correspond with each other; the posterior one remains beneath, and the anterior one above, the spermatic cord.

If the inguinal hernia is a congenital one it has no sac but forms in the peritoneal prolongation and in the tunica vaginalis of the testicles. It may stop at the spermatic cord (hernia congenita funicularis) or may descend into the testicle (hernia congenita testicularis). In the first instance, I extirpate the prolongation of the peritoneum of the tunica vaginalis which becomes transformed into a hernial sac; in the second instance I take off the prolongation of the peritoneum and the tunica vaginalis (hernial sac and neck) and leave only that part of the serosa which is sufficient to cover the testicle. This part I tack to the testicle with sutures. In both instances the operation is concluded as above. If there is ectopy of the testicle, I separate, stretch and unfold the spermatic cord as much as possible, pull the testicle down and fasten it with sutures to the bottom of the scrotum.

If the inguinal hernia should be internal, i.e. direct, a so-called Hesselbach hernia, one has to modify the treatment of the hernial sac, because the conditions are different than in external or oblique (indirect) hernia. The internal or direct hernia originates from the medial or internal inguinal groove and is internal to the epigastric vessels. Usually the hernia opening is small or of medium size, rarely voluminous. The hernia opening consists of the superficial or subcutaneous inguinal ring. The sac has a wide entrance of a short neck which goes obliquely from posterior to anterior over the spermatic cord. I observed that the majority of cases show that the vertical (transversalis) fascia is not penetrated, but is pushed forward by the sac and extended in the form of an envelope of the hernia. As soon as the direct hernia reaches a certain size the inner circumference of the neck pushes against the outer edge of the rectus abdominis muscle. If it enlarges further the mouth and neck of the hernia will be found pushed against the epigastric vessels and finally part of the sac will be outside of the epigastric artery, in such a manner that the sac itself in its external part is separated into two parts by a fold formed by the epigastric vessels. Because of these conditions it is difficult and at times impossible to ligate the sac of a direct hernia at its internal border. It is necessary, therefore, after separating the parietal peritoneum proximal to the opening of the hernial sac, to open the latter, replace the intestines, and sew up the peritoneum and excise the edges of the sac distal to the suture. Because of the relation of the sac to the epigastric vessels, it is necessary when operating on voluminous hernias to divide the vessels between two ligatures; to open the sac and sew it up as described above; and to cut the edges of the sac distal to the suture, otherwise the part external to the epigastric vessels would not be altered at all. The sutured peritoneum retracts by itself into the iliac fossa.

In women the operation on inguinal hernia is simpler since no spermatic cord is present, and the round ligament is removed in either the congenital (Nuck's) or acquired form. I have not seen any disadvantage result from the extirpation of the round ligament.

In both the indirect or direct hernia the inguinal canal is reconstructed according to its physiological formation. Under the influence of abdominal pressure the new posterior wall of the canal is forced against the anterior wall; they support one another and can resist the pressure of the intestines, and they allow the spermatic cord to pass through the middle without squeezing it. Both the new abdominal opening and the new posterior wall are covered by muscular and aponeurotic tissue which has function and therefore will not disappear through absorption.

[*Ed. Note:* Bassini then reports his statistics and case reports (omitted here) of 262 operations performed on 216 patients, the youngest being 13 months old and the oldest 69 years old; 251 hernias were reducible and 11 were incarcerated; 232 were indirect and 19 were direct. His follow-ups were remarkably complete, including all but 4 of the 251 cases of reducible hernia. Though he reports a mortality of zero, there was 1 death from pneumonia on the fifteenth postoperative day. His cures numbered 239 cases followed for 1 month to 4½ years. Of the entire group of 251 operations for reducible inguinal hernia, he reported only 7 recurrences. In the 11 cases of incarcerated hernia he had an operative mortality of 2, one 4 hours after operation, of shock, and one 21 days after operation, of septicemia.]

CONCLUSIONS

The operation which I advise for radical cure of inguinal hernia, and which I might call a rational procedure, is absolutely without danger. That one actually achieves radical cure with this operation in such way that the patient is not only cured, but does not have to wear a truss, is shown by:

1. the mechanics of the operation.
2. 108 patients operated on and followed for 1 to 4½ years after operation were cured and do not wear a truss.

3. 12 men now serve in the army and are able to take the strain of army life.

Aside from that, the method leads to a fast cure and the patient recuperates in 10 to 20 days. Although there are recurrences, the percentage is so small and they occur under such exceptional circumstances that the value of the method cannot be denied.

Padova, July 30, 1889

8. Surgery of the

Gastrointestinal Tract

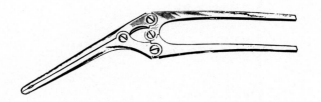

PREFATORY COMMENTS

The vast majority of major surgical procedures done today are centered on the gastrointestinal tract. The historical background is very interesting. In antiquity the prime interest in the gastrointestinal tract was the induction of vomiting. The techniques of "court vomiters" included passage of cloth tubes toward the stomach. During the Renaissance interest shifted to treating patients with strictures or malignant lesions of the esophagus. Willis devised a whalebone instrument for feeding, and metal tubes soon followed. The famed John Hunter exceeded all ingenuity with the passage of an eel-skin. During the nineteenth century flexible tubes came into use for evacuation of poisons, and washing of the stomach became a health fad. It is claimed that Kussmaul's paper on stomach tubes in 1869 was the stimulating impetus to the development of Billroth's interest in gastric surgery.

The earliest reference to gastric surgery was in 400 B.C. On the second pillar in the Temple of Aesculapius at Epidaurus, Greece, is inscribed the case of a man with a stomach ulcer. A god ordered the patient's followers to seize and hold him while Aesculapius opened his stomach, cut out the ulcer and sewed him up again.

Péan (1879) and Rydygier (1880) did pylorectomies, but their patients died.

The milestone article that is reproduced in this section is Billroth's first successful partial gastrectomy for carcinoma, performed in 1881. The discouraging results of this procedure were emphasized by Welch four years later with a report of 37 cases without a cure. However, many patients lived long enough after operation to encourage surgeons to continue their attack upon the stomach. In 1881, Anton Wölfler, an assistant to Billroth, performed the first successful gastroenterostomy. This operation was accomplished so skillfully that the technique did not change materially in the ensuing seventy-five years. It was inevitable that other surgeons would describe minor variations in technique. One brilliant modification, Roux's en–Y anastomosis, helped prevent regurgitation of the intestinal current into the primary anastomosis. With the development of blood transfusions, antibiotics and safer anesthesia, more radical surgery could be performed with decreasing risk to the patient.

The recognition of acute appendicitis was delayed for many years by Mikulicz and others who called the disease entity "perityphlitis," an inflammation around the cecum which would not lend itself to a surgical attack. Although it is not our primary purpose to establish priorities, the misconceptions about the first successful appendectomy are worth mentioning. Mestivier, Kronlein and Fitz have been erroneously singled out as the first to have performed appendectomy. The performance of an appendectomy was first described by Claudius Amyand at St. George's Hospital, London, in 1735 under the impressive title: "Of an Inguinal Rupture, with a Pin in the Appendix Coeci, incrusted with Stone: and some Observations on Wounds in the Guts." This was a ruptured appendix in an incarcerated hernia. What a lesson in humility for the aspiring young surgeon to read the following excerpts from the original article, if he recalls that anesthesia was not yet discovered: " 'Tis easy to conceive that this operation was as painful to the patient as laborious to me: It was a continued dissection, attended with dangers on parts not well distinguished: It lasted nearly half an hour, and the patient bore it with great courage."

The earliest colonic surgery was performed to eradicate malignancy. In 1903 Mikulicz described his exteriorization procedure. Soon afterwards, Murphy described the interlocking hard-rubber button which heralded a dynamic era of intestinal anastomoses. His method was simple, rapid, and had a great appeal since it eliminated tedious suturing. It consisted of a male and female plug arrangement, each of which was attached to the open bowel by a purse-string suture. The plugs were then snapped together, closed into the lumen and allowed to slough. Today the Murphy button has become obsolete and is an object of historical curiosity, but it saved many lives while gastrointestinal surgery was coming of age.

By the turn of the century more than 120 methods of intestinal suture had been described. It is now recognized that a simple, open method of anastomosis has stood the test of time. It is appropriate to emphasize that simplicity in surgery should be the keynote. The surgeon should not depend on special gadgets and intricate maneuvers. There are few gastrointestinal operations that cannot be performed safely and expeditiously with a few hemostats and proper suturing.

In 1908 Ernest Miles, stimulated by the disappointing results of perineal resection, reported his technique of abdominoperineal resection for cancer of the rectum. This procedure has stood the test of time and is considered by most surgeons the operation of choice today.

Other milestones in gastrointestinal surgery are so numerous that they would fill a separate volume. Surgery of the biliary tract, of the pancreas and of the bowel were all outgrowths of the development of safe intra-abdominal surgery. Codivilla, as early as 1898, described pancreatectomy by essentially the same technique as it is performed today. Halsted developed a method of inserting a metal hammer into the common duct so that it could be brought into the wound and sutured. Many other ingenious advances were made, but these are primarily of historical interest.

THEODOR BILLROTH (1829–1894)

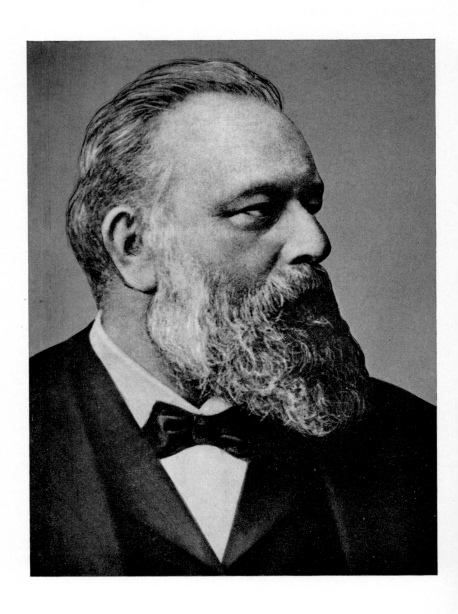

Theodor Billroth was born April 26, 1829, at Bergen on the island of Rugen. He was graduated from the University of Berlin where he later became an assistant to von Langenbeck, the director of surgery. His prime interest was pathology, but in 1860 he accepted the chair in surgery at Zürich. While there he published an admirable volume on surgical pathology which became a standard text and was translated into ten languages. After his return to Vienna in 1867, each accomplishment overshadowed the former one. He became a daring operator and an inspiring teacher. In 1872 he did an esophagectomy; in 1873 a total laryngectomy; in 1881 the first successful gastrectomy and a host of other intestinal resections and pioneer procedures. Despite this success, he remained humble and gave most of the credit to his assistants. He was a man of many talents who loved music perhaps better than medicine. His relationship with Brahms is well known and it is said that after hearing that master's compositions he burned many of his own.

The ultimate test of a good teacher is the quality of his pupils. If he had made no personal contribution at all, Billroth would deserve tribute for his entourage of students which included Mikulicz, Czerny, Wölfler, Gussenbauer and Eiselsberg. His influence on continental surgery and on Halsted and the many Americans who observed him is immeasurable. A book on How to Teach and Study the Medical Sciences resulted from research into the best teaching methods. Notwithstanding this remarkable history, we owe to Billroth an even greater debt. He was the first to publish his total surgical experience, including all of his unsuccessful as well as his successful cases. Thus he encouraged others to stand unashamed but humble before their colleagues and report their statistics honestly. The world has been enriched by his family's decision to stop his musical career and to encourage him to study medicine. He died of heart failure on February 6, 1894, at Abbazia in Istria.

He was guided and inspired by these mottos:

Nunquam retrorsum
Per aspera ad astra
Durch klarheit zur wahrheit

OPEN LETTER
TO DR. L. WITTELSHOEFER
BY PROF. TH. BILLROTH

Vienna, Feb. 4, 1881.

My Esteemed Colleague:

It is with great pleasure that I comply with your request to relate to you the details of the stomach resection I performed on Jan. 29 of this year. It is essentially a question dealing with the problem of whether the all-too-frequent stomach cancer, against which all internal therapy is helpless, can be cured surgically.

Seventy years have passed since a young physician, Karl Theodor Merrem, published a dissertation in which he proved, through experiments with dogs, that the pylorus can be extirpated and that the stomach can be joined with the duodenum; two of three animals so operated upon survived. He was heroic enough to propose that this operation could be carried out on human beings with incurable pyloric carcinoma. However, on the one hand, the opinion that the processes of life, its disturbances and its equilibrium is the same in animal and human bodies had not yet been established; on the other hand, the operative technique was not yet advanced enough for the meaning of these experiments to be grasped entirely and the physiological results correlated to humans. The question concerning the best technique of

Translated, with permission, from *Wiener medizinische Wochenschrift, 31*:162, 1881.

combining stomach and intestinal wounds has perplexed surgeons for some time and comes up again and again in discussions. The leading anatomists and surgeons of France, England and Germany have busied themselves with this topic in the course of this century since Lembert found the only proper principle for this operation (exact apposition of serosa to serosa). After this came many successful utilizations of this suture for intestinal lacerations. As regards extirpation of diseased intestinal portions, certainly no one as yet has had the courage to do so. Only in the course of the last decade were new and satisfactory advances ushered in in this field.

In 1871 I proved that one can extirpate pieces of the esophagus in large dogs. The esophagus healed well with a slight narrowing which could be dilated easily. Czerny was the first to perform this operation successfully in man. Then followed Czerny's experiments on the extirpation of the larynx, a few years after which I successfully removed a carcinomatous larynx in a human being. There followed the experiments of Gussenbauer and Al. v. Winiwarter of resections of pieces of bowel and stomach, which in turn were proven and enlarged upon by Czerny and Kaiser. Martini's and Gussenbauer's success in resection of the sigmoid and my successful gastrorrhaphy (1877) proved that further advances in this realm would be feasible. The last-mentioned operation also eliminated the question of whether the gastric juices would dissolve the scar of the stomach thus formed. That is why I closed the report of that operation with these words, "It is only a courageous step from this operation to the resection of a piece of carcinomatous degenerated stomach."

In order to quiet the opinions of those who think of my present operation as being an extremely heroic experiment on humans, I have given the foregoing introduction. It is not bold by any means. The basis for resection of the stomach is anatomically and physiologically sound, as shown by my students and myself. Every surgeon who has had personal experience in these animal experiments and similar operations in humans comes to the conclusion that resection of the stomach in the human also must and will succeed. Péan, a Parisian surgeon with the greatest experience in laparotomy, came to this same conclusion. In 1875 he resected a carcinomatous pylorus having a spread of 6 cm. in a patient who was cachectic and died four days postoperatively. The method of operation he used and also the suture

material (catgut) seemed to me to be ill-chosen so that I do not esteem
his failure too highly. The operation did, however, discourage Péan
himself since otherwise he would have repeated it; but so far as I
know he did not. Also, as far as I know, no other surgeon dared this
difficult operation. The few cases which I chanced to see in the last
few years did not seem to lend themselves for the first operation of
this kind. It was not until last week that my clinical assistant, Dr.
Wölfler, showed me a female patient who suffered, without a doubt,
of a movable carcinoma of the pylorus. After a few days of observation
and repeated examinations I was prepared to undertake this operation
to which the patient consented, since she felt that because of her increased debility and inability to retain food, her end would be near.

This 43-year-old woman had always looked pale but had been
healthy and well-nourished in the past. In October, 1880, she rather
suddenly took sick with vomiting. Soon the symptoms of a carcinoma
of the stomach with stenosis of the pylorus developed, the characteristics of which I shall not describe since they are well known. She
vomited coffee-ground stomach content only a few times; the extraordinary pallor and loss of weight, as well as the thin, rapid pulse,
had occurred only in the last six weeks. Because of the small amount
of food and the continuous vomiting the only thing that saved her
from complete starvation was the ability to retain some quantity of
sour milk. Preparation for the operation consisted of getting the patient used to peptone enemas and washings of the stomach with the
well-known method of injection and pumping out. I shall not now
mention all the preliminary plans we considered in the event that
during its course, the operation as such would prove not to be feasible,
or that the union of stomach and duodenum after the excision should
be impossible. I also reserve for a later, more detailed report the
mention of especially important details of the operative technique. Because of the great debility of the patient and the expected long duration of the operation (Péan's took 2½ hours), I asked H. Barbieri,
my well-versed private assistant, to administer the anesthesia. You
understand that I wanted to apply myself solely to the operation without having to fret about the anesthesia. The operating room, especially
equipped for laparotomies, was for well-known reasons heated to 24°
Reaumur. All my assistants were aware of the great importance of our
undertaking; there was not the slightest interference nor a single

minute of unnecessary stoppage. The movable tumor, the size of a medium apple, was situated just above and to the right of the umbilicus. A tranverse incision about 8 cm. long was made over the tumor through the thin abdominal layers. The tumor was difficult to deliver because of its size—it proved to be a partially nodular, partially infiltrated carcinoma of the pylorus involving more than one third of the lower portion of the stomach. Separation of the adhesions to the omentum and the transverse colon. Careful separation of the greater and lesser omentum—ligation of the blood vessels before cutting them. Extremely small loss of blood. Complete exteriorization of the tumor outside the abdominal wall. Cut through the stomach 1 cm. proximal to the infiltrated part; at first only posteriorly, then also through the duodenum. The cut ends could be brought together. Six sutures through the edges of the wound but not yet tied, the thread being used only to keep the edges of the wound *in situ*. Further incision through the stomach obliquely from above and inferiorly to below and exteriorly, always 1 cm. removed from the infiltrated part of the stomach wall. Next, union of the oblique wound of the stomach from below to above until the opening was just big enough to fit the duodenum. Thereafter complete removal of the tumor from the duodenum 1 cm. distal to the infiltration, by means of an incision parallel to the incision in the stomach (oval amputation). Exact fitting of the duodenum to the remaining opening in the stomach. Altogether about 50 sutures with Czerny's carbolized silk, cleaning with 2 per cent carbolic lotion. Review of the entire suture; a few more auxiliary sutures in apparent weak spots. Reposition into the abdominal cavity, closure of the abdominal wound, dressing.

The operation lasted, including the slowly induced anesthesia, 1½ hours. No weakness, no vomiting, no pain after the operation. Within the first 24 hours only ice by mouth, then peptone enema with wine. The following day, first every hour, then every half hour, 1 tablespoon of sour milk. Patient, a very understanding woman, feels well, lies extremely quiet, sleeps most of the night with the help of small injections of morphine. No pain in the operative area, subfebrile reaction. The dressing has not been changed.

Broth was tried but denied by the patient so that only sour milk in the quantity of 1 liter was taken. The peptone and pancreas enemas gave mild flatulence and colic and were therefore discontinued. An

injection of a little wine two or three times daily by rectum is agree-
able to the patient. Yellow pasty stool as with nursing babies. The
pulse is by far quieter and stronger than before the operation. Thus it
goes without the slightest setback. As proof of the well-being of the
patient I want to tell you that the day before yesterday, I had to bring
her from her isolated room to a general room because she couldn't
talk enough with another patient who had had an oophorectomy the
same day.

The excised piece was (terrible to say) 14 cm. at the greatest curvature, and through the pylorus one can just about force the shaft of a
feather. The shape of the stomach is little altered—it is only smaller
than before.

I am happily astounded over the extremely smooth course; I expected more local and general reaction; I might almost say I expected
more naughtiness from the stomach. I still cannot quite believe that
everything will continue as well. There could be a relapse into the
prior debility—this would be the most fatal complication since nothing
more could be done about it. The wound and everything around it
must be by now, after a six-day course, without reaction so that even
if one or the other of the sutures should suppurate a general peritonitis
should not be expected. There could be circumscript suppurations—
abscesses around the scar. We hope we shall discover them early
enough so that we can drain them.

The course thus far proves the feasibility of this operation. The objective of further studies has to be the indications and contraindications and the techniques for different cases. I hope we took a good step
in the right direction to cure some of the unfortunates who have been
thought to be incurable thus far, or at least to alleviate the pains of
those who finally will succumb to carcinoma and its metastases. Please
forgive me if I have a certain pride in the works of my pupils which
made this progress possible.

Nunquam retrorsum! was the watchword of my teacher, Bern-
hard v. Langenbeck—it shall be mine and that of my pupils.

ANTON WÖLFLER (1850–1917)

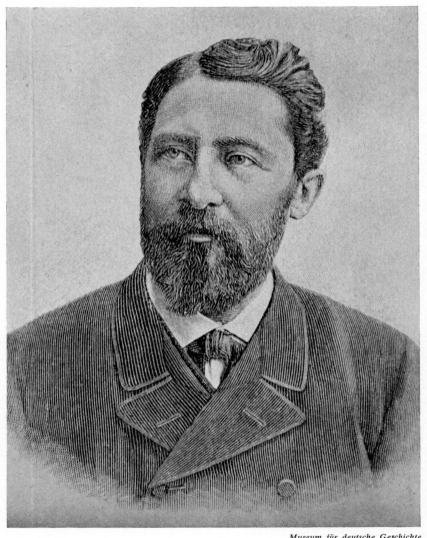

Anton Wölfler was born in Kopenzen, Bohemia, on January 2, 1850. He studied in Vienna and became assistant to Billroth in 1876. In 1881, at the age of 31, he performed the first gastroenterostomy. He did pioneer work in surgery of the thyroid, tongue and kidneys. He also served as recorder for many of the developments in Billroth's clinic. In 1886 he became Professor of Surgery at the University of Graz and in 1895 attained the chair at the German University of Prague.

He died on February 1, 1917.

GASTRO-ENTEROSTOMY

BY DR. ANTON WÖLFLER

Assistant, Professor Billroth's Clinic

With the name of gastro-enterostomy, I would designate an operation which I performed on September 28th, 1881, on a patient who was suffering from an inoperable carcinoma of the pylorus. A 38-year-old man named Michael Gold who had been suffering for 6 months with a stomach carcinoma was referred to Dr. Billroth's clinic by Dr. Kauder, who is an assistant in Dr. Bamberger's clinic.

The patient was extremely weak and emaciated due to vomiting of almost all his food in the previous 3 months. More recently he could only take small quantities of fluids provided that a daily lavage of his dilated stomach was done.

Under chloroform anesthesia a lemon-sized mass could be palpated in the pyloric region. The mass was mobile in all directions and this led me to do an exploratory laparotomy.

After opening the abdominal cavity it was evident that the pyloric carcinoma was mobile but there was infiltration of hepatoduodenal ligament and the head of the pancreas. Although pylorectomy was possible there was no hope for complete extirpation. If I didn't wish to close the abdomen without any treatment, I would have to think of performing a feeding fistula to the small bowel so that the patient could be nourished.

The disadvantages of such operations are apparent:

1. If the fistula cannot be placed at the upper, approachable portion of the duodenum one loses the bile and pancreatic secretions.

Translated, with permission, from *Zentralblatt für Chirurgie*, XLV, 1881.

2. Nourishment by such a fistula is a miserable situation for the patient.

Therefore, I decided to make a direct communication between the stomach and the jejunum and accomplished this in the following manner: I opened the stomach one finger's breadth above the insertion of the gastro-colic ligament on the greater curvature with a longitudinal incision 5 cm. long. Then I split a loop of the jejunum for an equal length at the part adjacent to the mesentery. By means of a previously described internal circular silk suture, I sewed the posterior edges of the lumen of the jejunum to the posterior edges of the lumen of the

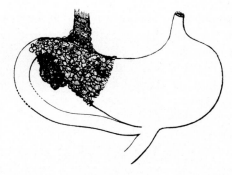

Fig. 1.—First recorded posterior gastro-enterostomy (1881). Wölfler.

stomach. The anterior edges of the stomach and intestinal lumen, first the mucosa, then the serosa and muscularis, were approximated by modified Lembert sutures.

After meticulous disinfection of the entire operative field with carbolic acid, the abdomen was closed and the wound covered with iodoform dressings.

During the entire operation the stomach and anastomosed bowel were lying on sponges saturated with disinfectant solution. During the operation, in order to insure that no spill would occur, I ligated the proximal and distal portions of the bowel very loosely with silk sutures passed through the mesentery. It appears to me that this type of temporary closure described by Schede is the simplest and most sensible.

The operation was performed along the lines of strict antiseptic precautions without the use of a spray. No drainage of the peritoneal cavity was used.

The postoperative course was smooth. The patient remained afebrile and from the day of operation felt progressively better. The disturbing vomiting ceased and the patient was able to ingest progressively larger quantities of, at first, fluid, and from the eighth day on, solid food without damage.

The abdominal wound healed *per primam* with the aid of a dressing. To date, four weeks postoperatively, the patient is passing a firm brown stool.

With the gastro-enterostomy I excluded the carcinomatous pylorus from the digestive stream. I have made a new pathway for food to pass without influencing the entrance of bile and pancreatic juice into the afferent loop. The complex, primarily physiological questions connected with this operation will probably be resolved at a later date. Though there are many theoretical objections, the success of the operation speaks for itself. Perhaps future experience will show that this type of intestinal plastic will be used not only for carcinoma of the stomach but will also supersede the enterostomy for other forms of intestinal carcinoma.

On Oct. 2nd of this year Professor Billroth performed the same operation on a 45-year-old patient named Georg Stadler who also suffered from an inoperable pyloric carcinoma which extended along the lesser curvature to the head of the pancreas. The operation ran smoothly and was completed after an hour. There were no postoperative symptoms of peritonitis. There was no obstruction, as evidenced by the fact that the patient passed several stools. However, from the first day of operation there was biliary vomitus which lasted till the tenth day when the patient expired. The post-mortem showed no peritonitis. The area of small-bowel anastomosis which was only 11 cm. from the duodenum was solidly healed to the stomach wall. The reason for the biliary vomitus is found in the fact that a spur was formed which divided the 4-cm. gastro-enterostomy opening into two unequal halves, the larger half belonging to the afferent loop. The unequal smaller half belonged to the efferent half of the intestinal portion and lay hidden under the right, somewhat overlapping edge of the stomach wall. Instead of the bile and pancreatic juices passing into the efferent loop, they emptied into the stomach.

These instructive findings show us that for future cases our task will be:

1. To choose a portion of small bowel which we are assured contains bile and pancreatic juice; then we will

2. Sew the intestinal loops in such a manner that each margin of the afferent lumen be covered by stomach wall. On the other hand, the efferent loop must communicate with the stomach by a lumen of 2 to 3 cm. That adequate nutrition can be carried out has been proved by the results of the first case.

W. ERNEST MILES (1869-1947)

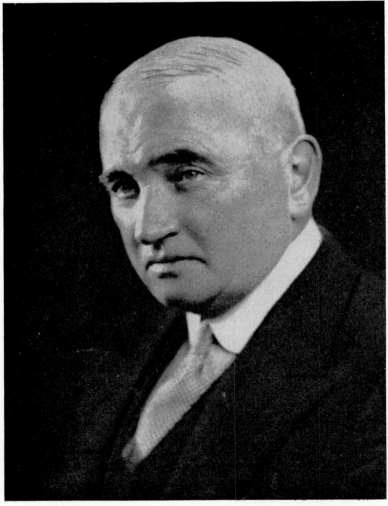

W. Ernest Miles was born in Trinidad in 1869. He received his training at St. Bartholomew's Hospital in London where he became interested in rectal surgery. His early work under David Goodsell stood him in good stead.

He did much to clarify the pathological anatomy and the operative treatment of hemorrhoids and fistula-in-ano. He spent many years studying the spread of cancer of the rectum in postmortem specimens and finally devised the abdominoperineal resection. He was a master technician who gradually cut his operating time for that procedure from 1 ½ hours to less than 30 minutes.

Dr. Miles earned the deep admiration and affection of his surgical colleagues. The British Journal of Surgery had this to say in his obituary: "He loved his fellow-men; he never said an unkind word of anyone; with his happy nature he lived to the Horation prescription: 'Ut quocunque loco fueris, vixisse libenter Tu dicas.'" Mr. Michael Smyth wrote the following: "To see Miles at work with his assistants was to see British surgery at its best. There was a calm, unhurried atmosphere about the theatre, and the lesiurely manner in which he went about his work made the whole performance seem at first somewhat slow. This was deceptive, of course, for there was an economy of movement and an effortless ease which only skill and experience could bring about. There was no delay, no hitch, everything looked simple, and the operation moved on quietly to a close. A glance at the clock showed that it had all taken place in an incredibly short space of time—in fact, as Lord Moynihan remarked, "the clock stood still." And after that there was the chat about the operation; the cup of tea and the cigarette—all very friendly, for Miles was the most approachable of all men and was kindness itself to visiting surgeons and students."

A METHOD OF PERFORMING ABDOMINO-PERINEAL EXCISION FOR CARCINOMA OF THE RECTUM AND OF THE TERMINAL PORTION OF THE PELVIC COLON

BY W. ERNEST MILES, F.R.C.S. ENG., L.R.C.P. LOND.

Surgeon to the Cancer Hospital, Brompton, S.W. and to the Gordon Hospital for Diseases of the Rectum, Vauxhall Bridge-Road, S.W.

Removal of the rectum by a combined abdominal and perineal operation was first performed by Czerny in 1884. Since that time several other surgeons, notably Maunsell, Chaput, Gaudier, Chaliot, Weir Boechal, Giodino, Quenu, Reverdin, Tuttle, Gant, Mathews, Sir Charles Ball, Wallis and Aldrich-Blake have employed the method with certain modifications of procedure and with varying success in regard to mortality. So far as I have been able to gather from the literature of the subject, however, the technique of these operators seems to have failed in one important respect—namely, the complete eradication of the zone of upward spread of cancer from the rectum, whereby the chance of recurrence of the disease, above the field of operation, can be diminished if not entirely obviated.

Until the close of the year 1906 I had relied solely upon the perineal methods of excision of the rectum, but I found that, even after the most complete and extensive removal possible, recurrence of the disease was a rule to which there were few exceptions. In fact, from a personal experience of 57 such operations, my records showed

From the *Lancet*, December 19, 1908. Reprinted by permission.

the disquieting fact that recurrence took place within periods ranging from six months to three years in 54 instances. Moreover, I found that although perfection of technique had reduced the proportion of recurrences in the immediate vicinity of the field of operation recurrence nevertheless appeared in situations that were beyond the scope of a removal from the perineum. Post-mortem examination showed that these situations were (a) the pelvic peritoneum (b) the pelvic mesocolon, and (c) the lymph nodes situated over the bifurcation of the left common iliac artery. Bearing these facts in mind I made observations upon the course taken by the upward spread of cancer among patients who had died from inoperable cancer of the rectum and found that the disease invariably extended by continuity of tissue along the parietal attachment of the pelvic mesocolon and in the adjacent parietal peritoneum for about one inch on either side of it as far as the group of lymph nodes situated over the bifurcation of the common iliac artery. In one case the disease extended by continuous spread to the suprarenal capsule of the left kidney. In all the cases thus examined the infiltration of the parietal border of the pelvic mesocolon had caused shrinkage of the pelvic mesocolon itself, whereby the pelvic colon appeared to be bound down, a condition which readily explains the difficulty in obtaining a satisfactory spur when performing colostomy in an advanced case of cancer of the rectum.

From these observations it is obvious that the above-mentioned structures constitute the zone of the upward spread of cancer from the rectum, the removal of which is just as imperative as is the thorough clearance of the axilla in cases of cancer of the breast if freedom from recurrence is to be hoped for. The appreciation of this important fact induced me two years ago to abandon the perineal methods of excision of the rectum as inadequate for the purpose of obviating recurrence and to endeavour, by utilizing an abdominal method of procedures to bring the operation of excision of the rectum into line with those methods of performing abdominal hysterectomy known as the Wertheim and the Kronig–Wertheim.

The study of the spread of cancer from the rectum has led me to formulate certain essentials in the technique of the operation which must be strictly adhered to if satisfactory results are to be obtained— namely: (1) that an abdominal anus is a necessity; (2) that the whole of the pelvic colon, with the exception of the part from which the colostomy is made, must be removed because its blood-supply is contained in the zone of upward spread; (3) that the whole of the pelvic mesocolon below the point where it crosses the common iliac artery, together with a strip of peritoneum at least an inch wide on either side of it, must be cleared away; (4) that the group of lymph nodes situated over the bifurcation of the common iliac artery are in all instances to be removed; and lastly (5) that the perineal portion of the operation should be carried out as widely as possible so that the lateral and downward zones of spread may be effectively extirpated.

THE OPERATION

This is one of the most formidable operations in surgery, entailing, as it does, the removal of practically the whole of the pelvic colon as well as the rectum. I have now performed it 12 times with a mortality of 41.6 per cent. Nine of the patients were males, of whom four died, and three were females, of whom one died. The surviving seven patients are all at present free from recurrences, the first three having been operated upon in January, March and May of 1907 respectively.

Preparation of the Patient—In all cases in which there is marked stenosis of the bowel, a preliminary left iliac colostomy should be performed at least two weeks before the operation. If there be no abdominal distension and if the lumen of the bowel be not much encroached upon the colon should be thoroughly emptied of its contents by the aid of enemata and mild purgation.

Method of Operation—The patient having been placed in an exaggerated Trendelenburg posture, a median incision is made from the umbilicus to the symphysis pubis and a self-retaining abdominal claw retractor is placed in position. The pelvic colon is then drawn out into the wound and a left iliac colostomy, if one does not already exist is established in the usual situation through a second incision. I usually do this by simply pushing a loop of the uppermost part of the pelvic colon through an incision in the abdominal wall and fixing it in position in the ordinary way. Some operators advocate first dividing the bowel and then establishing the colostomy from the proximal end only, but I think that by so doing there is a greater tendency to protusion afterwards. As soon as the knuckle of colon has been fixed in position in the manner indicated, the pelvic colon is divided transversely about two inches below it and both ends are closed firmly by means of purse-string sutures. The closure of the distal end should be done carefully, so as to avoid leakage from that part of the bowel during the subsequent steps of the operation. The peritoneal covering of the pelvic mesocolon is then divided transversely backwards on either side to the point where the pelvic mesocolon crosses the common iliac artery, the incisions extending into the parietal peritoneum for the distance of about one inch. The inferior mesenteric artery is then ligatured below the point where it gives off its uppermost branch to the pelvic colon. When this has been done the pelvic mesocolon itself is divided completely as far backwards as its parietal attachment, the inferior mesenteric artery being divided below the point of ligature. The upper and remaining portion of the pelvic mesocolon is now turned upwards for the distance of an inch or more and all the cellular tissue containing the group of lymph nodes situated over the bifurcation of the left common iliac artery dissected carefully away. All bleeding vessels in the cut edge of the pelvic mesocolon are caught and tied. The remainder of the operation is now practically bloodless and should be rapidly proceeded with. The peritoneum is next divided by incision which extend downwards into the pelvis, one on either side of the parietal attachment of the pelvic mesocolon and at least one inch distant from it, until the recto-vesical pouch is reached, when they are carried round the lateral aspects of the pelvic wall to meet again in front just behind the base of the bladder. In the female the left broad ligament should be detached, together with the left ovary and tube. This having been done, the pelvic mesocolon together with the adjacent strip of peritoneum on either side of it is detached from the hollow of the sacrum. By keeping close to the anterior sacral ligaments, the cellular tissue containing the lymph nodes in that situation is detached with the pelvic mesocolon in one piece. This separation is continued downwards in the middle line as far as the sacro-coccygeal articulation. A similar method of blunt dissection is then carried out anteriorly, by which means the bladder is detached as far as the prostate gland. Attention is now paid to the separation of the lateral aspects of the rectum and it is here that great care must be exercised to avoid injuring the left ureter, which adheres closely to the peritoneum as it skirts the wall of the pelvis. When the ureter has been defined it should be carefully freed as far as the base of the bladder. On the right side the ureter need not be seen. The dissection is then carried downwards on either side and the lateral ligaments of the rectum are divided with scissors. In these structures the middle haemorrhoidal arteries are found but seldom require a ligature. This lateral dissection is carried down to the upper surface of the levatores ani. When the rectum has thus been freed on all sides as far as the points indicated, the whole of the detached structures are crowded down into the pelvis and covered with sterilized gauze. Provided that the divided end of the colon has been firmly closed considerable pressure may be made upon it from above without fear of leakage. The edges of the pelvic peritoneum are now sutured so as to re-establish the pelvic floor. This having been done, the pelvis is thoroughly flushed with saline solution and the abdominal wound closed. The patient is now turned over and placed in the right lateral and semi-prone position so that the perineal portion of the operation can be proceeded with. A purse-string suture having been inserted round the anus to prevent escape of its contents, a transverse incision is made at the level of the sacro-coccygeal joint and from the centre of this a median incision is carried down to within an inch of the anus. From the lower-most extremity of the latter a semicircular incision is made round the anus on either side, meeting anteriorly at the central point of the perineum. These last incisions should include as wide an area of skin as possible so as to insure excision of the zone of downward spread. After reflecting the skin on either side to the requisite extent, the coccyx is removed and the interval between the levatores ani defined. These muscles should be divided as far outwards as their origin from the "white line" so as to include the lateral zone of spread. The remainder of the fascia propria of the rectum is then detached from the lower part of the sacrum when the pelvic colon and the rectum, which lie loose in the hollow of the sacrum, can be drawn out of the wound. The lower part of the rectum is then dissected from the prostate or the vagina, as the case may be, care being taken to remove the cellular tissue in its vicinity as freely as possible. The resulting chasm is then irrigated with saline solution and all bleeding vessels are tied. Finally, the skin margins are brought together with sutures and a large drainage-tube is inserted in the anterior and the posterior extremities of the median incision. The patient is now turned upon his back and as the final step of the operation a small opening is made into the extruded bowel to allow of the escape of flatus.

The operation thus performed takes from an hour and a quarter to an hour and a half and, so far as my experience goes, the patient suffers from no more shock than after an ordinary perineal excision.

The mortality after the operation appears to be high, but it must be remembered that the disease for which it is performed claims a mortality of 100 per cent if left alone and of over 90 per cent from recurrence when operated upon by the perineal methods. The causes of death in my cases have been; one from hypostatic congestion of the lungs, one from strangulation of a knuckle of small intestine which had become herniated through a rent in the peritoneal pelvic floor, one from gangrene of the stump of the pelvic colon below the colostomy, and two from peritonitis. With the exception of the first named I regard all these causes of death as preventable with further experience of the operation and with improved technique, and therefore hope that in a future series of cases I shall be able to show a lower degree of mortality than 41.6 per cent.

9. Intestinal Obstruction

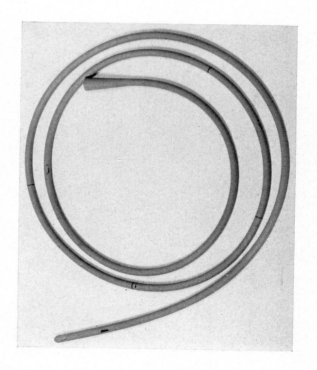

PREFATORY COMMENTS

No advance was made in the treatment of intestinal obstruction until MacCallum (1909) and Hartwell and Hoguet (1912) recognized the fact that the lives of dogs with pyloric obstruction could be prolonged by the administration of saline solution. Gamble (1925) gave further impetus to the solution of the problem of electrolyte imbalance by recognizing the fact that with high intestinal obstruction a state of hypochloremic alkalosis usually ensues. Furthermore, he pointed out that this derangement could be controlled by the administration of appropriate amounts of saline solution. For many years the problem of relieving the mechanical aspects of distention secondary to obstruction seemed to rest unchallenged. With the advent of appropriate drainage tubes, e.g. Levin and Miller-Abbott, the treatment of intestinal obstruction became more dynamic. Finally the introduction by Wangensteen of the proper use of suction to deflate the distended bowel represented a milestone advance. Despite his admonitions concerning its shortcomings and limitations, the customary wave of enthusiasm that accompanies new discoveries encouraged an unjustifiable reliance on suction drainage as the sole method of treating intestinal obstruction. It was soon recognized that this method of deflating the intestinal tract could not be employed to the exclusion of surgical intervention. Suction drainage is a valuable part of the surgeon's armamentarium but, except in rare cases, surgery remains the treatment of choice for intestinal obstruction.

In general, operations for simple mechanical obstruction should be performed within twenty-four hours after admission to the hospital. In a series of cases studied at the Massachusetts General Hospital, Mc-

Kittrick and Sarris reported that no deaths occurred in those patients who were relieved of their obstruction by surgical means within twenty-four hours after admission. This period of time affords one ample opportunity to start correction of the fluid and electrolyte losses, to deflate the intestine by passage of a tube and the employment of suction, to make x-ray examinations, and finally to decide whether the obstruction has been relieved or whether an operation should be performed. The diagnosis of gangrenous or inflamed bowel which would necessitate early surgery may be difficult to make. Repetitious and careful observations of the patient's condition pay extremely high dividends. All other findings, e.g., laboratory tests, x-rays, are of little significance when compared to meticulous examination of the abdomen. An intermittent, colicky abdominal pain which corresponds to the sound of loud borborygmus is almost irrefutable evidence that the patient has a mechanical obstruction. These telltale signs may disappear after aspiration through a tube and one may be lulled into a false sense of security in the belief that the obstruction has passed. At this point the surgeon must rely upon other signs, symptoms and laboratory procedures to establish the diagnosis. These include the amount and type of drainage, ability to tolerate clamping of the tube, passage of flatus or stool spontaneously per rectum and the insertion of a small amount of barium through the tube to delineate the probable site of obstruction.

Localized tenderness denotes impairment of circulation of the bowel or the formation of an abscess. Under these circumstances early surgical intervention becomes mandatory. In this situation it is appropriate to emphasize that light percussion can help elicit the exact site of tenderness much more efficiently and less painfully than the heavy, sharp thrust of the examining hand.

It is well for the reader to keep all these points in mind when he reads Wangensteen's article and to establish for himself a proper *modus operandi* in the treatment of intestinal obstruction.

OWEN HARDING WANGENSTEEN (1898–   )

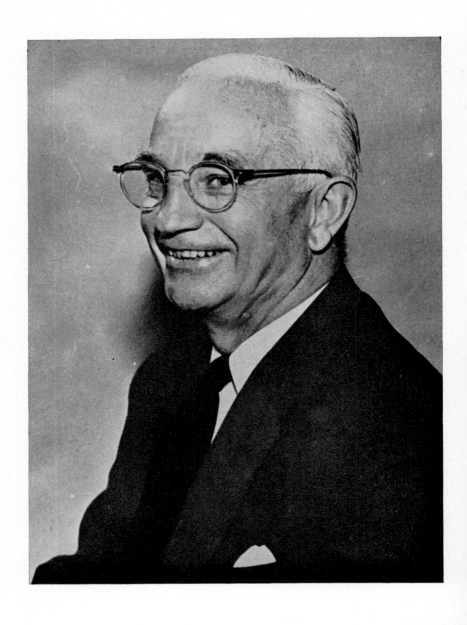

Dr. Wangensteen was born in Lake Park, Minnesota, in 1898 and received his early training at the University of Minnesota, where he earned a Ph.D. as well as an M.D. degree. He interned at the University Hospital at Minnesota and was surgical resident at the Mayo Clinic. In 1925 he was Assistant in Prof. F. de Quervain's Surgical Clinic in Berne, Switzerland, and in 1927–28 served as Voluntary Assistant to Professor Leon Asher at the Physiological Institute in that city. He ultimately became Professor of Surgery at the University of Minnesota. He is co-editor of the journal Surgery and a member of many surgical societies. Many honors have been conferred upon him in recognition of his great advances in the field of gastrointestinal surgery.

THE EARLY DIAGNOSIS OF
ACUTE INTESTINAL OBSTRUCTION
WITH COMMENTS ON PATHOLOGY
AND TREATMENT

With a Report of Successful Decompression of
Three Cases of Mechanical Bowel Obstruction by
Nasal Catheter Suction Siphonage

BY OWEN H. WANGENSTEEN, M.D.

From the Department of Surgery, University of Minnesota

I. PATHOLOGY

All cases of bowel obstruction at the onset, with the exception of primary thrombosis or embolism of the mesenteric vessels, may be regarded as instances of simple obstruction. Release of the obstruction before the anatomic changes consequent upon prolonged interference with the blood supply of the segment have occurred obviates the necessity of dealing with a non-viable bowel. Many types of bowel obstruction are potentially instances of strangulation obstruction from the beginning, in which the nutrition of the bowel is compromised as well as its lumen obstructed. Strangulated external hernias, intussusception, and volvulus constitute well known examples of this. In adhesive types of obstruction, encirclement of the bowel may eventuate in

From the *Western Journal of Surgery, Obstetrics and Gynecology*, vol. 40, January, 1932. Reprinted by permission.

Figures 3 and 5 have been omitted.

strangulation such as may also occur in kinking with secondary volvulus, the adhesive band serving as a fulcrum for the torsion. A number of instances of adhesive obstruction continues as simple obstruction throughout their course. Most cases of narrowing of the lumen of the bowel, whether due to an intrinsic lesion in the bowel wall, such as a benign or malignant stricture, or an obturative type of obstruction, due to a lesion within the lumen such as a gallstone; or narrowing due to compression from without upon a relatively fixed portion of the bowel, such as the pelvic colon by a carcinomatous mass in the pelvis—most of these, as well as most instances of bowel stasis due to nervous causes, whether inhibitive (paralytic) or spastic, remain instances of simple obstruction. An obvious exception is carcinoma of the colon, and especially carcinoma of the sigmoid flexure, in which a signet-ring type of constriction in the presence of a competent ileocolic sphincter eventuates in enormous distension, deprivation of blood supply, gangrene and perforation, and usually in the cecum, the most distensible portion of the bowel. With this single exception, however, mere narrowing of the lumen of the bowel with resultant distension of the proximal gut rarely eventuates in strangulation obstruction. Not uncommonly, however, local effects in the bowel wall at the site of pressure may become manifest, as directly over a large gallstone incarcerated within the lumen of the ileum.

Every surgeon doing enteroanastomoses of one sort or another with clamps, takes advantage of the fact that the bowel will tolerate with impunity brief exclusion of blood flow. That it is hazardous to permit sufficient time to elapse to permit of a potential strangulation becoming an actuality is best demonstrated in the comparative mortality rates in dealing with viable and non-viable bowel in strangulated external hernias.

The presence of a non-viable bowel in intestinal obstruction obviously magnifies considerably the risk assumed by the patient. It need not be emphasized, however, that in those instances in which the obstruction is due to narrowing of the lumen alone, and in which strangulating effects are unusual, continued obstruction is equally dangerous.

Delay and procrastination in arriving at the diagnosis of bowel obstruction and instituting adequate treatment are undoubtedly the most significant factors, contributing to the present prohibitive mortality of acute intestinal obstruction. Early diagnosis and immediate treatment in most instances would preclude the development of a nonviable bowel from a potential strangulation such as is at first present in strangulated hernias, volvulus, intussusception and certain varieties of adhesive obstruction. Early diagnosis in cases of simple obstruction would permit the performance of operations of election rather than of necessity, with a considerable saving of life.

With the years, a very striking improvement in the results of operation for most acute abdominal disasters has obtained. It is less than 50 years ago since the first successful operation was done for closure of a perforation of an ulcer. It would appear that the potential menace to life in this dramatic catastrophe would be greater than that afforded by obstruction to the continuity of the intestine by an adhesive band. Actually, however, the danger incurred by a patient with bowel obstruction, as judged by the comparative mortalities of these two disasters, is at least twice as great. The risk to which a patient with acute intestinal obstruction is liable is equal to that borne by ten patients with acute appendicitis. The threat to life in acute intestinal obstruction today, as manifest in current reports from large municipal hospitals, would appear to be almost as great as it was at the opening of the present century. In a series of 1000 cases operated upon at various hospitals for intestinal obstruction reviewed by Gibson in 1900, the mortality was 43.2 per cent. Van Beuren and Smith in 1925 published a collected report on 1089 operations for bowel obstruction performed since 1900 with a mortality of 41.8 per cent.

A number of statistical studies indicate that the mortality varies fairly directly with the time lost between the onset of the obstruction and the institution of effectual therapy. The chief problem in dealing with cases of bowel obstruction therefore would appear to be the elaboration of criteria of the disease upon which its recognition might be made early.

II. DIAGNOSTIC FEATURES OF BOWEL OBSTRUCTION

Pain, vomiting, constipation and meteorism have been the usual standards on which judgment has been based as to whether or not obstruction of the bowel exists. All of these phenomena may be observed at some time during the course of intestinal obstruction but their importance as measures of diagnostic value must be properly appraised.

In his nonpareil text on the "Principles and Practice of Medicine" the late Sir William Osler says, "The sequence of gastric, bilious, and finally stercoraceous vomiting is perhaps the most important diagnostic feature of acute obstruction." That this is in part true must be freely concluded, but it is decidedly unsafe to await confirmation of this succession of events. Similarly, absolute constipation, meteorism, and collapse may establish the diagnosis, but at a time when the patient is beyond hope and remedy.

Factors Contributing to Delay in Diagnosis

1. *Absence of Local Physical Findings:* Unlike other acute surgical lesions of the abdomen, simple obstruction of the intestine produces no local signs that help to corroborate the suspicion that obstruction may be present. Appendicitis, biliary colic and perforation in the gastrointestinal tract occasion definite physical findings that are of immense value in deciding the nature of the condition present. The recognition of the existence of acute inflammation of the vermiform appendix, without the occurrence of local tenderness and rigidity, would enhance the difficulties of diagnosis enormously; the number of cases coming to operation with peritonitis would be manifoldly increased, should such difficulties exist.

The significance of local physical findings in establishing the presence of an acute surgical lesion is attested in the value of such findings in strangulation of external hernias. Bower found that whereas a group of strangulations of external hernias came to operation within 37 hours after the onset of symptoms, in obstructions within the abdominal cavity this interval was 76.6 hours, or 177 per cent greater.

Undoubtedly the absence of definite local physical findings, more than any other factor, accounts for the delay in the recognition of simple bowel obstruction. Were this point continuously borne in mind, the occurrence of crampy intermittent pain without abdominal tenderness would not be so lightly considered. At the same time, the absence of local symptoms should be of distinct diagnostic value, inasmuch as it obtains in no other serious surgical emergency that affects the abdominal viscera.

2. *Mistrust in Enemas:* A diagnostic criterion upon which too much emphasis has been placed in the recognition of acute bowel obstruction is the inability of the patient to expel gas or feces following

the administration of an enema. There exists a general tendency to disbelieve the presence of a complete obstruction as long as gas or feces continues to be returned with the enema. It is not an uncommon thing to see patients admitted with enormous intestinal distension, in whom operation has not been advised because of the continued expulsion of gas after enemas.

In the experimental laboratory it was found that, even after complete division and inversion of the ends of the intestine, enemas were returned with gas as long as there was any present in the distal bowel. By placing balloons in the bowel distal to the obstruction, it was noted that the peristaltic activity compared favorably with that of the normal. The bowel distal to the obstruction is physiologically as well as anatomically normal. Why should not the bowel distal to the obstruction expel gas or feces following the administration of an enema? In high obstructions gas will continue to be expelled as long as rectal irrigations are given, and in partial obstructions as long as some of the content of the bowel proximal to the obstruction finds its way into the distal segments.

It is, of course, a good plan to give enemas when a patient is suspected of having obstruction, and I like to observe the following plan in their administration. An enema, preferably of soapsuds, is first instilled into the rectum and a responsible attendant is present to evaluate the results. Should the patient expel gas and feces but the pain continue, another enema, usually a Noble's, is given twenty to thirty minutes later. If intermittent pain continues, even though gas is expelled, and the other signs point to the presence of an obstruction, the institution of effectual therapy is urgently indicated. The evacuation of gas and feces does not militate against the presence of bowel obstruction.

3. *Danger of Morphine:* A serious evil in the management of all acute abdominal disorders is the administration of morphine before the diagnosis has been made. Frequently both patient and physician are pleasantly lulled into a sense of temporary security by this disguise, and the significant sentinel warning of intermittent collicky pain is silenced until physician and patient are apprised by the increasing distension, regurgitant overflow vomiting, and other sinister warnings that bowel obstruction is present, but also too late to undo the harm wrought by the irremediable delay. Even following the administration

of morphine, however, loud intestinal borborygmi may be heard on auscultation of the abdomen, significant of abnormal peristaltic activity of the intestine. Morphine enhances the tone of the normal as well as the obstructed bowel, but when pain is gone the significance of loud intestinal borborygmi is difficult to evaluate.

4. *Deception of Apparently Effectual Catharsis in Partial Obstruction:* Occasionally one hears the oral administration of a vigorous laxative such as castor oil vaunted as an important aid in determining the necessity for operation in bowel obstruction. In suspected postoperative obstructions, many surgeons place considerable significance on the results of such catharsis in deciding whether or not obstruction is present. Not infrequently unreliable or equivocal information is obtained through this practice. Only complete obstruction will be recognized by this therapeutic test. That it is decidedly unsafe to continue expectant treatment in partial obstruction is a matter of common knowledge among surgeons of experience.

Criteria upon Which the Diagnosis of Bowel Obstruction May Be Made Early

The occurrence of intermittent colicky abdominal pain, in a patient presenting no local physical findings, is strongly suggestive of obstruction to the continuity of the intestine. Too frequently, postoperatively, the pain factor is not given adequate consideration in evaluating whether or not a mechanical obstruction exists. Often such patients, after having denied the presence of pain, if interrogated concerning occurrence of gas pains, express themselves forcibly and freely about this complaint.

Establishment of Presence of Intestinal Colic: Auscultation of the abdomen often lends the most valuable of all physical signs of obstruction. Visible peristalsis, though regularly present in subacute and chronic obstructions, is rarely observed in acute bowel obstruction. Its presence is synonymous with hypertrophy of the bowel wall. Loud peristaltic rushes, like the bubbling sound produced by pouring water out of a bottle, may be heard with the stethoscope when a mechanical obstruction exists. A dilated intestine in which considerable fluid and air are present is necessary to elicit these bubbling sounds. Near the point of intestinal occlusion these intestinal noises may attain an explosive force. Frequently a metallic tinkle may be heard—a sign of conclusive significance of the existence of a bowel under tension. As the fluid and air are carried downward toward the point of obstruction by peristaltic rushes, their progress is suddenly arrested and fluid and air, which are intimately mixed in their advance, tend to separate as the onward movement is halted. As the air rises to the surface, a sound like drops of water falling in a rain barrel may be heard. The metallic character of the sound has a high pitch, imparted by the tension of the dilated intestine. Loud intestinal noises with maximum intensity at the height of the pain corroborate strongly the suspicion of mechanical occlusion. Just as the degree of obstruction may vary considerably, so also may the pain and the intestinal noises. It is an item of exceeding importance to see the patient often and to auscultate the abdomen over relatively long periods of time. In a patient who is not complaining of much or frequent pain, considerable progression may occur if this is not done. A patient suspected of having bowel obstruction should be under hourly scrutiny and preferably in a hospital. The coincident occurrence of gurgling sounds and intermittent pain is very significant. Only colics of the intestine are heralded by crampy pain and concomitant loud gurgling noises.

Roentgenographic Evidence: It has long been recognised that x-rays are of value in detecting bowel obstruction, but this agent has not been accorded the importance that it deserves in the diagnosis of acute intestinal obstruction. Case early described the significance of gaseous shadows in the small intestine as significant of the presence of bowel obstruction and has since been insistent in emphasizing the value of this aid in diagnosis.

When a single plate of the normal abdomen is made in the adult, gaseous shadows are usually observed in the stomach and colon. Gas is also present in the small intestine, but the intimate admixture of gas and fluid in the small bowel precludes distinguishing the gas from its immediate surroundings. The demonstration of gas in the small intestine on the x-ray film is therefore decidedly abnormal and is indicative of the presence of a mechanism interfering with the normal rapid rate of transit through the small intestine. The ladder "patterns," described as the typical x-ray picture of bowel obstruction, need not be awaited to make the diagnosis. Visible collections of gas in the small intestine of the adult are synonymous with intestinal stasis.   In the small intestine of the normal infant and child up until past two years of age, gas can regularly be visualized. In the experimental laboratory it has been found that definite x-ray evidence by the single plate method may be obtained within four or five hours after the obstruction. In doubtful cases, progression of distension as revealed in subsequent films made at two hour intervals reveals significant information. When the plate is taken in the erect posture, "fluid mirrors" can be made out in which air is layered over the fluid. The plate made in the prone or supine position, however, gives the most valuable information. From this plate alone the degree of distension and the location of the distended coils can most easily be made out. However, the surgeon cannot depend on finding the obstructing mechanism at operation exactly where it would appear to be on the roentgenographic film. Nevertheless, the localizing evidence afforded by the location of the distended coils designates better than any other method whether the obstruction is high or low in the small intestine.

The oral administration of barium is to be deprecated in all cases of acute intestinal obstruction, for the diagnosis can be made without its use. Frequently, in instances of acute intestinal obstruction when given, it fails to leave the stomach and it oftentimes takes considerable time before the barium goes down far enough in the small intestine to be of any value in locating the point of obstruction. It is far safer to locate and determine the nature of the obstruction at operation, at which time it can be done with much less risk to the patient.

The determination of whether the visualized gas is in the large or small bowel is occasionally a difficult matter. Gas in the small intestine is characterized by its central location; the long axis of the shadow is transverse, and, when the loops are considerably dilated, the two intestinal walls separating adjacent loops are seen as a very thin and narrow wall. The occurrence of a fairly thick wall separating greatly distended loops suggests the presence of fluid or exudate between the loops. Gas at the lateral borders of the abdomen is ordinarily in the colon; the long axis is usually vertical and the intestinal walls are thicker and haustral markings are occasionally in evidence. The typical appearance of the gaseous shadows in the obstructed small intestine may be described as a step-ladder arrangement of the coils; the mucous folds of Kerkring within the bowel lend a feathery appearance. However, it must be emphasized that this step-ladder-like arrangement is not necessary to make the diagnosis. Visible gas in the small intestine of adults is synonymous with intestinal stasis.

Verdict of the Stethoscope: The stethoscope serves to distinguish the type of intestinal stasis. When mechanical in nature, the occurrence of intermittent, colicky pain associated with loud intestinal borborygmi, establishes the obstruction as mechanical interference with the continuity of the intestine. If, however, gas is distributed throughout the colon as well, and the abdomen is silent on auscultation, it is almost a certainty that the obstruction is paralytic in character.

How many lives would be saved by the more frequent employment and judicious use of these two simple agents, the stethoscope and the roentgen ray! In many instances the diagnosis can be made over the telephone. The story of a previous operation with the occurrence of intermittent colicky pain, attended with nausea and vomiting, but no local tenderness or rigidity, is as suggestive of bowel obstruction as the pain, food-relief sequence in duodenal ulcer. The verdict of the roentgen ray determines whether intestinal stasis is present and the stethoscope tells whether it is mechanical or inhibitive (paralytic) in character.

Functional Spastic Obstruction: There is a group of cases, fortunately small, which may lead to confusion. We all recognize these patients when they do not present the symptoms of bowel obstruction. They have considerable difficulty with gaseous distension and exhibit in high degree the features of a neurogenic complaint with reference to the bowel. I have seen seven such patients in whom the clinical picture in every way simulated an organic obstruction of the bowel. They complain of intermittent, crampy pain, at the height of which loud intestinal noises may be heard on auscultation. They exhibit, usually, considerable distension, and vomiting is a prominent feature. The roentgenographic film of the abdomen, however, indicates that the gas is practically entirely in the colon and stomach. If a mechanical obstruction in the pelvic colon, such as a carcinoma of the sigmoid flexure, can be ruled out, the presence of gas in the colon contradicts the presence of a mechanical obstruction. Following the administration of enemas, with an organic obstruction in the small intestine, the gas in the colon should disappear. I have come to place so much reliance on the significance of the presence of the gaseous distension of the colon in such cases, that I believe they can be identified by this criterion, despite the other manifest signs of a mechanical obstruction. One of these patients previously operated upon six times for acute intestinal obstruction elsewhere has since been watched through two such attacks.

Postoperative Obstruction: In the trying situations that occur in the immediate convalescence after operation, when it is debated whether a paralytic ileus or an adhesive obstruction is present, the stethoscope and roentgen ray are equally dependable agents. Postoperative obstruction due to adhesions invariably concerns the small intestine. Roentgenographic examination in its presence reveals gaseous shadows in the small intestine, with an empty colon. The stethoscope indicates the mechanical nature of the obstruction. Paralytic ileus is usually heralded by a uniform distension of colon and small intestine on the roentgenographic film, and a death-like silence pervades over the abdomen.

General Condition

Early in the course of simple obstruction the general condition of the patient is good. The crampy, intermittent pain and nausea and vomiting make him ill at ease, but he may not appear especially sick. General abdominal distension is a late occurrence in acute intestinal obstruction and regurgitant vomiting, significant of a block in the bowel, occurs even more tardily. The vomiting which occurs early is of a reflex character, much like that observed in gall-stone or kidney colic or in acute appendicitis. The body temperature is normal and continues so until late in the disease, when subnormal, or, less often, elevations of slight degree may be recorded. There is ordinarily but slight quickening of the pulse and no change in blood pressure until prolonged continuance of the obstruction ushers in circulatory collapse as manifested by hurried, feeble pulse, cold and livid extremities, pinched and sunken features, anxious expression and great restlessness. Late in the disease, the tongue is parched and great thirst is complained of; the urine is scant and of high specific gravity and may contain albumin and indican. Alterations in respiration are dependent largely upon the presence or absence of distension. Late in the course of intestinal obstruction rapid superficial respirations are the rule. The sensorium remains clear until near the end, when the sinister warnings of euphoria, delirium and coma portend the approach of impending death.

Laboratory Data

Leucocytosis is absent early. Later, incident to the dehydration brought about by vomiting, high leucocyte counts may be obtained with similar increases in the hemoglobin and red blood cells. It is to be emphasized that, though blood urea elevation, plasma chloride decrease and an alkalosis occur with regularity in high obstruction, they are not early signs of acute bowel obstruction. In low obstructions, these changes are usually absent, and in high obstructions are observed only after about two days of vomiting.

Symptoms of Strangulation Obstruction

When in addition to a block in the continuity of the bowel, the intestine is deprived of its source of blood supply, a different clinical picture obtains than is observed in simple obstruction. Such a patient is more acutely ill; the pain is often agonizing in character; the pulse is usually quickened early in the course of the ailment and fever of 100° to 101° F. is not unusual. Higher temperatures may be recorded. The breathing is superficial and more frequent than normal. When a long segment of intestine is involved in the strangulating mechanism, symptoms of collapse may occur, due to loss of blood into the infarcted loop. Urinary suppression during the continuance of the strangulation is not uncommon.

The clinical picture is determined by the degree of arrest of blood flow to and from the strangulated segment. When this is marked, symptoms of strangulation predominate; when the deprivation of blood flow is less prominent, the symptoms of mechanical obstruction dominate the picture. Every gradation from mimicry of the picture of simple obstruction to profound shock may be manifest.

In strangulation obstruction local physical findings in the abdomen are almost invariably present. Consequent upon the infarction of the intestine, peritoneal irritation may usually be elicited by the demonstration of rebound tenderness. It must be conceded, however, that hemorrhagic infarction of the bowel or torsion of an ovarian cyst do not give rise to local physical findings in the abdomen as quickly as do intraperitoneal lesions of an inflammatory character. In the same manner, the degree of rigidity and tenderness is never as great. Occasionally, and especially in volvulus, the infarcted coil may become very prominent in the abdomen.

The demonstration of such a coil in strangulating types of obstruction has been described by Wahl as "Darmsteifung" or stiffening of the bowel. Contrary to general opinion, however, such an infarcted segment does not contain much gas, except in strangulations of a chronic nature, such as some types of volvulus, in which the obstructive rather than strangulating features predominate. When a short segment of small intestine is concerned in the strangulation, this sign may be absent, due to the concealment of the involved intestine by other coils of the bowel. Tenderness is usually present over the mass and the latter imparts to the palpating hand an elastic resistance. The coil is usually fixed, and exhibits no peristalsis. The intestine above the obstruction distends gradually but it has been found in the experimental laboratory that the gaseous shadows in the small intestine do not appear as early in strangulation obstruction as in simple obstruction and that the roentgen ray is, therefore, not as valuable in the early diagnosis.

Comparative studies have shown that the quantity of gas accumulating above the point of occlusion in simple obstruction is far in excess of that observed within the loop in closed or strangulated loops. Loud, peristaltic rushes may be heard from the contractions of the intestine proximal to the obstruction. The bowel below the obstruction being normal may evacuate feces and gas on the administration of an enema. Later in the course of the ailment an inhibition ileus, such as may be seen in kidney colic or peritonitis, may supervene and the abdomen becomes relatively silent, and enemas are not expelled.

Vomiting of a reflex nature sets in early after the onset of pain, but ordinarily does not continue in the same degree, as seen in simple obstruction. Blood in the stool is infrequent except in intussusception of children. Blood in the vomitus in high strangulation has now and then been observed. If the course of the disease continues uninterrupted, the beginning of the end of life is heralded for the sufferer by extreme restlessness, a feeble thready pulse, a cyanotic appearance of the skin, which is cold and moist with sweat, and general signs of circulatory-failure.

If the strangulated bowel becomes nonviable, peritonitis supervenes and hiccough frequently manifests this occurrence. It is to be remembered, however, that although the course of strangulation obstruction is ordinarily unusually rapid, owing to the deprivation of blood supply to a portion of the intestine, such is not the invariable occurrence. When the strangulating features are less prominent, the progress of the disease simulates the picture seen in mechanical obstruction at the same level, and it has not been an extremely rare observation to find that a short infarcted loop, as a consequence of thrombosis of the vessels in a segment of the mesentery, has gone entirely unsuspected for more than a week's time, manifesting some abdominal discomfort, but not sufficient to warn the surgeon or patient of the lurking danger.

Differential Diagnosis: Briefly, it may be stated that cases of simple obstruction are most closely simulated by colics that are unattended by physical findings. Strangulation obstructions must be differentiated from every abdominal colic that produces tenderness and rigidity of the abdominal wall.

Simple Obstruction: The lesion for which early simple intestinal obstruction is probably most often mistaken is the simple "bellyache," under which category one might list food indiscretions of one sort or another, abdominal allergic reactions and acute enterocolitis. In these, however, diarrhea is usually a prominent symptom; and vomiting is very much less in the foreground than in obstruction. Even though the early vomiting of intestinal obstruction is reflex in character, just as it is in gall-stone or kidney colic, the vomiting of obstruction is more frequent, urgent and copious than in other types of reflex vomiting. When gaseous distension occurs in "bellyache" it involves almost invariably the entire intestine, whereas most mechanical obstructions of the small intestine (except carcinoma of the left colon) cause only gaseous distension of a portion of the small intestine (the bowel above the occlusion). Progression of intestinal distension, as observed in obstruction to the continuity of the bowel, likewise does not occur in enterocolitis.

The absence of local findings and the presence of loud gurgling intestinal noises at the height of the colic account adequately for the mimicry of bowel obstruction by these colics. The high-pitched tinkling sounds, such as are heard in the presence of a dilated obstructed bowel under tension, rarely occurs in enterocolitis and its related types of intestinal pain.

Strangulation Obstruction: As has previously been pointed out, strangulation obstructions present a block in the bowel with the addition of infarction of the imprisoned segment of bowel. Venous obstruction of the circulation permits of a more rapid accumulation of blood within the lumen of the bowel as well as within its wall, and consequently signs of peritoneal irritation develop more rapidly than when the arterial inflow, as well as the venous egress, of blood is occluded. The lesser grades of venous block, however, may be somewhat tardy in giving rise to peritoneal irritation and, as has already been stated, either the symptoms of obstruction to the continuity of the bowel or the strangulating features may dominate the picture, contingent upon how much the circulation is interfered with.

When the signs of bowel occlusion predominate, the sequence of intermittent colic, at the height of which loud intestinal borborygmi may be heard, serves to distinguish the condition. Even in fear of reiteration to the point of being wearisome, I repeat, other abdominal colics do not give rise to increased peristaltic activity of the intestine. In strangulation obstructions, accompanied by tenderness and slight rigidity, this occurrence is of extreme importance in diagnosis.

A large number of conditions must necessarily be thought of in the differential diagnosis of strangulating obstructions, including all the abdominal colics, such as gall-bladder and renal seizures; the inflammatory conditions such as appendicitis, salpingitis, peritonitis and kidney infections; pancreatic necrosis and diaphragmatic pleurisy; purpura and other skin lesions with hemorrhage in the bowel wall, as well as the torsion of other organs, especially ovarian cysts and the testis.

The very presence of local physical findings will indicate on casual examination the probable presence of a surgical lesion, a warning signal which unfortunately the early case of simple obstruction does not present. Many of the conditions that have to be differentiated present gaseous distension of the bowel on roentgenologic visualization, but usually it concerns the entire bowel. It must be admitted, however, that there are instances among the causes of reflex ileus accompanying the conditions enumerated, in which localized gas accumulation may only concern part of the bowel. However, the progression of distension is different. Even in the atypical instances mentioned above there is a tendency to rather rapid and uniform, even though not great, gaseous distension of the entire bowel. As has been mentioned previously, however, the strangulated segment contains relatively little gas and instances have come to my attention in which we have been able to make preoperatively, from viewing the roentgenographic film, the diagnosis of strangulation obstruction by the interruption of continuity of the "ladder-pattern" of the distended coils.

Employing the criteria outlined above, it is my firm conviction that most cases of bowel obstruction of both the simple and the strangulating variety can be detected early. If the functional neurogenic ileus displaying spastic features referred to above be properly identified, no great anxiety need be had lest cases be operated upon that do not exhibit obstruction of the bowel, when operation is advised in the absence of general distension and absolute obstipation. Though I have not as yet experienced such an embarrassment, I am prepared to meet it and will not feel particularly chagrined, supported by the belief that an unnecessary exploration which is not accompanied by operative risk and which wipes out the dilemma of the existence of a potential serious lesion is the lesser evil.

J. B. Murphy's statement that procrastination kills more patients than cancer is truer of acute intestinal obstruction than of any other disease. Too often the diagnosis is delayed by seeming improvement. But how many patients die of it? It is the physician who makes the diagnosis early in bowel obstruction who saves most lives. Not infrequently unwarranted delays occur after admission to a hospital, and in the past year several cases have come to my attention in which patients with bowel obstruction were in a hospital almost continuously from the onset under a surgeon's care and came to necropsy with the diagnosis suspected but not made during life. Such caution can only be attributed to negligence or ignorance! No campaign need be carried on with the laity to acquaint them with the seriousness of the problem. Their complaint in most instances brings them to the physician adequately early. It is upon ourselves, as a profession, that we must focus our attention and efforts at education in order that bowel obstruction may be early recognized.

III. ESSENTIALS OF TREATMENT

The most significant factor in determining the extent of the agency of relief necessary in dealing with acute bowel obstruction is the elapse of time since the onset of the obstruction. Whether a nonviable segment of gut will be found in a potential strangulation type of obstruction depends naturally in large measure upon the rigidity of the constricting agent, but as much upon the time lost between the occurrence of the disaster and the intervention of the surgeon.

In internal hernia, intussusception, volvulus, and adhesive strangulations in which the constricting agent is more yielding and flexible than in external hernias, deprivation of blood supply does not result as quickly in devitalization of the incarcerated segment. Most strangulations are essentially venous in character, in which there is an incomplete obstruction to venous outflow.

Experimentally, it may readily be shown that the more complete the venous occlusion and the longer the segment concerned, the greater is the loss of blood into the segment. Dogs in which the veins of a three-foot segment of bowel are ligated will die on the average in about five hours; if an encirclement ligature is placed about the bowel and mesentery to simulate a clinical type of strangulation, the animal will survive for about twenty hours. Ligation and division of both arteries and veins or arteries alone are also tolerated for about twenty hours.

There is adequate blood loss in the lumen and bowel wall in the venous ligations to account for the rapid death by shock alone. In the animal that survives longer the element of blood loss and shock in strangulation obstructions is also significant. The matter of absorption, whether through the blood or lymph vessels of the mesentery, or via the peritoneal cavity, after transudation through the bowel wall, here comes into question. Suffice it to say that when the circulation of a segment be damaged, whether it be by ligation of arteries or veins, absorption from the bowel is very seriously retarded. Whereas a few milligrams of strychnine placed within the lumen of the normal bowel or in the peritoneal cavity will cause convulsive spasms in a dog in a few minutes, if the blood supply of the segment be interfered with by an encirclement ligature or interruption of either arteries or veins, the strychnine effect can not be elicited even after hours of obstruction with the employment of many times the lethal dose. The peritoneal transudate from these animals gives no strychnine effect on injection into other animals.

Only in those instances of strangulation obstruction in which the peritoneal fluid exhibits characteristics of an exudate with foul odor, dark color, and high protein content and bacteria, does the item of transperitoneal absorption assume any significance. In such instances, the bowel wall is usually perforated or frankly gangrenous. The injection of peritoneal fluid exhibiting the physical characters of a transudate in strangulations into other animals is without effect.

In dealing with strangulation types of obstruction surgically, the important question is whether or not the bowel is viable. Return of normal color to the bowel and pulsation to its mesenteric vessels after release of the strangulating mechanism indicates a viable bowel. If the bowel is not viable, exteriorization with excision of the gangrenous segment on completion of the closure of the wound should be done. No attempt at enteroanastomosis should be made in the usual case, it being much safer to establish the continuity of the bowel secondarily. The combined risks of the two operations does not approximate the risk assumed by the patient if a gangrenous gut be excised and the enteroanastomosis be done simultaneously.

In early cases of simple obstruction the operation of election, viz., seeking and releasing the obstruction with immediate establishment of the continuity of the bowel, may be safely practiced. In instances in which there is considerable distension of the bowel, and in which free peritoneal hemorrhagic fluid and a discolored bowel are not found, the operative procedure of choice is enterostomy. In practically all obstructions occurring during the convalescence from operation, enterostomy is the safest operative procedure. Consequent upon the subsidence of intestinal distension brought about by enterostomy, the continuity of the intestine is usually automatically reestablished and the enterostomy opening closes spontaneously, when the safety vent has served its purpose upon withdrawal of the tube. All anastomotic operations upon the distended bowel in acute intestinal obstruction are fraught with danger and should be deliberately avoided.

I am not persuaded that there is any evidence that abnormal absorption occurs from a distended bowel that is still viable, whether through the mesenteric vessels or by transudation through the bowel wall into the peritoneal cavity. On the contrary, absorption of substances to which the normal bowel is permeable is delayed under conditions of distension and obstruction. When strychnine is placed in an obstructed loop under considerable hydrostatic or air pressure (130 mm. Hg) no effect will be observed over hours of observation. Only when the intraluminary pressure is lowered to about 70 mm. Hg can the strychnine effect be elicited. When histamine or hydrokollag (substances to which the normal bowel is impermeable) are placed in the obstructed and distended bowel, no evidence of their absorption can be demonstrated. Though the bowel grossly may appear hyperemic, when examined microscopically no interstitial hemorrhage is apparent. Erosion of the villi in killed dogs does not appear more frequent in the obstructed than in the distal bowel. Edema and congestion may be demonstrated but no alteration of structure is observed. Whereas, theoretically simple obstruction may partake of the features of strangulation obstruction, due to the increase in intraluminary pressure, this is a rare occurrence. Clinically it is observed in obstructions of the colon and usually in obstructions at the sigmoid flexure, the distension effects being found in the cecum. The competent ileocecal sphincter converts this simple obstruction into a closed loop obstruction in which the features of deprivation of blood supply regularly occur. Hollow, muscular viscera such as the bladder, stomach and intestines have the ability to alter their capacity materially without exhibiting significant changes in tension. Owings and his associates were able to demonstrate a sustained pressure of only 6 to 8 mm. Hg in experimental simple obstruction in dogs.

The tendency to perform operations of election rather than the adaptation of a procedure suitable to the precarious condition of the patient contributes in no small degree to the persistence of a forbidding mortality in late cases of simple obstruction. Many lives in this group of cases can be salvaged if the surgeon will observe the restraint practised by a lifeguard in saving a drowning man. He concentrates his attention upon saving the man's life; later he may be taught how to swim.

In the performance of enterostomy any dilated loop may be sought. The level of the segment presenting depends largely on the site of the incision. On the whole, the nearer the enterostomy is to the site of obstruction, the more efficient is the drainage. In postoperative obstructions, a short oblique incision over the left rectus, pulling the muscle medially, serves the purpose best; in other simple obstructions in which the exact site is unknown, I prefer the midline subumbilical incision. It is an item of extreme significance for the success of the

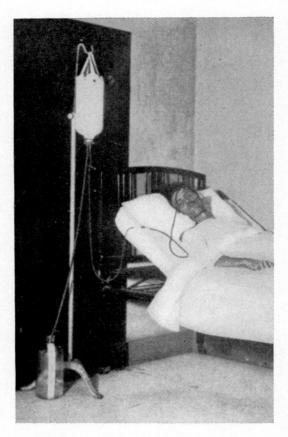

Fig. 1.—Photograph of a patient upon whom a successful decompression of the bowel was obtained for acute
mechanical obstruction (postoperative adhesive), showing
the apparatus in operation. The gas collects in the top of
the suspended bottle; the degree of negative pressure is
represented by the difference between the level of the end
of the catheter in the stomach (or duodenum) and the
height of the column of water in the bottle on the floor
(usually about 2.5 feet or about 75 cm. of water siphonage pressure).

operation that there be absolutely no spillage in doing the enterostomy. Whereas ordinarily the opening and suture of the small intestine may be done without great danger of contamination, under the influence of obstruction, bacteria multiply rapidly in the bowel to such a degree that the slightest spillage enhances greatly the peril of peritonitis. A number 14 or 16 French urethral catheter buried in the bowel wall by the Witzel technique serves the purpose well and a long peritoneal tunnel results that closes spontaneously when the continuity of the bowel has become reestablished after temporary drainage.

In computing the fluid output through the enterostomy tube in adhesive types of obstruction I have been astonished to note how surprisingly little fluid comes away in the majority of instances. Still, a dilated, distended bowel, following the decompression, establishes its continuity automatically (when no intrinsic obstruction is present in the lumen or wall of the bowel). Only in fairly complete persistent obstructions, or in external fistula does a large amount of fluid drainage continue through the enterostomy catheter. The amount of catheter drainage in adhesive obstruction in my experience has not been in any way correlated with the level at which the enterostomy has been done; I believe it depends almost solely on the degree of constriction present. The immediate drainage has often been fairly large in amount, but after the first 24 hours the daily escape of fluid through the catheter usually falls to a low level (50 to 250 c.c.). Persistent daily escape of 600 to 900 c.c. or more of fluid usually indicates considerable constriction of the bowel. In such instances it is always wise to clamp the catheter for several hours a day before withdrawing it, to be certain that pain will not recur. As yet I have found it unnecessary in adhesive obstruction, after performing enterostomy, to secondarily release the constricting agent. Only recently have determinations of the escape of gas been made in these enterostomies, and it is my impression that the measurement of gas, though somewhat greater in amount than the fluid drainage, will be correlated also with the degree of bowel constriction present. In a recent case with fairly complete obstruction, in which there was considerable persistent drainage for ten days after placement of the catheter, the total gas escape in ten days was 10,800 cc. and the fluid drainage was 7650 cc. In another instance in which the drainage of fluid through the catheter was negligible after the es-

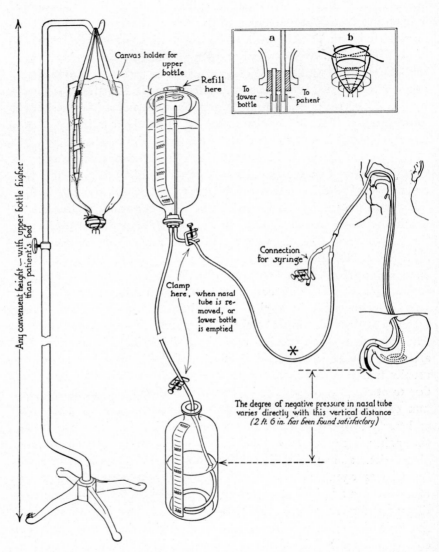

Fig. 2.—Sketch of the apparatus; the bottle is inverted so that the gas may be collected and measured as well as the fluid.

tablishment of enterostomy, the gas escape during the ten days during which time the catheter functioned was 1700 cc.

Nasal Catheter Suction Treatment

These observations led me to employ the nasal catheter (Levin duodenal tube) with suction obtained by water siphonage, in the treatment of acute mechanical bowel obstruction (Fig. 1). Considerably more gas and fluid of course is aspirated from the stomach with the nasal catheter than drains away through an enterostomy tube. To date three cases have been successfully treated by this means. One of these patients, a feeble old woman of 72 with a 72-hour obstruction, with considerable intestinal distension and in very poor condition, was thought to have a carcinoma of the cecum. Initial drainage with a nasal catheter and suction decompressed the bowel completely, with manifest improvement in the patient's condition. Because of the conjectured persistent nature of the obstruction, operation was then done (40 hours later) and a stricture (probably syphilitic) was found in the terminal ileum. It was invaginated into the cecum and a proximal enterostomy was made, following which the patient convalesced uneventfully (Fig. 3) [Ed. Note: Figure omitted].

The other two patients in which nasal catheter drainage alone proved successful were both instances of adhesive obstruction (Fig. 4); one of these occurred postoperatively during the convalescence from operation for a ruptured appendix with peritonitis. The method was tried unsuccessfully in one instance of adhesive obstruction in which enterostomy was subsequently done with recovery (Fig. 5) [Ed. Note: Figure omitted].

In adhesive types of obstruction in which the cause often ceases to operate following decompression of the bowel, the method should have its greatest field of usefulness, and in postoperative obstructions particularly, the method should prove to be an agent of therapeutic value. I have observed the caution of following the intestinal decompression by taking x-ray films of the abdomen (portable) every two or three hours until it is obviously apparent, from the degree of intestinal distension present, whether the method will be successful or not. The chief source of intestinal gas in bowel obstruction is swallowed air, which is only very slowly absorbed from the bowel. In the instance referred to above, in which the method proved unsuccessful, the dis-

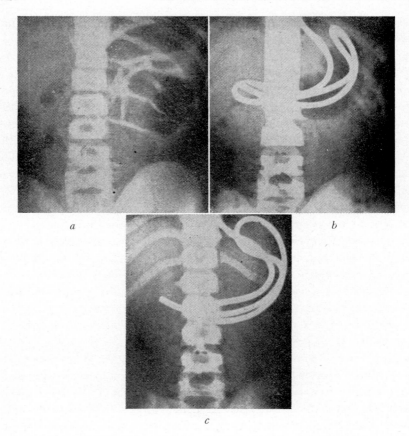

FIG. 4.—*a*. Intestinal distension in a boy of nine years admitted with an acute obstruction of 48 hours' duration, complaining of considerable crampy pain and vomiting.

b. After three hours' suction, when 550 c.c. of fluid and 650 c.c. of gas had been aspirated off.

c. Twenty hours after the institution of nasal siphonage; 1625 c.c. of fluid and 2250 c.c. of gas were aspirated meanwhile.

tension did not progress; all pain stopped with the institution of nasal siphonage, but I felt it unwise not to decompress the bowel by a more direct method. In all of these instances but one, the nasal catheter has remained in the stomach; in the one instance in which the method proved ineffectual, an unsuccessful attempt was made to pass the catheter under the fluoroscope into the duodenum. It is believed that spasm of the pylorus was in some measure responsible for the failure of the nasal catheter drainage in this instance.

The method undoubtedly has its shortcomings and is not to be recommended in the treatment of strangulation obstruction, which is to be recognized clinically in the occurrence of rebound tenderness and rigidity of the abdominal muscles. In carcinoma of the sigmoid flexure in which gaseous distension involving only the colon usually obtains, due to competence of the ileocecal valve, catheter drainage of the upper reaches of the bowel would be inadequate; and when the cause continues to operate as in the first patient referred to above, it is not to be expected that drainage through a nasal catheter alone will suffice.

In the management of all cases of bowel obstruction it is important to give enough fluid to insure a good urine output. Saline is in no sense a specific except in high obstruction. Only in so-called arterio-mesenteric ileus and the temporary mechanical obstructions that occur at the stoma following gastroenterostomy or the Polya type of gastric resection is one justified in temporizing with saline alone.

Mortality: Seventy-three operations for acute bowel obstruction have been done at the University Hospital during the last three years. There have been thirteen deaths attributable to the relief of the obstruction; a mortality of 17.8 per cent.

Amongst these fatal cases there were two due to intussusception. One of these patients was practically moribund at the time of operation, dying before the incision was made. Both were of more than 48 hours' duration. There were four deaths amongst twelve cases of carcinoma of the colon causing obstruction. In one of these (carcinoma of the sigmoid flexure) peritonitis was already present at operation, due to gangrene of the cecum consequent upon enormous gaseous distension. There was one fatal case of carcinoma of the small intestine with metastases to the liver and peritoneal fluid; one case of multiple myeloma with multiple fractures, the obstruction being due to a deposit of amyloid throughout the small intestines. Two cases of intestinal atresia were operated upon, both of which died (only nine successful cases are reported in the literature). There were three deaths in the adhesive type of obstruction. In one of these with frank gangrene, resection was done with subsequent peritonitis (exteriorization should have been done). One of the remaining two was a young boy whose bladder was full and was accidentally nicked as the abdomen was opened. An indwelling catheter was left in the bladder postoperatively and pyelonephritis developed, from which the boy died. (Since then we have always made certain that the bladder is empty, especially in youngsters in whom the bladder is often an extra-pelvic organ.) The other fatal case of adhesive obstruction was a post-abortal case in which plastic masses and a low grade peritonitis were both present. Three enterostomies were done on this patient at rather long intervals, necessitated, by progression of plastic masses. Enteroanastomosis was impossible at either of the subsequent operations, due to an obliteration of the normal anatomy of the peritoneal cavity by the plastic inflammatory masses.

Amongst late hospital deaths related to the initial obstruction may be enumerated one of carcinoma of the bowel following excision of the tumor at a secondary operation. Amongst late hospital deaths unrelated to the initial obstruction may be enumerated the four following: one due to peritonitis of unknown origin after withdrawal of the intestinal catheter and after the patient was ambulant; one case of intussusception due to bilateral middle ear infection three weeks after operation; one case of imperforate anus due to congenital heart disease; and one case of infectious diarrhea and enterocolitis several weeks after the relief of obstruction. The inclusion of these cases in the computation of the operative mortality would bring the total to 24.6 per cent.

In 19 cases (largely cases of adhesive obstruction) enterostomy alone was done with two deaths (two of the three fatal cases of adhesive obstruction referred to above); a mortality of 10.5 per cent, indicating the superiority of the indirect attack upon all late cases of simple obstruction. In this group there is one case of strangulation obstruction in which exteriorization and excision of the strangulated segment with secondary anastomosis was done.

There were 19 strangulated hernias operated upon without mortality. Aside from the two lethal cases of intestinal atresia in which the risk may be directly measured by the inherent difficulty of successfully establishing the continuity of the intestinal canal, and the operative accident referred to above in which the bladder was injured, all the other operative deaths were in very late cases in which operation was an eleventh hour expedient.

SUMMARY AND CONCLUSIONS

The present high mortality in acute intestinal obstruction is due in a large measure to late diagnosis. The absence of local abdominal physical findings in simple obstruction; misinterpretation of the significance of the expulsion of gas with enemas; indiscriminate administration of morphine before making a diagnosis; and the equivocal and oftentimes deceptive information obtained with apparently effectual catharsis in partial obstructions, are factors that contribute to delay in diagnosis.

Intermittent colicky pain, associated with nausea and vomiting but unattended by abdominal tenderness or rigidity, suggests a block in the continuity of the bowel. In strangulation types of obstruction local physical findings are usually present, though not as early as in peritoneal lesions of an inflammatory character. The bowel below the point of obstruction is physiologically, as well as anatomically normal, and will expel an administered enema with the return of gas and feces. Gaseous shadows in the small intestine, visualized by roentgenographic examination, demonstrate the presence of intestinal stasis. The stethoscope serves to distinguish whether the stasis is mechanical or paralytic in character.

The general condition of the patient is not significantly altered in simple obstruction. In strangulation types, there is often quickening of the pulse. Blood chemistry alterations obtain regularly only in high intestinal obstructions and occur late.

When the criteria upon which the diagnosis can be made early are properly evaluated and patients with acute intestinal obstruction come to operation at an opportune hour, the appalling mortality of the disease will cease to exist. In dealing with the late case of simple obstruction, enterostomy, an indirect procedure and an operation of necessity rather than of election, should be practiced. Decompression of the bowel with the nasal catheter, employing water siphonage, should prove to be a therapeutic agent of great value in many types of simple obstruction and especially in postoperative adhesive obstruction. In strangulation obstructions in which the bowel is not viable, exteriorization and excision, with the temporary establishment of a complete fistula, followed by secondary anastomosis, is to be preferred to primary resection.

10. Thoracic Surgery

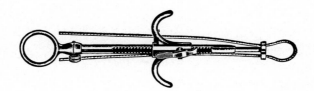

PREFATORY COMMENTS

Thoracic surgery prior to 1925 was confined, mainly, to drainage of empyema and to the removal of lesions of the chest wall. Two text-books appeared in the English literature: Stephen Paget's *Surgery of the Chest,* published in 1896, and Carl Beck's *Surgical Diseases of the Chest* in 1907. Paget wrote in a pessimistic vein: "There are signs that we have reached the stage in this position of our art beyond which on our present lines we cannot advance much further." Similar state-ments of defeatism have been made in regard to other aspects of sur-gery, only to be disproved by the inventiveness of man. Although Meltzer and Auer had introduced a simple and practical method of administering endotracheal anesthesia in 1909, Bevan decried the use of the method nine years later when he stated, "Endotracheal anes-thesia has little place in practical surgery." The published results of the Empyema Commission in World War I gave new impetus to the field of thoracic surgery. The combined efforts of Keller, Bell, Dun-ham and Graham resulted in a more profound understanding of the physiological aberrations secondary to open pneumothorax. They rec-ognized the fact that patients ill with streptococcal empyema could not tolerate open pleural drainage because of the mobility of the mediasti-num. By substituting the simple expedient of needle aspiration or closed-tube drainage for open drainage, they reduced the mortality rate from about 40 per cent to 4.3 per cent. They also pointed out the fact that once the abscess became localized in the postpneumonic phase, open drainage could be performed with impunity.

We have included Franz Torek's description of the first successful esophagectomy for carcinoma in 1913 because it opened up the entire

333

field of esophageal surgery, albeit belatedly. He removed the lesion, closed off the lower end of the esophagus and performed a cervical esophagostomy which later was connected by a tube to a gastrostomy opening. That patient survived for eleven years. The mortality and morbidity rate for esophageal resection was so high that the Torek operation fell into disrepute until 1924, when Carl Eggers reported the second successful removal of an esophageal carcinoma. However, operations of this type were attempted with "tongue in cheek" until 1940. The main reason for the many failures was ascribed to the fact that the esophagus has no serosal covering and therefore watertight anastomoses would be difficult to attain. Adherence to the admonition of Edward Churchill that the esophagus should be sutured as carefully as the vermilion border of the lip resulted in a safe method of esophageal surgery. Again the adages of the past were challenged by the questioning spirit of the present and were discarded.

Advances in the field of thoracic surgery had to await the development of more exact techniques of localization. The techniques were crude until 1917 when the modern Coolidge tube was invented. In 1922 Sicard and Forestier introduced lipiodol as a satisfactory method of visualizing the tracheobronchial tree. Later laminography, angiocardiography and Bucky films yielded more exact information concerning the configuration and localization of pulmonary lesions. These developments were the natural outgrowth of the scientist's attempt to obtain more detailed information.

In 1921 Lloyd summarized the current viewpoint of the surgeon regarding operations on the lung: "For tuberculosis, if a collapse of the cavity is possible by pneumothorax it is preferable, if not, extrapleural thoracoplasty should be performed in one or several stages. For bronchiectasis, extrapleural thoracoplasty may be performed as advocated by Hedblom, although excision and drainage or lobectomy offers a better chance of a radical cure. Foreign bodies should be removed through the bronchoscope; if impossible, thoracotomy with direct removal may be necessary. For lung abscesses, the best results may be obtained by thoracotomy and drainage. Tumors of the chest wall, including ribs and pleura, should be treated by completed removal and the use of pedunculated skin grafts from the abdomen, if the defect is too large."

In 1922, Lilienthal reported 31 cases operated upon for suppurative disease. His mortality was 4.2 per cent for lobectomy cases and 70 per cent for those requiring more than a lobectomy. He described both the one-stage and the two-stage technique requiring abrasion of the lung and the parietal pleura as the first stage and removal of the diseased lung as the second procedure. He employed a water-seal drain much in the manner of today's use.

Because of Lilienthal's shockingly high mortality rate, Graham employed the technique of "pneumonectomy with cautery" in 1923. If the lung was not adherent at the first operation, he placed an iodoform pack on the pleura. Once the visceral and parietal pleural became adherent, a large soldering iron heated to red heat was applied to the diseased lung, which was removed piecemeal and often in many stages. A few years later, Lilienthal made the following remarks concerning lobectomy: "It is also right to counteract the effect of the depressing mortality with the picture of a successful result and restored health. In reply to the question as to the probable period of convalescence, we may look forward to two months in the hospital and seven to twelve months longer for the patient's convalescence. After the interview, the patient ought to take a day or two to make up his mind and only in the acute progressive cases should we insist upon a more prompt decision."

At first lobectomies were performed by the tourniquet technique. It was not until the present era that the technique of individual ligation of the hilar structures was elaborated as an outgrowth of the work of Churchill and Belsey, Brock, Huber, Jackson, Overholt and others. In 1931, Rudolf Nissen of Berlin successfully removed a bronchiectatic left lung in a 12-year-old girl. He employed the tourniquet technique and allowed the lung to slough. The second successful pneumonectomy was performed by Cameron Haight of Ann Arbor, Michigan, who used the same method. In 1933 Evarts Graham, employing individual ligation of hilar structures, removed the entire lung for carcinoma at one stage and performed a simultaneous partial thoracoplasty to diminish the size of the pleural space. The physician upon whom he operated is still alive and free of the disease. The technique of individual ligation was practiced by Rienhoff and Overholt during the ensuing years. It is a tribute to their astute observations and meticulous technique that pneumonectomy is being performed today by the same method and with a gratifyingly low mortality.

The treatment of pulmonary tuberculosis consisted almost entirely of bed rest before 1920. If bed rest failed, pneumothorax was instituted. To ensure complete collapse of the lung, Jacobeus in 1913 designed a thoracoscope which enabled him to divide intrapleural adhesions under direct vision. Thoracoplasty was employed sporadically before 1920. The pioneers in the development of this operation were Sauerbruch in Germany and Alexander in this country. The latter's book, *The Collapse Therapy of Pulmonary Tuberculosis,* became a surgical bible after its publication in 1937. The more daring surgeons attempted resection of the tuberculous lung but the high incidence of spread of the disease, bronchial fistula and empyema discouraged them from pursuing that approach for many years. Finally, with the advent of antibiotics, streptomycin, para-aminosalicylic acid and later isoniazid, the pendulum swung toward resectional surgery. It soon became obvious that by using a more accurate and fastidious anatomical approach, diseased segments of lobes could be removed safely. We are indebted to Overholt, Chamberlain and many others for these more recent developments. This chapter on the surgical management of tuberculosis exemplifies the tremendous effect of progress in one field of investigation upon another. The high incidence of complications following resections for tuberculous lesions as reported by Overholt and Sweet in 1946 would have been perpetuated if Waksman and other microbiologists had not discovered efficacious antibiotic agents. In less than one generation, the forbidding aura surrounding thoracotomy has disappeared. Endotracheal anesthesia, the accurate replacement of blood losses, meticulous technique and the administration of appropriate antibiotics have all contributed to make chest surgery safe.

FRANZ JOHN A. TOREK (1861–1938)

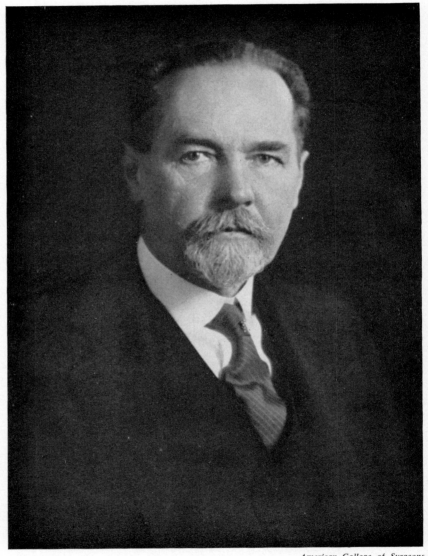

Dr. Torek was born on April 14, 1861, in Breslau, Germany. He attended City College of New York and later received his medical degree from Columbia University in 1887. He interned in New York at the German Hospital now known as the Lenox Hill Hospital. He has been described as an extremely versatile general surgeon who planned most of his difficult operative procedures by cadaver practice. He did considerable work on radical procedures for cancer and originated the Torek procedure for undescended testicle. He was an accomplished musician as well.

Torek was President of the American Association for Thoracic Surgeons, the New York Society for Thoracic Surgeons and the German Medical Society. He wrote the chapter on thoracic surgery in Johnson's Operative Therapeusis and a section on esophagectomy in Cyclopedia of Medicine. He died in Vienna on September 19, 1938, of bronchopneumonia.

THE FIRST SUCCESSFUL CASE OF RESECTION OF THE THORACIC PORTION OF THE OESOPHAGUS FOR CARCINOMA

BY FRANZ TOREK, A.M., M.D.

*Surgeon to the German Hospital and the New York Skin and Cancer Hospital;
Adjunct Professor of Surgery in the New York Post-Graduate Medical School*

The resection of the thoracic portion of the oesophagus for carcinoma has been one of the greatest problems of modern surgery. It is not the object of this paper to give the history of oesophageal surgery; much less could I mention the notable achievements of any one surgeon without injustice to others not named. But I must call attention to the view expressed by one of the most competent representatives of this branch of surgery, not only because it exerted a far-reaching influence on the efforts of others, but especially because my case does not substantiate this view. I refer to the standpoint of Sauerbruch that operations for carcinoma of the oesophagus should be undertaken only if the new growth is either high up near the neck or low down, where an anastomosis with the stomach could be made, but that the growths in the middle portion of the oesophagus are not removable. The reasons for excluding these cases from the realm of operative interference were, first, the inaccessibility of that portion of the oesophagus which passes behind the arch of the aorta, and secondly the danger arising from injury to the pneumogastric nerves, which in that location branch in front of the oesophagus like a plexus. Division of both vagi

From *Surgery, Gynecology and Obstetrics, 16:*614, 1913. Reprinted by permission of *Surgery, Gynecology and Obstetrics.*

Figure 4 has been omitted.

at a place before they reach the heart causes instant death, and at operations in that region it has been repeatedly observed that tugging at a vagus, or pinching it, was promptly followed by collapse of the heart, as manifested by the pulse, which persisted for a longer or shorter time, until death set in. Finally, the uncertainty of the closure of the upper stump of the oesophagus, and consequent infection of the pleural cavity, has been a source of great danger after resection in any part of the oesophagus where an anastomosis could not be made. The leakage from that stump was doubtless due to the tension in the oesophagus from swallowed saliva. Every contraction of the constrictors of the pharynx would temporarily increase the tension in this blind pouch, until the suture finally was unable to withstand the pressure from within. The patients who had escaped death either from injury to the vagus or from shock, pneumothorax, or pneumonia, all died from the giving way of the oesophageal closure, no matter how skillful the operating surgeon had been.

Statistics show that carcinoma of the oesophagus is most frequently found in the middle third, the location in the lower third coming next, while those in the upper third are comparatively rare. On the other hand, metastases are found most frequently with those situated in the lower third, near the cardia. Since, therefore, the carcinomata at the cardia are not only numerically less frequent than those in the middle third, but are also more frequently associated with metastases that render the cases incurable, the most important role in the problem of cancer of the oesophagus seems to belong to the carcinomata in the middle portion, the very ones that Sauerbruch and others advised leaving untouched.

In a case operated at the German Hospital on March 14, 1913, I succeeded in demonstrating the feasibility of resection of the middle portion of the oesophagus for carcinoma. The patient, a woman 67 years old, had a carcinoma of the oesophagus beginning just below the lower border of the transverse portion of the arch of the aorta and extending from there downward for about 1¾ inches. A pair of very beautiful steroscopic X-ray pictures taken by Dr. William H. Stewart demonstrated the condition before the operation. A reproduction of one of these is seen in Fig. 1. I had performed a gastrostomy upon her some time previous to the resection of the oesophagus. Knowing the difficulties of the case, the problem was to plan the ways and means of overcoming them. It was necessary, first, to afford better access; secondly, to perform more careful dissection of the vagi, avoiding rough handling of them; and thirdly, to do away with the danger of leakage from the proximal stump after resection.

The method of access to the field of operation was as follows: Instead of going through two different intercostal spaces and dissecting

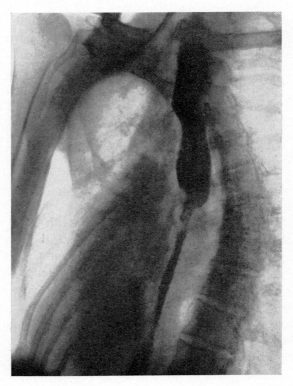

Fig. 1.—The bismuth shadow shows where the constriction of the oesophagus begins.

off the scapula, or of resecting several adjacent ribs, as recommended by others, the incision was carried through the whole length of the seventh intercostal space, from the posterior end of which it was extended upward by cutting through the seventh, sixth, fifth, and fourth ribs near their tubercles, which gave a much better exposure and is far simpler. The photograph (Fig. 2) shows the scar from the incision, the upper end of which is almost at the level of the shoulder; the front end of the incision is seen in Fig. 3. The black line accompanying it is a marking with nitrate of silver made on the day before the operation.

Extensive adhesions between the lung and the parietal pleura were present, the greater part of the lower lobe being attached both to the costal and the diaphragmatic pleura. The firmest adhesions were at the

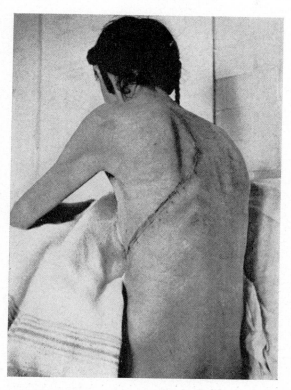

Fig. 2.—Photograph taken 12 days after the operation. The black line accompanying the incision is a nitrate of silver marking made the day before the operation. The upper end of the incision is almost at the level of the shoulder. The anterior end of the incision is seen in Fig. 3.

apex. All these were separated. The tumor was found to be fairly fixed in the position above described, viz., just below the lower border of the transverse portion of the arch of the aorta, allowing only very slight mobility. The portion of the oesophagus below the tumor, between it and the diaphragm, was exposed in the usual manner by incising the pleura, drawing the vagi aside, and lifting the oesophagus out of its bed. At the site of the tumor the dissection of the vagi was more difficult, and some of the branches crossing over in front of it had to be cut in order to permit liberating the tumor without undue

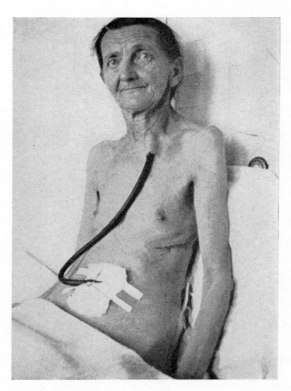

Fig. 3.—Photograph taken 12 days after operation. The incision at the anterior border of the left sternocleidomastoid muscle, through which the oesophagus was taken out is scarcely recognizable. The oesophagus has been placed under the skin of the chest and its end sutured to an incision in the skin. The gastrostomy tube is introduced into the oesophagus whenever the patient desires to swallow.

roughness in handling the vagi. To my great satisfaction the pulse never wavered during this procedure, remaining between 93 and 96. The dreaded vagus collapse had, therefore, been safely avoided.

The dissection of that part of the oesophagus which passes behind the arch of the aorta offered great difficulties, which were finally overcome by dislodging the aorta at that site and lifting it forward, having ligated and divided a number of its thoracic branches. Getting the aorta out of the way, where it crosses the oesophagus, is of considerable help in liberating the latter; in simple cases, however, I feel certain that the dissection could be done without ligating the thoracic branches of the aorta. The tumor was attached to the left bronchus, which sustained a longitudinal cut during the progress of the separation of the tumor from it. The cut in the bronchus was afterward sutured with silk.

The oesophagus had now been detached from its bed, beginning at a point about an inch above the diaphragm, up to about an inch above the arch of the aorta. The resection of the carcinoma *in situ* could therefore have been easily performed. But my plan was different. I had come to the conclusion that the rational way to deal with the danger of leakage from the upper stump of the oesophagus was to eliminate that organ from the pleural cavity altogether. I therefore dissected the oesophagus loose from its attachments all the way up to the neck, divided it with a cautery at a safe distance below the carcinoma, after double ligation, and brought the oesophagus with the tumor out through an incision in the neck at the anterior border of the left sterno-cleido-mastoid muscle. Thus the pleural cavity could not possibly become infected from that course. The ligation of the lower stump had been made after first crushing the oesophagus at that site. This stump was invaginated like an appendix stump, only with the difference that two successive purse-string sutures of silk were used instead of only one, as in the case of the appendix.

The thorax was now closed, silk threads being used to hold the seventh and eighth ribs together, chromicized catgut for the muscles, and silkworm gut for the skin. No drainage was employed. Now the oesophagus which was hanging out from the wound in the neck was placed under the skin of the chest. For this purpose a transverse incision was made in the skin at a place corresponding to what was going to be the free end of the oesophagus after the carcinoma was cut off, for at the time this was still attached. The site of that incision in this case corresponds to the second intercostal space. The skin between the incision in the neck and the new incision was tunneled, the oesophagus drawn through, the carcinoma cut off, and the fresh rim of the oesophagus, sutured to the skin. The neck wound was closed.

As regards other details of the operation. I may say that the incision through the skin and muscles was made under local anesthesia, one half per cent novocain with suprarenin being used. The general anesthesia was given by tracheal insufflation according to Meltzer–Auer, the apparatus constructed by Dr. Hermann Fischer being used. It worked very satisfactorily. The employment of a differential pressure chamber, either positive or negative, could not be considered, as the rubber cuff around the patient's neck used in such an apparatus to separate the air about the head from the air about the body would have interfered with the operation at the neck.

From the notes taken by Dr. Carl Eggers, who administered the anaesthetic, I extract the following: For the induction of anaesthesia, 15 cc. of anaesthol was used. Then intubation was performed, a woven silk catheter, No. 18 French, being introduced with the aid of the finger. The catheter was fastened to the upper lip by a suture, as the patient had no teeth to which to tie it. Ether was used now for anaesthesia, 100 cc. sufficing for the entire operation. The pulse was regular and of good quality throughout the operation except when the aorta was strongly pulled over for the purpose of suturing the cut bronchus. At that time it became weak and rose to 102. Strychnin, caffein, and camphor were used for stimulation. A hot coffee enema with whiskey and strychnin was also given at the end of the operation. The intrathoracic portion of the operation, from the incision of the pleura to the closure of the thoracic cavity, took 1 hour and 45 minutes; the whole operation, from the first incision to complete closure, 2 hours and 43 minutes; the general anaesthesia, 2 hours and 27 minutes.

The microscopic examination of the specimen made by Dr. Frederick B. Humphreys proved the new growth to be a squamous celled epithelioma. From his description I quote the following: In the center of the specimen (Fig. 4) [Ed. Note: Figure omitted] there is a ragged indurated ulcer, roughly circular in form, measuring 4.6 cm. across and 4.3 cm. from above down. The ulcer extends over the entire circumference of the mucosa, excepting a small strip about 0.8 cm. in width. The floor of this ulcer is ragged, reddened, and firm, the edges raised and nodular and fairly well circumscribed. The adjacent portions of the oesophageal mucosa show a few small, non-ulcerated, raised nodules, but at the lines of section the mucosa appears entirely free from invasion. The outer surface is rough. The external coat is slightly lacerated, but nowhere has the tumor macroscopically grown through, excepting in one region where there is a nodule about 1 cm. in diameter. Immediately over this nodule is a soft anthracotic lymph node attached to the muscle.

My assistants at the operation were Drs. Frederick H. Dieterich, Martin Bry, and Albert Barge, members of the house staff of the German Hospital. The patient made a good recovery. The stitches were removed, some on the fourth day and the remaining ones on the seventh day, when the wound proved to be completely closed. The pulse, respiration, and temperature had become normal by the fifth day. The highest point that the temperature had reached was 102° F., on the third day after the operation.

Up to the eighth day after the operation the patient was nourished in the same manner as before the operation, through the gastrostomy tube with a funnel attached. After that time the free end of a gastrostomy tube was introduced into the cut end of the oesophagus for the purpose of feeding the patient (Fig. 3). The rubber tube being of somewhat smaller caliber than the oesophagus, the patient has to make slight pressure upon the skin to one side of the tube to prevent leakage. This is accomplished by the patient without the slightest trouble, and she now swallows all varieties of food that can be chewed into an almost fluid state, such as bread, cereals, potatoes, eggs, spinach, etc. As she had not been able to take any bread for about nine months before her operation, she feels very happy with her rubber oesophagus.

A number of methods of oesophagoplasty have been devised, the most promising of which at the present time seems to be that of Jianu, utilizing the greater curvature of the stomach to form an oesophagus. This is placed under the skin of the thorax and in favorable cases may reach up to the end of the divided oesophagus so as to render a union of the two ends possible.

Now that the way for a successful performance of this operation has been shown, it is our evident duty to advise operation as soon as the presence of a carcinoma of the oesophagus is recognized, remembering that success depends to a great degree upon early diagnosis and early operation, and that it is not wise to wait until the difficulty in swallowing becomes marked before our suspicion of the presence of cancer is aroused.

EVARTS A. GRAHAM (1883–1957)

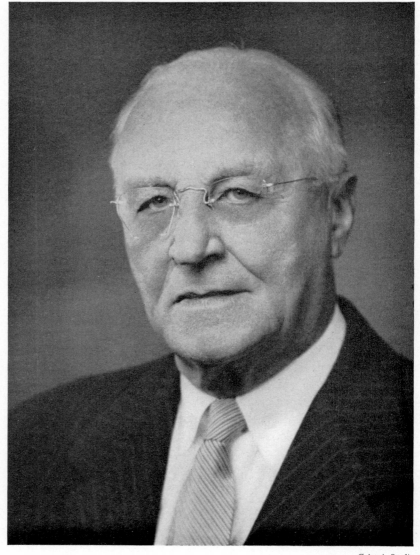

Evarts A. Graham was born in Chicago, Illinois, on March 19, 1883. He attended Princeton and was graduated from Rush Medical College in 1907. His activities were centered about Washington University School of Medicine, the Barnes Hospital and the St. Louis Children's Hospital. He was a founding member of the American Board of Surgery and the Board of Thoracic Surgery. His curriculum vitae filled four typewritten pages and included 16 honorary degrees, 18 awards, 23 lectures, 16 distinctions and a great number of memberships in societies. He was co-editor of Annals of Surgery and Archives of Surgery and was editor of the Year Book of Surgery and of the Journal of Thoracic Surgery.

Dr. Graham's appointment to the Empyema Commission in 1918 was the beginning of a glorious career which was concomitant with the development of thoracic surgery. The men who served on that commission were the fathers of thoracic surgery in this country. Dr. Graham made numerous contributions to the surgical literature and to medical education, including an epoch-making method for cholecystography which has been rated his most important work. Nevertheless, he will best be known for having performed the first successful pneumonectomy for cancer with individual ligation of the hilar structures. The patient, an obstetrician, is alive and well today, thirty-four years later.

The following quotation from Dr. Blalock's memorial oration gives us some insight into Dr. Graham's character: "Warren Cole once said that Dr. Graham instilled so much pride in the mind of the young surgeon that he would become ashamed not to have the proper information on questions related to his research problem." Nathan Womack stated that Dr. Graham expressed complete confidence in the members of his house staff, and, as a result, there developed a spirit among them that looked upon a failure of performance as a break of confidence. Like Billroth and like Halsted, Dr. Graham developed a school of surgery.

He died in March, 1957, of, ironically, carcinoma of the lung.

SUCCESSFUL REMOVAL OF AN ENTIRE LUNG FOR CARCINOMA OF THE BRONCHUS

BY EVARTS A. GRAHAM, M.D.,

AND

J. J. SINGER, M.D.

*From the Medical and Surgical Chest Service of Barnes Hospital
and the Washington University School of Medicine*

Carcinoma of the bronchus in recent years has become a problem of major importance. It is now known that primary carcinoma of the lung, which almost always arises in a bronchus, constitutes between 5 and 10 per cent of all carcinomas. In frequency, therefore, it is comparable with carcinoma of the large intestine, and it is much more frequent than the malignant tumors of some other organs that have received much more comment. The problem of primary carcinoma of the lung is of special importance, since up to the present time at least the prognosis has been almost uniformly bad because of the complete futility of any methods of treatment other than surgical excision. There is no record in the literature of the successful treatment by radiotherapy of a single case in which the pathologic evidence has been incontrovertible and in which a five year interval without recurrence has elapsed between the treatment and the time of reporting the case, despite the fact that many cases have been treated according to the most modern methods of using both x-rays and radium. It would seem, therefore, that unless some entirely new general principle in the treatment of carcinoma is devised, the only method that at

From the *Journal of the American Medical Association, 101:*1971, 1933. Reprinted by permission.

Figure 5 has been omitted.

present can offer any hope is the wide surgical removal of the tumor and the surrounding tissue.

In a recent extensive review of the literature, Carlson and Ballon of the Barnes Hospital have discussed the reported cases in which surgical removal has been accomplished or attempted. In all, there are apparently six cases in the literature in which a patient has survived the surgical removal of the carcinoma and has been well at the time of the report, a year or more later. Two of these patients were operated on by Sauerbruch, one by Churchill, two by Tudor Edwards and one by Allen and Smith. In these reported cases only a limited removal of lung tissue has been performed, amounting, however, in most cases to the removal of one lobe of the lung. In Churchill's case, the lower and middle lobes of the right lung were removed. There have also been six cases reported in which malignant tumors of the bronchi have been removed by means of the bronchoscope. In practically all the latter cases, however, there is no evidence that survival has extended beyond one year. The case about to be reported is apparently the first one in which an entire lung has been successfully removed for a carcinoma. In fact, it is apparently the first time in which the whole lung has been deliberately removed at one stage. It is possible that Kümmell removed the whole lung for a carcinoma, but the description of the case is so meager that it is difficult to be sure. At any rate, the patient died. There are two instances in which an entire lung has been removed for bronchiectasis, one by Nissen of Berlin and the other by Haight of Ann Arbor, Mich. In both the latter cases, however, the lung was allowed to slough out after ligation of the hilus. It seems particularly important to call attention to the fact that an entire lung has been successfully removed for carcinoma of the bronchus because if this should prove to be a feasible operation in properly selected cases it is probable that many patients would be saved who otherwise would die of carcinoma.

REPORT OF CASE

J. L. G., a man, aged 48, a physician, admitted to the Barnes Hospital, Feb. 27, 1933, had had repeated attacks of cough and fever with pain in the left side of the chest for a period of seven months. Other complaints were loss of weight and general lassitude. In January, 1929, he had a pneumonia of the lower lobe of the right lung (the other lung). The pneumonia in the right lung was said to have spread and to have

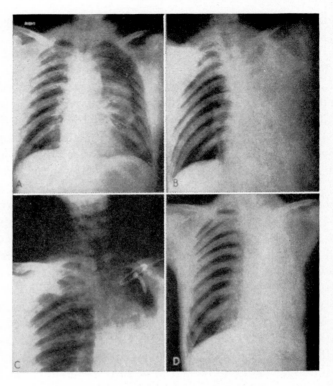

Fig. 1.—Carcinoma obstructing the bronchus of the left upper lobe: *A,* atelectasis of the left upper lobe with the surrounding pneumothorax; *B,* after removal of the entire lung and all but the first two ribs. The air-tight catheter leading to the stump of the bronchus is seen. *C,* drainage of the empyema cavity that was caused by leaving the first two ribs in place. *D,* at time of discharge from the hospital and after the removal of the first two ribs: the empyema cavity is completely obliterated and the wounds are solidly healed; the trachea is in the midline.

involved the entire lung. After several weeks, however, he stated that he recovered fully from the attack of pneumonia until his symptoms appeared insidiously in the left lung more than three years later.

In July, 1932, he complained of malaise with chilly sensations and a temperature of 104 F. At that time nothing was found on physical examination to explain his symptoms. The leukocytes numbered 17,000. August 11, a roentgen examination revealed a fan-shaped shadow with the base outward in the region of the left axilla. By August 20, his symptoms had subsided and the x-ray shadow had become smaller. October 7, he had a repetition of his former symptoms with a return of the former x-ray shadow. These symptoms subsided in a few days but recurred again

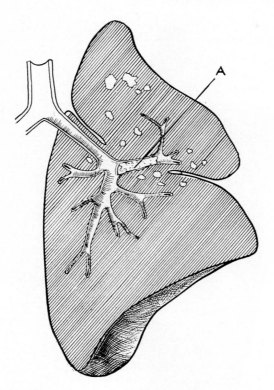

Fig. 2.—Diagram of lung showing (*A*) location of the tumor in the bronchus of the upper lobe but extending so far medially as to project slightly into the bronchus of the lower lobe. For this reason it was impossible to attempt to save the bronchus of the lower lobe. The location of numerous small abscesses is also seen on the diagram as well as the incomplete interlobar fissure.

about October 20. At this time there was some dullness, and a diagnosis either of interlobar empyema or of lung abscess was made. When an attempt was made to aspirate pus, December 5, a pneumothorax developed, after which a marked improvement in his symptoms was noted, although there was a complaint of some pain in the left side of the chest. Artificial pneumothorax was then continued and the patient showed steady improvement until ten days before his admission to the Barnes Hospital (Feb. 17, 1933), when he had a recurrence of fever and dis-

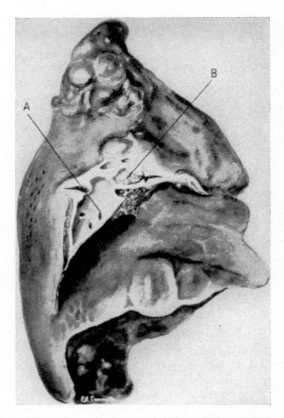

FIG. 3.—Mesial aspect of lung after removal. The main bronchus of the lower lobe (A) has been split open. The tumor (B) is seen projecting from the bronchus of the upper lobe.

comfort. At no time was there any actual pain and never any bloody sputum.

The patient was of medium build with a suggestion of loss of weight and a rather pale complexion. The left side of the chest moved less than the right, and the breath sounds were diminished or absent on that side.

A roentgen examination showed the left upper lobe to be atelectatic with pneumothorax present. The lower lobe seemed to be fully expanded and adherent to the chest wall. The blood examination showed 4,800,000 red cells, 11,500 leukocytes and 85 per cent hemoglobin. Because of the presence of the atelectasis of the upper lobe and in view of the patient's history of an insidious onset, a diagnosis was made of an obstruction of the bronchus of the upper lobe, probably by a tumor. Bronchography with iodized oil substantiated the diagnosis of obstruction of the bronchus

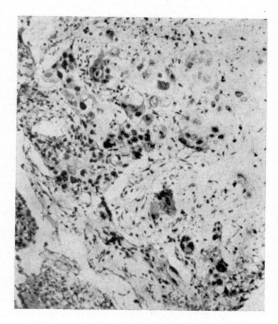

Fig. 4.—Specimen obtained at biopsy through a bronchoscope.

of the left upper lobe. A bronchoscopic examination was accordingly advised and performed by Dr. Arbuckle, March 1. At this time tissue was removed which seemed microscopically to be only granulation tissue. The patient's symptoms improved following this examination, because the obstruction of the bronchus had been somewhat relieved. A bronchoscopic examination was repeated on March 14 and again on March 21, and specimens were removed again at both examinations. Both of these specimens revealed a squamous cell carcinoma of the bronchus. The patient was advised to have the left upper lobe removed because of the presence of the carcinoma obstructing the bronchus of that lobe.

At the operation, however, which was performed, April 5, with intra-tracheal anesthesia of nitrous oxide and oxygen, it was found that the carcinoma extended so closely to the bronchus of the lower lobe that it was impossible to save the latter bronchus. Moreover, there were many nodules in the upper portion of the lower lobe about which uncertainty existed as to whether they were tumor tissue or areas of inflammation. Finally, also the interlobar fissure was not complete. For all these reasons it was decided to remove the entire lung. The adhesions between the lower lobe, chest wall and diaphragm were separated without great dif-ficulty. A small rubber catheter was tied tightly around the hilus as close to the trachea as possible. Crushing clamps were placed on the hilus be-low the catheter and the lung was cut off with an electric cautery knife. The open end of the left main bronchus was carefully cauterized with the actual cautery as far up as the catheter would permit in order to destroy the mucous membrane thoroughly. A transfixing double ligature of number 2 chromic catgut was tied around the stump just distal to the catheter and the latter was then removed. No bleeding occurred. Another transfixing ligature of number 2 chromic catgut was placed where the catheter had been. The stump of the pulmonary artery was then ligated separately with catgut, and seven radon seeds of 1.5 milli-curies each were inserted into various parts of the stump. Several en-larged tracheobronchial glands were removed from the mediastinum, and seven ribs, from the third to the ninth, inclusive, were removed from the transverse processes of the spine to the anterior axillary line. The ribs were removed for the purpose of allowing the soft tissues of the chest wall to collapse against the bronchial stump and therefore to obliterate as much as possible the pleural cavity. The first and second ribs were not removed at this time merely because it was desired not to do too much operating at once. Nevertheless, it was felt that there would be some danger of the development of an empyema in the upper part of the pleural cavity because of the failure to obliterate that space. The wound was closed tightly, but provision for drainage was made by the use of an air-tight catheter brought out through a stab wound. [*Ed. Note:* Fig. 5 omitted.]

The patient left the operating room in excellent condition but was nevertheless given a transfusion of 500 cc. of blood. The closed drainage yielded about 800 cc. af serosanguineous fluid during each of the first two days. After that period the drainage rapidly diminished and practically ceased on the fifth postoperative day. The catheter was gradually with-drawn. The wound healed by primary intention. There was surprisingly little immediate postoperative reaction of any kind except for a moderate amount of dyspnea on exertion and deep seated pain in the back, which was controlled with opiates. On the ninth postoperative day there was a collection of air and pus in the extreme upper portion of the pleural cavity. The rest of the pleural cavity was completely obliterated by what seemed to be solid healing of the soft tissues of the chest wall against the mediastinal pleura. The small empyema cavity in the upper part of the thorax was drained through a stab wound made posteriorly just below the second rib. It was evident, both from the previous accumulation of air in the unobliterated portion of the cavity and also because the patient

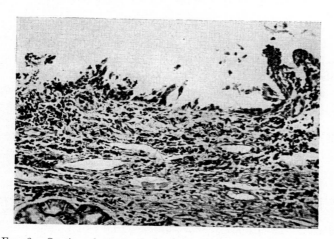

Fig. 6.—Section through the wall of the bronchus about 0.5 cm. mesial to the tumor. There is no evidence of carcinoma at this place. Evidently, therefore, the tumor was confined to its original location.

was coughing up pus, that there was a small communication between the unobliterated portion of the pleural cavity and the bronchial stump. After about two weeks the drainage tube slipped out of the cavity and was found on the dressings. The wound had healed sufficiently so that it was difficult to replace the catheter. It was therefore decided to re-establish drainage anteriorly in order to have the back free from infection when the first and second ribs should be removed. A small drain. therefore, was placed through the first interspace, anteriorly, for a few days. The patient's temperature and pulse had been normal during the entire time of the drainage of the empyema cavity. May 22, through a posterior incision, the first and second ribs were removed in almost their entire length. There was almost no reaction after this operation. The small remnant of pleural cavity was completely obliterated at once.

The pain in the back subsided and within three weeks the wounds were all solidly healed. The patient's strength gradually increased, his appetite was excellent and he was discharged from the hospital, June 18, looking and feeling better than he had for many months previously. His only complaint was some dyspnea on exertion, but he had been walking about the hospital for two weeks before his discharge. His vital capacity on admission was 3,500 cc.; at his discharge it was 1,650 cc. Also, at the time of discharge an examination of the blood showed 5,100,000 red

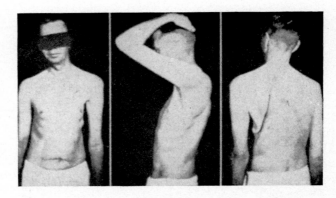

Fig. 7.—The patient at time of discharge from the hospital. The wounds are solidly healed and he has good movement of the left arm.

cells, 8,500 leukocytes and 90 per cent hemoglobin. An electrocardiogram was essentially normal and a roentgen examination showed the left pleural cavity to be completely obliterated. A report received from him, July 25, five weeks after his discharge, stated that he had gained 8 pounds (3.6 Kg.) at home, that he was able to walk about a mile without much dyspnea, that he was driving his automobile and that his strength was rapidly improving. The dyspnea was rapidly becoming less.

COMMENT

The examination of the lung after its removal was encouraging, because it showed no evidence of any extension of the carcinoma beyond the original site. The whole tumor measured only about 1 cm. in the long diameter, but it was situated almost at the bifurcation of the main bronchus into the bronchus of the upper lobe and that of the lower lobe. The nodules, which had been felt in the lung at operation, were small abscesses that showed no evidence of carcinoma on microscopic examination. Likewise, the enlarged tracheobronchial glands, which had been removed from the mediastinum, showed no evidence of carcinoma. The tumor itself was definitely a squamous cell carcinoma. A feature of it, which is probably important, was that it had not invaded the bronchial cartilage. By analogy with what is well known concerning carcinoma of the larynx, the failure of the tumor to invade the bronchial cartilage in this case would seem to be of excellent prognostic significance.

Several features about this case warrant special comment. In the light of the experience derived from this first case of complete removal of a lung, together with many of the mediastinal tracheobronchial glands, for carcinoma, the operation would seem to be one that is entirely feasible in properly selected cases. Just as experience with carcinoma in other parts of the body has taught that the number of cures is, in general, directly proportional to the extent of radical removal, so it may be inferred, perhaps, that if the entire lung is removed the patient will have less chance of a recurrence than if only one lobe or a smaller portion is removed. In order, however, to have a creditable number of successes, surgeons who are properly qualified by experience in this special field to perform such an operation must receive the patient before extensive metastases have occurred. There is now little excuse for the common failure to diagnose a carcinoma of the bronchus in its early stages. Certainly the majority of such tumors can be diagnosed before demonstrable metastases have occurred.

Another feature of peculiar interest in this case is that, despite the fact that the hilus of the entire lung was suddenly shut off by a tight ligature, none of the signs or symptoms of pulmonary embolism appeared. The sudden obstruction of the pulmonary artery of the left lung by the ligature was analogous to the sudden obstruction of it by an embolus. Nevertheless, not the slightest change in the character of the patient's respiration could be noted immediately following the application of the ligature. Possibly the fact that he was receiving intratracheal anesthesia was of importance.

SUMMARY

The left lung and many of the tracheobronchial mediastinal glands were removed in a one stage operation because of a carcinoma that originated in the bronchus of the upper lobe but which was so close to the bronchus of the lower lobe that, in order to remove it completely, it was necessary to remove the entire lung. This is apparently the first case in which an entire lung has been removed successfully at one stage.[1]

[1] A letter from the patient written on Sept. 19, 1933, four and one-half months after the operation, states that his weight has increased by 16 pounds (7.3 Kg.) since leaving the hospital and that he is constantly gaining in strength and energy.

11. Cardiovascular Surgery

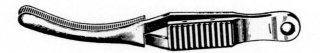

PREFATORY COMMENTS

References to cardiovascular surgery date back to antiquity. The classic Antyllus operation for aneurysm was performed in the first century A.D. However, the groundwork for the astounding developments in the last few decades dates back only to the end of the last century. Although Eck, Jasinowsky and Heidenhain had done blood vessel suture and anastomoses, their methods were not satisfactory. In 1896, in France, Jaboulay and Briau performed vessel anastomoses and grafts in the dog, using through and through, intima to intima interrupted sutures. Later that same year, in the United States, J. B. Murphy, the designer of the rubber button for intestinal anastomosis, independently described what we believe to be the first planned resection and anastomosis of an artery in the human. He standardized his technique after doing 34 animal experiments and thereby emphasized the importance of the experimental method. He was singularly well-prepared to operate upon a patient whose femoral artery had been lacerated by a bullet. Murphy resected one-half inch of the patient's artery and performed an end-to-end suture by invaginating one end into the other. He also started working with grafts composed of tubes of magnesium and caramel, forerunners of plastic prostheses.

The most monumental piece of surgical investigation emanated from the efforts of Alexis Carrel. His primary interest was in the transplantation of organs which depended in great measure on his ability to successfully anastomose blood vessels. Like many other developments in surgical technique, the keynote of his success was simplicity. His method of triangulating the cut ends of vessels before su-

363

turing has stood the test of time. Carrel had limited success in his attempts at transplanting organs but a preliminary step, viz., successful anastomosis of blood vessels, constituted a major contribution to the development of surgery.

In New Orleans the incidence of arterial aneurysm was high primarily because of the high rate of syphilis in the Negro population. Here flourished a progressive school of surgery led by Rudolf Matas, whose contributions to the development of an "intravenous drip" apparatus and of thoracotomy under endotracheal anesthesia were far-reaching. His technique of endoaneurysmorrhaphy opened a new era in surgery of the blood vessels. One can appreciate his misgivings at the time of his first operation when he stated, "I found myself in a dilemma and it occurred to me that the best way out of my trouble was to close the orifices through which blood was coming at me."

During the past decade there has been a phenomenal increase in the advances in the field of vascular surgery. Among the many contributors, Gross and Hufnagel, Blakemore, Harkins, DeBakey, Cooley, Julian and Bahnson are prominent. This is an era alive with great discoveries, when scarcely a month goes by without the appearance of a startling new development in the surgical literature. In 1948 Gross successfully resected a coarctation of the aorta and employed a homologous graft to close the defect. In March, 1951, Dubost resected an abdominal aortic aneurysm and bridged the gap with a homologous graft. These epoch-making events acted as catalysts in setting off a number of reactions which were to contribute heavily to the welfare of mankind. In 1919 Guthrie reported the successful use of formalin-fixed arterial grafts in the experimental animal. More recently, plastic materials like nylon, orlon, vinyon N, and dacron have been employed with a high incidence of success in bridging the ends of large arteries but with limited success in the treatment of occlusive disease of the smaller arteries. These tremendous advances were accomplished about fifty years after Carrel's work. The delay was unduly long when one considers that blood replacement and safe anesthesia had been in vogue for many years.

The direct attack upon the heart was also delayed more than twenty years since the first finger "fracture" of a mitral valve was successfully performed by Sir Henry Souttar in 1925. Prior to that, in 1913, finger dilatation of a stenotic pulmonary valve was attempted by Doyen, and a year later Tuffier dilated an aortic valve through the invaginated aortic wall, with survival of the patient but with only temporary success. Because of the contributions to this field made by Smithy, Bailey, Harken, Glover and many others, mitral commissurotomy has become a safe and efficacious procedure.

It was a logical outgrowth of this work on the mitral valve for the more enterprising and ingenious surgeon to attack the anomalies of the other valves. Now all four valves have been successfully operated on but the aortic valve has been the most difficult and the mortality rate in the treatment of aortic stenosis and insufficiency remains high. As in the treatment of disease of the other three valves, the mortality rate associated with direct attack on the aortic valve will undoubtedly decrease as the experience of the surgeon grows. The extracardiac anomalies defied treatment until 1937 when Greybiel, Strieder and Boyer made an unsuccessful attempt to ligate a patent ductus arteriosus. In the following year Gross reported the first successful operation for closure of a patent ductus. In 1945 Blalock reported improvement in the condition of "blue babies" manifesting the tetralogy of Fallot after anastomosing the subclavian to the pulmonary artery. During the same year, Crafoord and Gross almost simultaneously reported curing coarctation of the aorta by resection and anastomosis. One year later, Potts described an ingenious clamp which he designed to enable him to create an aortic–pulmonic "window" for treatment of the tetralogy of Fallot. Now attempts are being made to cure this anomaly by eradicating all the defects rather than by the institution of another defect in the form of an artificial patent ductus arteriosus. How these advances are being made will be discussed more fully in the final chapter entitled "Milestones on the Horizon."

The development of improved technique in the anastomosis of veins was slow since there were so few diseases which required this procedure for their amelioration or cure. In 1879 Eck had described an elaborate method of creating an opening between the portal vein and the vena cava in dogs. The efficacy of diminishing the pressure in the portal bed of humans by a side-tracking procedure can be attributed to the painstaking labors of Blakemore, Whipple, Rousselot, Linton and many others.

The reader should be imbued with the feeling that this chapter of surgery is opening and constitutes our heritage. It is an exciting era in which we live because so many major developments are unfolding and will continue to unfold before our eyes. They are awaiting the understanding, the integration, the experience and the insatiable curiosity of the prepared mind.

NIKOLAI VLADIMIROVICH ECK[1] (1849–1908)

Nikolai Vladimirovich Eck was born in Petersburg, on November 9, 1849. From 1865 to 1871 he was a student of the Medical and Surgical Academy, from which he graduated with distinction. His name was entered on the marble board in the conference hall and he was awarded the Busch Prize. For his work on "polypus of the Larynx" presented in his last university year, N. V. Eck was awarded a gold medal.

On January 7, 1872 N. V. Eck started work as an interne in the 1-st therapeutic department of the Military Hospital, where he worked until March 31, 1878. From 1872 to 1875 he worked as an externe in the maternity hospital of the St. Petersburg foundling home. On May 22, 1877 he was appointed reserve surgeon of the army.

From June 20, 1877 to March 31, 1878 N. V. Eck worked on the Balkan front in divisional hospitals and dressing stations. He also did some important work in connection with the organization of hospitals in Sofia. On March 1st, 1880 N. V. Eck was dismissed from the army at his own request.

On August 14, 1883, he was appointed delegate of the Russian government to the international sanitary council in Alexandria for observations on the progress of cholera. On his return from Egypt in February 1884 he handed in two articles: "The Results of a Mission to Egypt in Connection With the Epidemic of Cholera in 1883–1884" and "Quarantine in Egyptian Waters," which were published in the collection of works of the Society of Russian Physicians.

On April 1, 1885 N. V. Eck was appointed physician to the Ministry of Finance.

On April 12, 1885 he was sent as delegate to the international sanitary conference in Rome.

---

[1] This is an exact copy of the biography sent us by the Soviet Information Bureau in Moscow following our request to the Russian Embassy in Washington, D.C.

N. Eck was a member of the Society of Russian Physicians in Petersburg, The Russian Surgical Society named after prof. Pirogov and the Physicians' Society of Plotsk and member of the Medical Academy of Rome.

The idea of porto-caval anastomosis in cases of scirrhosis of the liver belongs to Nikolai Eck, who was also the first to perform this operation on a dog. He was the first author who described in medical literature a case of interstitial myoma of the womb and the first surgeon in Russia to remove a cancerous womb.

N. Eck was also the first in Russia to perform a resection of the cancerous forepart of the stomach.

N. Eck suggested an original method of urano-plastics, which is used to this day and named after him.

Towards the end of his life N. V. Eck abandoned medicine and took up mining. He has left some works on geology.

N. V. Eck died on April 2, 1908.

N. V. Eck wrote the following works: "Grafting Normal Epithelium," "Three Ovariotomies," "Two Histerotomies with a Favourable Issue, Performed in a Temporary Rural Hospital," "Dressing Neck Veins," "A New Method of Staphylorraphy," "Making Ligatures in Cases of Nose Polypus," "The Sanitation of Russia," "Experience in Working Out Statistical Data on Mortality in Russia," and a number of other works.

ECK'S FISTULA

BY CHARLES G. CHILD, III, M.D.

*Department of Surgical Research of the Department of Surgery
of the New York Hospital-Cornell Medical Center*

With the recent renewed interest in the treatment of portal hypertension by means of portal decompression, no article has been quoted more often than has that of Nikolai Eck. Because Eck's original article was published in Russian in the *Military Medical Journal* it has never been readily available to those in this country interested in this field of vascular surgery. It has seemed worth while, therefore, to publish a translation of this classic essay. A photostat of the original was obtained from the Surgeon General's Library and translated by Dr. Ilia N. Kovarsky, Recording Secretary of the Russian Medical Society of New York City.

In reviewing this article, two facts are of especial interest. First, Eck suggested that his shunt might prove useful in man for the control of ascites, not in the management of patients with esophagogastric hemorrhage from a varix. Second, Eck stated that his inspiration to devise this venous shunt was derived from an abstract of an article by B. F. Lautenbach of Philadelphia entitled "On a New Function of the Liver." The original article appeared in the *Philadelphia Medical Times*, 1876–1877, 7:387. The abstract to which Eck refers appeared in the July issue of the *Military Medical Journal*. This was also translated by Dr. Kovarsky who stated that the abstract follows faithfully Lautenbach's original article. For this reason, there is little purpose in publishing a translation of this abstract.

From *Surgery, Gynecology and Obstetrics,* 96:275, 1953. Reprinted by permission of *Surgery, Gynecology and Obstetrics.*

CONCERNING LIGATION OF THE VENA PORTA

Preliminary Notification by Dr. N. Eck

If the portal vein of a dog is ligated after making sure that the blood from this vein flows freely into the inferior vena cava, then this change in the direction of the blood flow and deprival of the liver of the portal blood does not cause any serious disturbance to the body. The animal recovers after such an operation, its nutritional status improves gradually, and it remains in perfect health thereafter.

By means of several experiments, including more than 60 vivisections, I have worked out a convenient method for establishing a fistula between the above mentioned veins.

With 3 longitudinal fine silk sutures, I sew the left side of the anterior surface of the inferior vena cava to the left side of the posterior surface of the portal vein. Thereafter I sew the right side of the posterior surface of the portal vein to the right anterior part of the vena cava by means of a line of sutures alike and symmetrical with the first 3 sutures.

Sutured in this way, the veins oppose one another on approximately equal surface. Upon these surfaces which are delimited by 2 rows of sutures, a fistula between the sutured veins is formed by means of a longitudinal cut of the walls. The intravascular tension presses the edges of the gash of one vein to the edges of the gash of the other vein so that any outside hemorrhage is prevented.

For the incision of the veins, I invented small scissors curved under an angle on the same plane. To each point of the scissors, a thin, long, silver wire is soldered with a steel needle at each end.

After application of the first row of sutures, by means of which the left sides of the veins are sewed, and before putting in the second row of sutures, one establishes approximately the site of the eventual incision of each vein. Throughout the entire length of this incision we introduce into either vein the wires from the ends of the scissors in such a way that the needle with the wire which is introduced at the level of the inferior suture is brought out from the lumen of the vein opposite to the superior suture. When these wires have been introduced, the right sides of the veins are sewed up. By pulling at the wires, the slightly opened scissors are introduced from below into the space between the veins. The blades of the scissors follow the wires and enter into each vein. The walls of the veins are cut by gently moving the blades of the scissors from the point of the entrance of the wires to their exit. The completion of the incision is indicated by the fact that the scissors now move freely between the veins. Afterward, the scissors with the wires are pulled out. The portal vein is ligated at the entrance into the liver by means of previously set ligature. The abdominal cavity is cleaned of blood and sewed up carefully.

According to this method, I operated on 8 dogs. Among them, 1 did not survive 24 hours, and 6 survived from 2 to 7 days. One, which was operated upon on May 28, recovered completely and lived in the laboratory for 2½ months. Because of lack of attention, he ran away on August 10. The cause of death in the 7 cases mentioned was peritonitis or strangulation of the intestines and omentum.

Formation of clots in the splenic vein was found in 2 cases only in which the length of incision did not exceed 1 centimeter; in 1 of these cases there was occlusion of the vein with enlargement of the spleen. Occlusion does not occur when the fistula is 1½ to 2 centimeters long, and the outflow of the venous blood from the abdominal organs goes on undisturbed.

This preliminary communication was stimulated by the work of Lautenbach, "On a New Function of the Liver," which I read in the "Journal Review" in the *Military Medical Journal* of July of this year.

I am conducting these experiments with the purpose of clarifying some physiological problems as well as to determine whether it would be possible to treat some cases of mechanical ascites by means of forming such a fistula.

I consider the main reason to doubt that such an operation can be carried out on human beings has been removed because it was established that the blood of the portal vein, without any danger to the body, could be diverted directly into the general circulation and this by means of a perfectly safe operation.

I made the above mentioned 8 experiments in the laboratory of Professor I. R. Tarchanow. I had to postpone further experiments because I was called to join the active army.

September 25th
October 7th, 1877

ALEXIS CARREL (1873–1944)

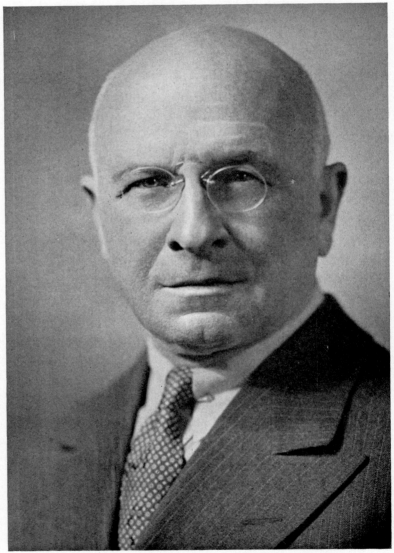

Alexis Carrel was born at Sainte-Foy near Lyons, France. He received his M.D. degree in 1900 and in 1902, at the age of 29, published his classic paper on blood-vessel anastomosis. He came to America in 1905, where he later joined the Rockefeller Institute and eventually became its director. His work on tissue culture and transplantation of organs has provided the basis for present-day and future milestone accomplishments. There are few experiments which are done today on organ transplantation that were not previously described by Carrel. In the first decade of the twentieth century, he transplanted kidneys in dogs with technical success. Other contributions include the Carrel–Dakin treatment of wounds and studies on the altered characteristics of in vitro tissue cultures as regards acceleration or inhibition of growth. His work on the artificial cultivation of whole organs, done in collaboration with Col. Charles Lindberg, gained wide recognition. In 1912 he received the Nobel Prize "for his work on vascular suturing and on the grafting of blood vessels and organs."

He died in Paris on November 5, 1944.

THE OPERATIVE TECHNIQUE OF VASCULAR ANASTOMOSES AND THE TRANSPLANTATION OF ORGANS

BY DR. CARREL

During the latter months of 1901 I began researches on the operative technique of vascular anastomoses with the objective of accomplishing the transplantation of certain organs.

This transplantation consists of taking a gland, thyroid or kidney, for example, removing it with its artery and vein, then to graft these vessels to another point in the circulatory mechanism. Though a simple operative curiosity today, the transplantation of a gland may some day have a practical application.

We studied only those techniques necessary to accomplish good union of blood vessels, often very small in size.

The method I wish to describe is very simple. It works equally well for arteries and veins; for large vessels or those of small calibre. It respects the integrity of the endothelium. The anastomosis is absolutely watertight and does not cause narrowing in the calibre of the vessel. It is as easy to do an end-to-side anastomosis as an end-to-end. It is performed simply.

None of the methods presently employed have all of these advantages. This superiority is due to the use of *extremely fine needles,* and a maneuver which permits *dilation of the vessel* at the time of suture and prevents constriction.

Translated, by permission, from *Lyon Medical,* vol. xciii, 1902.

We have availed ourselves of Kirby number 13 or number 14 needles and of linen threads, used in the manufacture of Valenciennes lace, or more simply number 500 Alsatian cotton. These solid, round, very sharp needles, finer than any used by surgeons up to the present time, allow penetration of the venous or arterial walls without fear of oozing. On the other hand, their tenuousness permits easy insertion into the wall without disturbing the arterial endothelium. The only drawback is the smallness of the eye, which makes it difficult to thread. Practice with the needle overcomes this difficulty. The dilation of the vessel at the time of suture is accomplished by a very simple stratagem. Three supporting sutures are applied at equidistant points around the circumference of the vessel. Traction on each of these threads converts the circumference to a triangle, the sides of which can be elongated as far as the elasticity of the coats will permit. A closely placed overcast suture is then carried out rapidly on the three sides.

With the same objective of preventing narrowing, we have tried anastomotic tubes or rods. Some were of magnesium, which are absorbable according to Payr, others were of a blood soluble substance, caramel.

The magnesium tube was introduced into the lumen of the vessel; one could gently overlap the coats of the two ends and join them with a linen thread. This procedure did not seem very advantageous to me; it is difficult to insert a large enough tube into the lumen, and the embarrassment of the circulation produced by this foreign body makes coagulation probable.

The caramel tubes or rods were used with the aim to facilitate a circular overcasting suture while the wall of the vessel was stretched. I have never had fear of impeding the circulation because the caramel is embedded in a few minutes as soon as the forceps which are used for temporary hemostasis are removed.

I have renounced their use as well because introduction of a large enough rod is difficult and because dilation by traction on three equidistant points about the circumference is so effective and makes suture so much easier.

A vascular anastomosis can be end-to-end or end-to-side depending upon whether the calibre of the vessels to be united is almost equal or quite different. For example, it is possible to do an end-to-end union of the common carotid and renal arteries in the dog; on the other hand, it is necessary to do an end-to-side anastomosis of the thyroid artery to the carotid. Because of their thinness and their great expansibility, veins of quite different size can often be united end to end.

We will describe the end-to-end procedure. We will indicate the variations employed for end-to-side suture.

The operation requires several phases.

1st phase:—*Temporary hemostasis.* Between one and two centimeters from their free end, the vessels are grasped with rubber-shod forceps. The assistant takes a clamp in each hand and holds the ends of the vessels in view.

2nd phase:—*Preparation of the ends of the vessels.* The operator frees the area of section by sharp scissor dissection. If the external coat has slid like a veil over the lumen of the vessel so as to obstruct it, it is necessary to resect it a little distance further. This phase of the operation is delicate especially when it is a question of very small arteries or veins.

3rd phase:—*Passage of supporting sutures.* At one extremity, at three equidistant points on the circumference, three needles are embedded into the external coat toward the endothelium. If the calibre of the artery is sufficiently large, the point of the needle can go through the wall without penetrating the endothelium.

The three needles are removed, leaving three loops of thread in the wall of the vessel (Fig. 1).

On the other vascular pedicle, the three needles are passed from within outwards at three equidistant points around the circumference.

They are removed.

The assistant brings the vascular ends together. The operator tightens and ties the three sutures. The two ends of the vessel now are found united at three equidistant points in their circumference.

4th phase:—*Conversion of the circumference of the junction into a triangle by traction on the guide sutures. Overcasting.* The guide sutures have been marked with forceps. With the help of these forceps eccentric traction is exerted on the arterial wall, so as to transform the circumference into an equilateral triangle, following which they are brought into juxtaposition and the ends of the vessels can be sutured (Fig. 1).

This maneuver permits the calibre of the vessel to be dilated as much as necessary before performing the overcasting. Well done, this wholly prevents constriction and greatly favors the suture.

The assistant successively presents each side of the triangle to the operator. It is then very easy to anastomose by a continuous over-and-over suture, closely approximated, the lips of the ends of the vessels being well spread (Fig. 2).

The operation is finished. The temporary hemostasis is released and the circulation is reestablished.

If it has been possible to stitch the interstitial tissues alone, the watertightness is absolute. In the anastomosis of small vessels where the

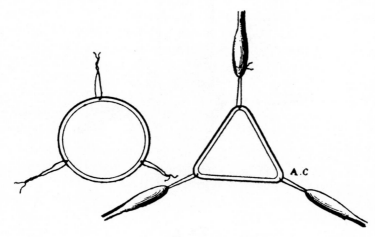

FIG. I.

stitches have perforated the mucosa, it produces a slightly bloody ooze which stops spontaneously in a short time, one or two minutes at the most.

The end-to-side anastomosis has an almost identical procedure. After temporary hemostasis and the preparation of the end of the smaller vessel, a small opening is made in the wall of the larger vessel. This orifice should be a bit larger than the calibre of the small vessel.

Then, the three guide sutures are applied and the rest of the operation follows the rules already established.

I have used this procedure for end-to-end union of large arteries and large veins and for the transplantation of certain organs.

The suture of an artery or vein which is cut transversely, gives no narrowing. When using a large artery such as the femoral in man, the endothelium remains intact, the sutures being entirely interstitial, and there is no constriction. On the living dog, circulation is reestablished very easily.

Thanks to M. le professeur Soulier, who placed his new laboratory at my disposal for these experiments, and the valuable collaboration of M.M. Morel and Marcel Soulier, I have been able to practice transplantation of organs in the dog, such as the kidney and the thyroid

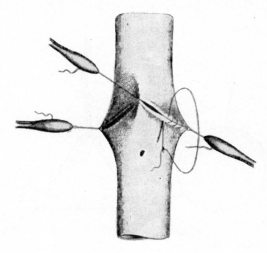

FIG. 2.

whose vessels were grafted to the common carotid artery and the external jugular vein.

Here is an example:

In a dog, one of the kidneys, removed by transperitoneal nephrectomy, was placed in the cervical region. The renal artery and vein were anastomosed to the carotid and the external jugular. With elimination of the temporary hemostasis, we have seen the renal arteries throb under the flood of arterial blood, the veins distend and fill with black blood, and the kidney loses its violaceous color to regain its redness and warmth. In about half an hour, a little red serum appears at the end of the ureter which is connected to the skin. But we do not wish to consider anything but the operative result; the arterial suture was excellent despite the fact that the renal artery was quite small. The vein suture oozed a bit of blood, but in a minute this stopped.

The experiments that we have pursued to this moment on the transplantation of the thyroid, the kidney, the pancreas, etc., are too little advanced for it to be possible to draw any conclusions whatever at this time.

We know only that the method I have described allows the accomplishment, in a simple enough fashion, of the difficult anastomosis which is demanded for the transplantation of an organ.

RUDOLPH MATAS (1860-1957)

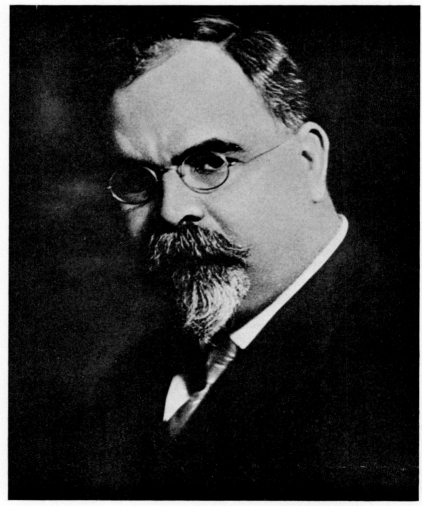

Biographical Sketch by Isidore Cohn, M.D.

*Rudolph Matas, described by William Osler as "our modern Antyllus"
and universally regarded as the father of modern vascular surgery, was
born in the United States of Catalonian parents, on September 1, 1860.
His mother's brother, an early emigré to the United States, persuaded his
newly married sister and her husband, Narciso Hereu y Matas, to follow
him to New Orleans.*

*There Rudolph was born, two months before Lincoln's first election as
president. When hostilities between North and South began, his father,
in cooperation with the Union occupation chiefs at New Orleans,
amassed a tidy fortune by bartering tobacco, medicines, and war ma-
tériel to the Confederacy for cotton, which was sold at a fantastic profit
in Liverpool, Boston and other markets supposedly closed by Union
blockade and embargo. Wealthy Narciso and his family returned to
Europe, where he studied ophthalmology in Paris under de Wecker, and
then settled in Barcelona. But a disastrous venture into railroad speculation wiped him out, and he returned to New Orleans in 1867 to amass
another stake.*

*He landed at the height of a yellow fever epidemic in which 7-year-
old Rudolph contracted a "benign" case; that is, one from which he recovered, with lifelong immunity against future infections. Later the family moved to Brownsville, Texas, and Matamoros, Mexico, where the boy
began his English schooling on the American side, but completed preparatory education at the Colegio de San Juan in Matamoros.*

*In 1877 he matriculated in the Medical College of Louisiana, now
Tulane University, and distinguished himself from the first in competi-
tive tests through which he secured and retained appointment as a resident student at Charity Hospital. When he was 19 Dr. Stanford Chaillé*

selected him to serve as clerk, laboratory assistant and interpreter of the U.S. Yellow Fever Commission to Havana. There Rudolph met Dr. Carlos Finlay, with whom he left a set of the commission's photomicrographs of blood smears and tissue sections from yellow fever victims.

The fact that these showed the blood corpuscles not disorganized in any way suggested to Finlay that yellow fever was an "inwardly eruptive malady" whose infection must therefore be transmitted by some bloodsucking insect. He published his then much-derided mosquito hypothesis in 1881, when his only convert was newly (1880) graduated Rudolph Matas; as associate editor of the New Orleans Medical and Surgical Journal, the young man translated, published and subsequently defended the Finlay paper. Meanwhile he was summoned to aid in checking a disastrous yellow fever epidemic in the Rio Grande Valley. One of his first patients at Fort Brown was a lieutenant recently commissioned in the Medical Corps, William Crawford Gorgas.

Dr. Matas' subsequent career was meteoric. At 23 he was made editor of the New Orleans Medical and Surgical Journal; at 25 he succeeded Dr. A. B. Miles as Demonstrator of Anatomy for Tulane's medical school, and at 35 he succeeded to the chair of surgery in which such men as Tobias Richardson and Samuel Logan had preceded him. In this same year, 1895, he married Adrienne Goslee. The only child of this union was stillborn, but one of Mrs. Matas' two sons by a former marriage, Lucian Landry, became a physician and was for many years closely associated with his stepfather.

Dr. Matas' first major contribution to the advancement of his profession was a monumental paper, published in 1885, categorically defining the cecum and appendix as intraperitoneal; but the greatest of his achievements was the development of the intrasaccular suture for the surgical relief of aneurisms. This was first done in May, 1888, as an operation of necessity, not of election, yet it succeeded beyond all expectations. The patient, who had been in extremis, lived out a normal life expectancy as a plantation hand engaged in heavy manual labor.

Dr. Matas was also the first surgeon in the United States to perform an operation under spinal anesthesia (1889) and his pioneer researches in the use of local anesthesia brought him and W. S. Halsted into close

*friendship. Among his other major contributions to medicosurgical prog-
ress were the intravenous drip, the indwelling catheter for siphon drainage of the gastrointestinal tract, and a positive-pressure apparatus to eliminate the hazards of thoracic surgery.*

*Many of his successes were achieved after 1908, when he lost one eye
through an infection which necessitated enucleation. His unfaltering
courage and his cheery assurances to others of what "we Cyclopeans can
accomplish in a binocular world" have heartened any number of those
who have suffered similar impairments.*

*Within the compass of this thumbnail portrait it is clearly impossible
to list even a tithe of the honors accorded him. He received the first Dis-
tinguished Service Medal (1938) bestowed by the American Medical
Association, the first Order of Carlos Finlay awarded in Havana by the
Cuban Government and the Academy of Sciences. He served as president
of the American Surgical Association, Southern Surgical Association,
American Society of Thoracic Surgery, Louisiana State and Orleans
Parish Medical Association, and in 1936 was elected* in absentia *to the
presidency of the International Surgical Society at that body's meeting in
Cairo.*

*Perhaps the best known of his writings was an address before the Mis-
sissippi State Medical Society, under the title "The Soul of a Surgeon."*

*In 1926 he became Tulane's Emeritus Professor of Surgery, devoting
himself thereafter to private practice and an active participation in civic
affairs; he remained extraordinarily vigorous until total blindess and the
growing debility of age compelled his withdrawal from such activities
after his ninety-second birthday. He died in New Orleans on September
23, 1957, at the age of ninety-seven.*

AN OPERATION FOR THE
RADICAL CURE OF ANEURISM
BASED UPON ARTERIORRHAPHY

BY RUDOLPH MATAS, M.D.

*Professor of Surgery in the Medical Department of the
Tulane University of Louisiana*

The radical cure of aneurism as classically described embraces two distinct procedures: (1) The old operation of Antyllus, in which the sac is left *in situ* after evacuation of the contained clot and ligation of the proximal and distal ends of the main artery outside of the sac, and (2) Purmann's operation, also attributed to Phillagrius, in which the sac is extirpated *in toto* or in its greater part. Numerous modifications of these procedures have been suggested at various times and by different operators, which affect details of technique, but do not alter the fundamental principles of these methods. In the original procedures, as well as in their subsequent modifications, from remote antiquity to the present time, the ligature has been relied upon almost exclusively as the haemostatic agent to arrest the circulation in the sac and to control the bleeding from the artery which feeds the aneurism.

In the operation described in this paper, the sac is, as a rule, not extirpated or disturbed, except in so much as is required to evacuate its contents and freely expose its interior, and in this way it may be regarded as a derivative of the old Antyllian operation. Apart from this it differs essentially from either of the classical procedures in the fact that no ligatures are applied to the main artery, and that the

From *Annals of Surgery,* 37:161, 1903. Reprinted by permission.
Figures 1, 4, 7, 11, 13, 14 have been omitted.

circulation in the sac is arrested, and haemostasis is secured, solely by suturing the arterial orifices found in the interior of the sac. Again, in suitable cases—that is, in the true sacciform aneurisms with a single orifice of communication with the parent artery—this method will allow the operator to obliterate the aneurism without obstructing the lumen of the artery or interfering with the circulation in the injured or diseased vessel,—a great desideratum which should never be lost sight of when operating upon this class of cases.

Finally, it differs essentially from the Antyllian operation in the fact that the cavity of the sac is not simply packed or drained and left to heal by granulation, but is at once obliterated by inverting or infolding the walls of the sac with the attached overlying skin. The flaps thus formed are sutured to the bottom of the cavity, so that no dead spaces are left to suppurate or favor secondary complications.

The operation now proposed by the writer is applicable to all aneurisms in which there is a distinct sac, and in which the cardiac end of the main artery can be provisionally controlled. It is especially applicable to all forms of peripheral aneurisms of the larger arterial trunks (carotid, axillary, brachial, iliac, femoral, and popliteal); and, while the author has had no experience with similar lesions of the large visceral trunks, the principle suggested would appear to be applicable to abdominal aortic and other accessible forms of abdominal aneurisms. It is particularly indicated in the treatment of traumatic aneurisms in which the wounded artery communicates with a well-developed and circumscribed sac, and in all fusiform and sacculated aneurisms, whether traumatic or idiopathic, in which the conditions for securing provisional haemostasis can be obtained. The method proposed does not contemplate the treatment of arteriovenous aneurism and the circumscribed or diffuse pulsating haematomas of recent origin, which result from arterial and arteriovenous injuries. These cases offer admirable opportunities for the conservative application of arteriorrhaphy, with the view of preserving the lumen of the injured vessel, and thus maintaining their functional value as blood-carriers. Notable illustrations of the value of arterial and venous suture in cases of diffuse traumatic aneurism, or, rather, pulsating haematoma, are the cases of simultaneous injury of the common femoral artery and vein, reported by Murphy, of Chicago, in 1897, and by Cammaggio in 1898. Murphy's case is especially notable as the first on record in which an artery was successfully united by suture after circular resection of the injured area.

Steps of the Operation As Applied to Peripheral Aneurisms of the Larger Arteries

1. *Prophylactic Haemostasis.*—The circulation of the limb should be controlled by preliminary elevation of the limb, followed by the application of the Esmarch elastic constrictor. Prophylactic haemostasis may also be obtained when the aneurism is situated high up near the root of a limb (or in the neck) by exposing the main artery near the cardiac pole of the tumor and compressing it with a traction loop passed under the artery and held by an assistant. Pressure may also be applied over the exposed artery by the finger of an assistant after duly protecting the vessel with a pad of sterile gauze. The artery may be still better controlled by direct pressure with padded forceps: Billroth's forceps, with broad blades and graduated catch, the blades covered with rubber (Murphy, Burci); with a special clamp for this purpose (Crile's, Allegiani's, J. Tilden Brown); by ordinary spring clamps, such as Langenbeck's Serre-Plat's (Tomaselli), etc. I have found the simple silk traction loop to be the most convenient, because it is always at hand; but I believe that a properly-made clamp, permitting a careful adjustment of pressure, such as the Crile or Allegiani compressors, would be preferable. In carotid and other cervical aneurisms the collateral circulation is so free on the distal side that both poles of the tumor should be controlled, if possible, before opening it.

2. *Incision of the Skin and Exposure of the Sac.*—After all perceptible pulsation in the tumor has been arrested by the measures previously described, a free incision, parallel with the long axis of the aneurism, should be made down to the sac, exposing it to view from one end to the other. When the tumor is deeply seated under the skin, the sac should be exposed by careful dissection for some distance on each side of the cutaneous incision in order to identify any important structures (nerves, arteries, and veins) that might be adherent to its superficial surface. In any event this dissection should not be carried beyond the more prominent or superficial portion of the sac. If any important nerves or other structures should be found attached to the sac and in the way of a free longitudinal incision, these should be carefully detached and held out of the way with retractors.

3. Opening of the Sac and Evacuation of its Contents; Recognition of the Type of Sac, Number of Openings, etc.—A free incision is now made into the sac, extending from one extremity of the tumor to the other in its longest diameter and in the line of the main artery. The contained blood and clots are evacuated and the interior of the cavity is freely exposed to view by vigorous retraction of its edges. This will expose all the orifices which open into the sac. The type of sac that is being dealt with will now be disclosed. If it is a *fusiform* aneurism, two large openings will be seen, usually at the bottom of the sac, separated by an intervening space of variable length, frequently marked by a shallow groove which represents the continuation of the floor of the parent artery. This is more often seen in the aneurisms of the extremities than elsewhere. If the aneurism is of the *sacciform* type, there will be a single opening of variable size, circular or ovoidal in shape, which connects the sac with the main artery. The differentiation of the sac into the two fundamental varieties just described is most important in its bearings upon the further aims of the technique. In the spontaneous aneurisms of the *fusiform* type the artery blends so completely with the sac walls that its continuity cannot usually be restored, at least in the present state of our experience. In these cases the object of the suture is simply to seal the openings leading to the artery for the purpose of haemostasis and obliteration of the sac. In the *sacciform* aneurisms, with a single opening leading to the main vessel, it is often quite possible to close the opening without encroaching upon the lumen of the parent vessel, thus maintaining the functional as well as anatomical continuity of the artery.

We shall now consider separately the treatment of the first variety, —the *fusiform* aneurisms with two main openings.

At this juncture, while the interior of the cavity is exposed and after the chief openings have been identified, careful search should be made in the floor of the sac (especially in the fusiform aneurisms) to discover the openings of any collaterals or branches springing from the sac, which, if not carefully sutured, would give rise to troublesome haemorrhage. Three of the cases operated upon by the author showed this peculiarity. If there is any bleeding from the orifices as a result of a free collateral supply, the closure of these openings by suture should be at once proceeded with. This kind of bleeding can only occur during the operation in cases in which the circulation of the

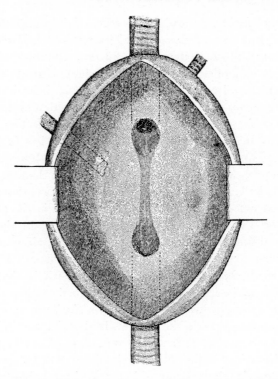

Fig. 2.—Interior of large anuerismal sac of the fusiform type exposed by retraction. The two openings lead respectively to the parent trunk on the proximal (cardiac) and peripheral sides, and the groove between them represents the continuity of the arterial walls blending with the aneurismal sac. This was the type of sac observed in Cases 1, 2, and 4, reported in the text. The orifice of one collateral or branch originating in the sac is shown, and a large collateral opening into the main trunk near the orifice of communication, on the cardiac side, is indicated by the dotted line.

sac is controlled solely by pressure on the cardiac side of the main artery, with a traction loop or other contrivance, and not by general circular constriction at the root of the limb. Whenever the tourniquet or constrictor can be used the ischaemia is complete. The mechanism by which these bleedings are produced in spite of the most perfect control of the artery on the cardiac side is plainly shown in Figs. 1, 2, and 3, and especially in Fig. 17, which is intended to explain the unusual condition encountered in Observation 1. [*Ed. Note:* Figs. 1, 4, 7, 11, 13 and 14 omitted.] In this case, as well as in Observation 4, the most important bleeding appeared to come from the collaterals which emptied into the main artery between the point of compression

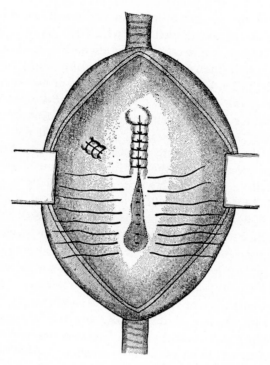

Fig. 3.—Shows the orifices in the aneurismal sac in process of obliteration by suture. The first plane of sutures may be made with fine silk, but chromicized catgut is preferred. The sutures are applied very much like Lembert's sutures in intestinal work; the first plane of sutures should be sufficient to secure complete haemostasis.

The orifice of the collateral vessel on the left upper side of the sac is shown closed by three continuous sutures.

and the orifices within the sac. Fortunately, this bleeding is readily controlled by pressure, which should be applied directly over the bleeding openings with the finger or sterile sponges until they are sealed by rapid, continued suture. When the haemostasis is complete the interior of the sac should be gently, but thoroughly, scrubbed with gauze soaked in sterile saline solution, with the view to clearing it of adherent laminated blood-clots, which interfere with the healing of the sutured surfaces. This toilet of the sac also improves the circulation of the intima and prepares it for prompt plastic reaction when the surfaces of the sac are brought in apposition. In this respect the serous lining of the aneurismal sac, which is simply an extension of the intima of the parent artery, closely resembles the peritoneal serosa, and this, as is well known, unites more quickly when sutured after a preliminary irritation by rubbing, scarification, or abrasion.

4. *Closure of the Aneurismal Orifices in the Fusiform Type of Sac.* After the interior of the aneurism has been carefully prepared by this preliminary toilet the systematic closure of all the visible orifices opening into the sac by suture should be proceeded with, if this has not been done already, as in the conditions previously referred to. The tissues about the margin of these orifices are usually strong, firm, resisting, and hold the sutures well.

The orifices in the sac attached to the parent vessel are often large enough to admit the index-finger of the operator, and the margins are so thick that comparatively few sutures will be required to bring them into apposition. The suture material may be either twisted, braided, or floss silk, chromicized catgut, or even the finest kind of kangaroo tendon; the size of the thread of whatever kind used should correspond with the size of the needle, and this in turn should vary in size according to the dimensions of the openings to be closed and the density of tissues to be sutured. I prefer absorbable sutures, and of these well-prepared chromicized catgut (Nos. 1, 2, and 3) is the best. This material is strong, and remains in the tissues long enough to accomplish its purpose. In applying the sutures the size and shape of the needle are important. The best needles are the round, full curved, with long eyes and prismatic points. Those designed for intestinal sutures are admirably adapted for the present purpose. The full curved needles, known as Mayo's, Kelly's, and Ferguson's, which are intended for intestinal work, are all excellent; but I have used the ordinary curved surgical needles, and even Hagedorn needles, with satisfactory results. As a rule, the continued suture will do well in all cases, especially when time is pressing. When the object of the suture is solely to seal the opening for haemostatic purposes, and not to restore

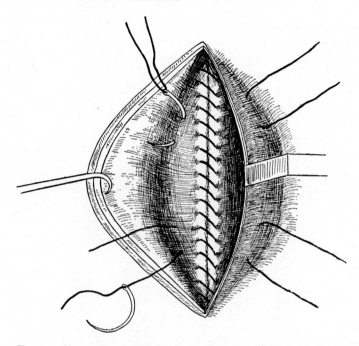

Fig. 5.—Shows the details of the method of obliteration after the floor of the sac has been raised by the second row of sutures. Two deep supporting and obliterating sutures of chromic catgut are inserted through the floor of the sac on each side. The number of these sutures will vary according to the size and length of the sac that is being treated. In the smaller aneurisms, one of the deep sutures on each side will suffice; in others, two or more on each side may be required to keep the surfaces in close contact. After the sutures are passed through the floor of the sac the free ends of the threads are carried through the entire thickness of the flap by transfixion.

The plate shows the mode of placing these sutures on the left side preparatory to transfixion of the flap. The two sutures on the right side have been carried through a flap and are in position.

the caliber of the vessel to which it is attached, as is the case in saccular aneurisms, then the continued suture will be found to be not only the most rapid but the most effective. The distance which should separate the suture points should be regulated by the size of the opening to be closed. Eight or ten sutures to the inch are more than sufficient.

In suturing wounds of *normal* arteries very fine needles and silk should be used, and the sutures should enter the vessel one-sixteenth to one-twentieth of an inch apart. In closing the orifices of aneurismal sacs the conditions are, however, altogether different, as aneurismal tissues are so much thicker and more easily approximated. What is more important is to secure a firm grip of the sac tunics so as to bring a broad

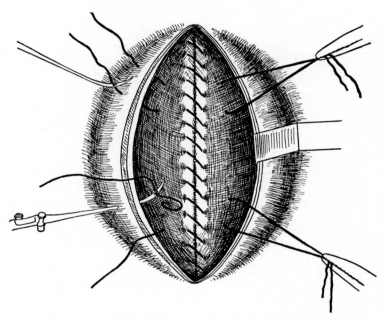

Fig. 6.—Shows the deep supporting sutures in position and the details of transfixion of the flaps. The Reverdin needle is used to carry the free ends of the threads through the flaps formed by the skin and aneurismal walls.

surface in confrontation. In dealing with the larger openings in this class of aneurisms (fusiform), the needle should penetrate at least one-quarter or one-sixth of an inch beyond the margin of the orifice, and then, after reappearing at the margin, dip again into the floor of the artery, and continue to the opposite margin as in the start (Fig. 3). This mode of occluding the orifice of the main artery will secure a very complete apposition of a large marginal area, including the floor of the artery which is visible under the orifice. When the open-

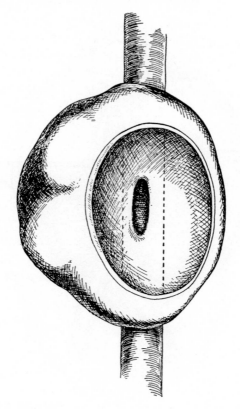

Fig. 8.—This shows a typical sacciform aneurism with one main orifice of communication opening into the sac. In this type of aneurism the lumen of the parent artery is maintained. It is possible in this class of cases to close the orifice of communication by suture without obliterating the lumen of the artery, and without interfering with the circulation in the main artery or of the distal parts supplied by it.

ings must be closed quickly, as in cases in which there is considerable bleeding from collateral vessels, the dip of the needle into the floor of the vessel may be omitted, and the margins of the orifices are brought together quickly with a continued suture. In suturing these orifices the operator should act precisely as in closing perforations of the bowel covered with peritoneum, and remember that the principle of the suture is here, intima to intima or serosa to serosa, as in applying

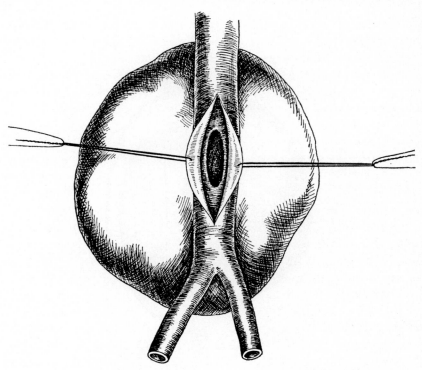

Fig. 9.—This figure is simply intended to show the same type of
sacciform aneurism, viewed from the posterior side. The parent artery
is continuous throughout, and is simply attached to the sac at the
orifice of communication. The artery has been laid open on its posterior surface, showing that the orifice of communication can be closed
on the aneurismal side, without occluding the lumen of the parent
artery. The drawing is taken from a pathological specimen, and is
utilized solely to show the favorable anatomical characteristics of this
class of aneurism for the conservative procedure suggested by the
author.

the Lembert suture to a perforated bowel. The one capital point of
difference in the analogy is that the membrane dealt with is practically all serosa and that it is continuous with the interior of the artery
to be closed; there is no mucosa or infection to be dreaded. Hence
the invariable tendency of the tissues to heal by primary union and
aseptic plastic endarteritis when brought together in broad and firm
apposition.

Continuing with the technique of suture as applied to the *fusiform* aneurisms with two openings, I have found it advantageous to extend the first line of suture from one orifice to another when the intervening space is not too long. These sutures include the floor of the sac (Fig. 3), and are applied on the Lembert plan. They fold up and bring together a considerable area of the floor of the sac, which is thus raised to the upper level of the orifices; in this way they diminish not only the transverse diameter of the sac, but lay the foundation for the obliteration of the cavity which is to follow. If the floor is dense, rigid, or bound down by adhesions to unyielding parts (which is not often the case) the suture should be limited to the orifices. The subsequent steps in the technique will be considered further on in the text.

5. *The Sacciform Aneurisms with a Single Orifice of Communication; Haemostatic and Reconstructive Suture with the View of Preserving the Lumen of the Parent Artery* (Figs. 8 and 9).—This type of sac is the most favorable for the display of the conservative value of arteriorrhaphy from every point of view. The intrasaccular suture of the orifice not only permits of the radical cure of the aneurism by closing its nutrient orifice, but also favors the restoration of the affected artery to its functional and anatomical integrity. The suture is here not only occlusive but reconstructive. The same material and needles should be used as in the previous case, the main point to bear in mind is that in introducing the sutures these should be inserted at a sufficient distance from the usually thick and smooth margins of the opening in order to secure a firm and deep hold of the fibrous basal membrane (Figs. 10, 11, and 12). The needle should be made to appear just within the lower edge of the margin, care being taken that when the sutures are tightened the caliber of the artery will not be encroached upon so as to obstruct its lumen, and that the threads will not be brought in contact with the blood in the lumen of the artery. Greater care must be exercised in securing accurate coaptation in this class of cases than in the fusiform type previously described. As shown in Figs. 10 and 11, it will be advantageous to begin the line of suture at some distance from the orifice, as this will secure a broader and stronger line of approximation. The larger the caliber of the parent vessel the more favorable will the conditions be for the restoration of the lumen of the artery and for the functional success of the operation.

6. *Removal of Constrictor and Test of Sutures.*—After all visible orifices in the sac have been closed by suture, the constrictor or other provisional means adopted to control the circulation are removed. The interior of the cavity should now be perfectly dry, and the only change

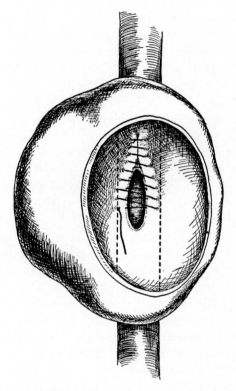

Fig. 10.—Shows the same sac opened. The dotted lines indicate the position and relations of the main artery to the sac and to the orifice of communication. The object of the operation in this case is to close the orifice of communication without obliterating the main artery. The closure of the orifice with continued suture is shown in the plate.

noticed by a return of the circulation should be an improved, more pinkish color of the sac. If there be any oozing capillary points these will be usually stopped by pressure and by the means subsequently adopted to obliterate the cavity.

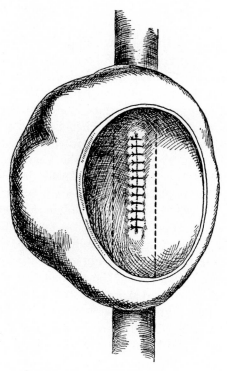

FIG. 12.—Shows the obliteration of the orifice of communication completed. The appearance following the application of interrupted suture is shown in this figure. If the suture has been properly applied, the haemostasis will be complete, and the circulation in the main artery restored. After this has been done, the second protective row of sutures shown in Fig. 4 [*Ed. Note:* Figure omitted] and other details of the technique of the obliteration of the sac (shown in Figs. 5, 6 and 7) [*Ed. Note:* Figure 7 omitted] should be carried out precisely as in dealing with aneurisms of the fusiform type. Anomalous orifices or collaterals opening into the sac, in addition to the main orifices, are less liable to exist in the sacciform aneurisms than in the fusiform aneurisms, in which a large area of the arterial wall is involved. In any event, however, should such additional orifices exist, they should be individually closed by a few continued sutures as shown in Fig. 3.

7. *Obliteration of the Aneurismal Sac* (Figs. 4, 5, 6, and 7).—This step of the operation is the same in all cases. In large sacs, where the floor of the cavity is deeply situated and there is an abundance or even redundance of material, it will be a good practice, as previously stated, to reinforce the first line of occlusive sutures by a second row, applied also on the Lembert plan at a higher level. This second row will raise up and bring together a considerable surface of the sac floor and lateral walls of the cavity, and when finished will not only bury the first plane of sutures, but will reduce the dimensions of the sac considerably (Fig. 4). The closure of the aneurismal space is now readily accomplished by turning the relaxed flaps of skin into the interior of the cavity. If the sac has not been previously dissected from its surroundings, the skin flaps will be lined on their inner surface with the smooth sac walls, thus constituting an aneurismo-cutaneous flap on each side. These flaps, in their relaxed state, can, as a rule, be made to touch the bottom of the cavity with comparative ease. One or two relaxation sutures on each side of the median line will usually suffice to tack down and hold the skin flaps in contact with the bottom and sides of the sac. The sutures are best applied with a large size, full-curved intestinal needle, which is made to grasp a considerable portion of the sac wall in its bight. The needle should penetrate through the entire thickness of the sac; by carrying it through in this way a loop is formed, the two ends of which are carried through the skin flaps by transfixion with a straight Reverdin needle, and tied firmly over a loose pad of gauze after the flaps have been carefully adjusted in position (Figs. 5, 6, and 7).

The principle adopted in the obliteration of the sac has been made familiar by Neuber's method of closing bone cavities with cutane-operiosteal flaps. After the relaxation sutures have been tied the edges of the skin should come in close contact in the median line, and all that will be required to finish the operation will be a few interrupted catgut sutures to complete the approximation of the skin margins (Fig. 7). When the operation is completed, the aneurismal cavity is obliterated without in the least disturbing the sac or interfering with its vascular relations. The collateral circulation, which is usually important in the vicinity of the aneurism, is also respected, and in this way the best condition for the maintenance of a healthy nutrition in the sac and in the parts beyond the aneurism are assured.

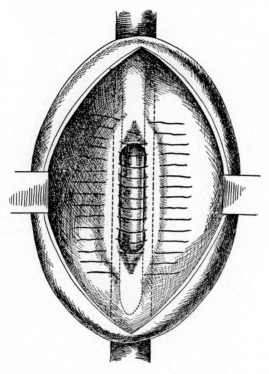

FIG. 15.—Shows a possible but not yet tried method of restoring the large lumen of the parent artery in favorable cases of fusiform aneurism with two openings in which the healthy and flexible character of the sac will permit of the restoration of the arterial channel by lifting two lateral folds of the sac and bringing them together by suture over a soft rubber guide. The principle of this operation is precisely like that adopted in a Witzel gastrostomy. The figure shows the soft rubber catheter lying on the floor of the sac and inserted in the two orifices of communication. The sutures are placed while the catheter is in position acting as a guide.

At the site where the bulging tumor previously existed there will be a depression varying in depth according to the size of the original sac, and presenting the appearance of an inverted hollow cone or ovoid. As no exposed or raw surfaces are left in view, there is no need for drainage, and union *per primam* can be confidently expected, thus greatly abbreviating the duration of the after-treatment.

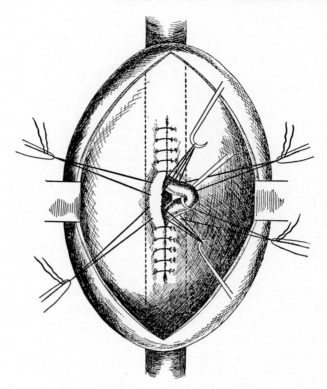

FIG. 16.—This shows a more advanced step of the procedure described in Fig. 15. The sutures are nearly all tied,
and the new channel is completed except in the centre. The
two middle sutures are hooked and pulled out of the way
while still in position, and the catheter is withdrawn. The
obliteration of the sac and final steps of the operation are
carried out precisely as previously described in Figs. 4, 5, 6
and 7.

Dressings.—A simple sterile gauze dressing is applied as a graduated compress to fill the hollow left in the place previously occupied
by the aneurism. This is held in position by a few strips of aseptic
rubber plaster. The limb is then wrapped up from the periphery to
the trunk in a thick layer of cotton-batting, over which a well-padded
splint is adjusted to secure the immobility of the entire limb, especially if the field of the operation occupies one of the flexures of the

extremity. If sufficient padding has been applied to protect the distal parts from undue pressure or exposure to cold, a starch bandage or a light plaster-of-Paris roller over the whole limb will complete the dressing. If there are no reasons to the contrary, the first dressing should not be disturbed for a period of a week or ten days.

[*Ed. Note:* A discussion of exceptional cases is deleted.]

My experience with this method of endoarteriorrhaphy, or, rather, to define it more accurately, endoaneurismorrhaphy, if I may be permitted such a neologism, is limited to four cases: two of direct traumatic aneurism of the brachial, caused by gunshot wounds, one of which involved the lower and the other the upper third of this artery; one femoral and one popliteal, and both of the so-called spontaneous variety. The first operation dates as far back as March, 1888, and was published in the *Medical News* in the issue of October 27, 1888. This case presented features of exceptional interest apart from the method of treatment employed. It is one of the cases of traumatic aneurism of the brachial caused by gunshot wound. In this case (a very large sac) indirect and direct compressions by Reid's method were tried unsuccessfully; then ligatures were applied above and below the sac at different sittings, and failed; the pulsation returned on the tenth day. Upon opening the aneurism its rebelliousness was explained by finding the openings of several large collaterals which kept up the circulation in the tumor after the main artery had been ligated above and below the sac. The anastomotic circulation which accounted for this unusual condition is explained by Fig. 17, which is reproduced from the original article. In this case (a large aneurism of the fusiform type) extirpation was attempted, but had to be abandoned because of the great risk of injuring adherent nerves which were incorporated in its walls. Under these circumstances, and without any previous knowledge of the practicability of suture in such cases, all the bleeding was immediately controlled by suturing the orifices with fine silk. A redundant portion of the sac which had been detached by dissection was excised, leaving the floor and lateral walls undisturbed, to heal by granulation. A long interval elapsed between this and the next case, which was operated by more advanced technique in the summer of 1900; several opportunities had presented themselves in the interval for the application of this method, but I had not yet overcome the dread of atheroma and secondary haemor-

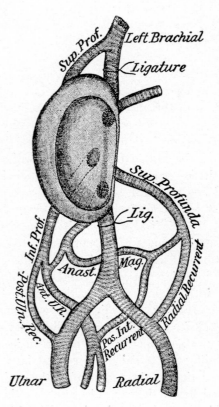

Fig. 17.—This is a reproduction of a diagram published in the *Medical News* (Philadelphia), October 27, 1888. It is intended to explain the condition found in a case of traumatic aneurism in which the author applied intrasaccular arteriorrhaphy for the first time. The abundance of the collateral supply in that case could only be accounted for by a distribution of the vessels such as shown in this figure.

The failure of the ligatures applied to the main artery above and below the sac and difficulties of extirpation were well illustrated in this case, and led to the suture of the aneurismal orifices which promptly secured their obliteration and an immediate arrest of the hemorrhage.

rhage. But the disastrous results which followed in a case of femoral aneurism treated by Hunterian ligation, in which the patient barely escaped with his life after an amputation at the thigh for gangrene, and also the vivid recollections of the great difficulties encountered in extirpating a femoral aneurism of Scarpa's triangle, followed also by gangrene of the toes, led me to revert to the method of incision and suture detailed in the previous case. After this experience I grew more confident, and applied the operation with more boldness, and added the modifications referred to in describing the technique of obliteration.

While this experience is too limited to justify any dogmatic or broad generalizations, the simplicity of the method and the favorable results thus far obtained are sufficient to encourage its more general application. The later suggestions and modifications made in this paper, which aim at the further conservation of the main trunk, and thus safeguarding the integrity of the circulation in the sacciform and fusiform aneurisms, are still waiting the test of clinical experience. But from a priori grounds and the experience thus far gained, it would appear quite reasonable to anticipate still greater gains in a conservative direction in a group of cases in which the classical procedure is still fraught with great uncertainty.

As the chief object of this paper has been to describe the technique of this procedure and to relate the author's personal experience in its practical application, no systematic effort will be made to study its comparative merits in relation to other methods of treating aneurisms. The indications for the application of this operation have been sufficiently stated. It is intended to meet the conditions which call for the radical operation by extirpation. It is not intended to supplant it altogether, because extirpation is still the method of election in dealing with the smaller aneurisms of the secondary arteries of the extremities, in which the question of mortification or gangrene does not enter into consideration on account of the certainty of an abundant vascular supply. Its chief object is to simplify the technique of the radical cure, to make it less bloody, to diminish the traumatism, to interfere less with the important neighboring structures, which are often damaged by extirpation (veins, nerves, and organs), and, above all, to reduce the dangers of gangrene of the distal parts to the strictest minimum compatible with the cure of the aneurism.

It is only just to state that after a careful inquiry into the literature of aneurism I have failed to find any reference to a procedure that resembled or suggested the method described in this paper. In the constantly growing list of contributions on the subject of arterial suture there are frequent allusions and suggestions as to the possible advantages of suture in the treatment of traumatic and arteriovenous aneurisms. These recommendations all refer to the direct suture of the artery in recent wounds or at the bottom of diffuse extravasations and pulsating haematomas in which no well-circumscribed sac exists. The three reported cases of arteriovenous aneurism in which the arteries had been detached from the veins and sutured by lateral and circular arteriorrhaphy have been mentioned at the beginning of this paper. These cases, however, represent conditions which are entirely different from those under consideration. A single exception that I have found in the literature of the subject is the notable contribution by J. B. Murphy, of Chicago, on the resection of arteries and veins injured in continuity (*Medical Record*, New York, January 16, 1897), in which he boldly and very originally discusses the practicability of obliteration of the orifices of an aneurism, and published a full account of the case nearly ten years before the publication of Dr. Murphy's experimental contribution.

It will be seen, however, by the quotations above given that Dr. Murphy's procedure, bold and brilliant as it is in its conception, is entirely different from that described in this article. Murphy's suggested operation is practically an extirpation of the sac, and as such is fraught with all the difficulties and undesirable features of this operation, with the added difficulty of suturing the openings in the vessel itself. He has also overlooked the fact that in fusiform aneurisms the continuity of the main artery is lost for a considerable distance in the sac, where it merges completely with the aneurismal walls; hence the impracticability of resecting the sac by the method he suggests. In the sacciform and the arteriovenous aneurism his procedure is perfectly feasible, but the same result can be accomplished by the much easier and safer plan described in this contribution.

In conclusion, the writer would submit the following propositions:

1. That the recognized advantages of the radical operation for the cure of aneurisms of the peripheral arteries, as demonstrated by the statistics of the last decade, can be greatly increased, and the sphere

of application of this operation can be broadened by the adoption of the method of suture and obliteration of the sac instead of the classical ligation of the arteries, with or without extirpation, as hitherto practised.

2. That the closure of the arterial orifices which supply the aneurismal sac, whether these be single or multiple, by means of suture, and within the aneurismal sac itself, greatly simplifies the technique of the radical operation, and is a reliable means of securing haemostasis.

3. That in favorable cases—and the saccular aneurisms with a single orifice communicating with the lumen of the larger arterial trunks are the most favorable—it is possible, by careful suture, to obliterate the aneurismal opening without obstructing the lumen of the parent artery, thus protecting the limb from the risk of gangrene.

4. It is also possible in favorable cases of fusiform aneurisms of traumatic origin, and in all those in which the sac material is healthy and pliable, to restore the lost continuity of the artery by building a new channel which will connect the two main orifices of communication and restore the interrupted circulation in the parent vessel. This result can be obtained by utilizing the sac in the manner previously described by the author.

5. That the fear that atheroma and other degenerative changes will interfere with the healing and repair of the arterial tunics has been greatly exaggerated is shown by the abundant experience of the aseptic period in the ligature of sclerotic arteries in continuity, in the absence of secondary haemorrhage in the amputated stumps of the aged, diabetic, and other arterially diseased subjects (Heidenhain, Webber, Barwell, and others), and is still demonstrated more fully by the observations and statistics of the partisans of the radical operation by extirpation (Delbet, Kubler, Ransohoff, Annandale, and others) who have reported numerous successful results in spontaneous as well as in traumatic aneurisms.

6. The fallacy and dangers of the old operation of Antyllus lie (a) in the fact that the preliminary ligation of the main artery above and below the sac will not always control the bleeding from the collaterals which often open into the aneurism or into the main trunks between the orifices in the sac and at the seat of ligature. This compels a more or less extensive dissection of the sac out of its bed as one of the necessary features of the procedure, in order to secure all the col-

lateral vessels that empty into the sac, unless the uncertain process of plugging the openings and packing the sac itself is resorted to. If the sac is dissected, as is usually done to secure the collaterals, the difficulties of the operation are increased, and the vitality of the limb is endangered by interfering with the collateral circulation which, in many types of aneurism, is most freely developed in the neighborhood of the sac.

(*b*) Another serious objection to the old Antyllian operation as usually performed is that the sac is allowed to remain as an open cavity in the bottom of the wound, where it is packed or drained and allowed to heal by granulation. This invites infection, suppuration, and its attendant dangers of secondary haemorrhage; all that is obviated by the author's method of endo-aneurismorrhaphy, which does not disturb the sac from its vascular connections, and favors its prompt obliteration by suturing the infolded walls of the sac, and keeping them in direct and close approximation.

7. The uncertainties and dangers of extirpation of the sac (Purmann's operation) are even more apparent than those of the Antyllus operation, because, in addition to the greater technical difficulties of extirpation, there is much greater risk of injury to the accompanying satellite veins and nerves which blend most intimately with the sac, and often compel the operator to limit his intervention to a partial extirpation, leaving behind a considerable portion of the sac wall in order to avoid injury to important adherent structures. The greatest objection to extirpation, however, lies in the decided interference with the collateral circulation in the immediate vicinity of the aneurism, which entails a considerable risk of mortification in the distal parts. All these dangers are reduced to a safe minimum, and are largely eliminated by simply obliterating the sac, instead of extirpating it.

SIR HENRY S. SOUTTAR (1875–)

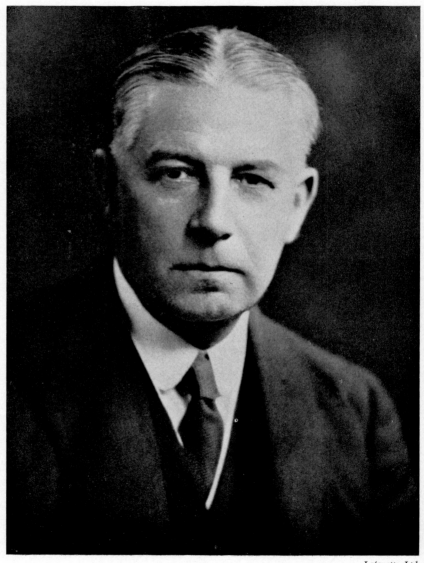

Lafayette Ltd.

Henry S. Souttar was born in England, in 1875, son of Robinson Souttar, member of Parliament for Dumfriesshire. His early education was at Queens College and Oxford. He entered the London Hospital in 1903 where he remained until the first World War. He saw active service as Surgeon in Chief of Field Hospitals at Antwerp and Furues and ultimately became Deputy Consulting Surgeon to the Southern Command. His numerous publications include articles on nerve injuries, radium, esophageal and cardiac surgery. His foresight in the treatment of mitral stenosis stands as a milestone in surgery and is a fine example of how a monumental advance may be buried in the literature. We are in receipt of a comment from Sir Henry which details the follow-up of the first case:

"It would probably interest them to know that the patient made an uneventful recovery; lived in very fair health for five years, and then had a cerebral infarct, probably from a clot in the left auricle, from which she died. I could get no other case as medical opinion was solidly against such attempts. In fact it was in America that someone discovered my article after 25 years and ventured another trial. I am told that about a hundred cases are now done every week in this country and it is odd that the original technique remains exactly as it was thirty years ago!"

THE SURGICAL TREATMENT
OF MITRAL STENOSIS

BY H. S. SOUTTAR, C.B.E., M.Ch., F.R.C.S.

Surgeon (With Care of Out-Patients), London Hospital

There can be no more fascinating problem in surgery than the relief of pathological conditions of the valves of the heart. Despite the consecutive changes to which these lesions may have given rise in the cardiac muscle, the relief of the lesions themselves would undoubtedly be of immense service to the patient and must be followed by marked improvement in his general condition. Expressed in these terms, the problem is to a large extent mechanical, and as such should already be within the scope of surgery, were it not for the extraordinary nature of the conditions under which the problem must be attacked. We are, however, of opinion that these conditions again are purely mechanical, and that apart from them the heart is as amenable to surgical treatment as any other organ. Incisions can be made into its chambers, portions of its structure can be excised, and internal manipulations can be carried out, without the slightest interference with its action, and there is ample evidence that wounds of the heart heal as rapidly as those in any other region.

The conditions which appear as fundamental are, first, that the operations have to be carried out on a structure in rapid movement; and secondly, that no interference whatever with the circulation must take place. The first is not quite so difficult as it sounds, for it is possible to fix the actual portion of the heart which is under operation, but it

From the *British Medical Journal*, 2:603, 1925. Reprinted by permission.
410

must obviously limit the possibilities of repair. In animals the second condition may sometimes be ignored, and the circulation has been clamped for as much as two minutes. This, however, would never be justifiable in a human being, in view of the extreme danger to the brain from even the shortest check to its blood supply. Any manipulations which are carried out must therefore be executed in the full flow of the blood stream, and they must not perceptibly interfere with the contractions of the heart.

The simplest valvular lesion for surgical interference is stenosis of one of the valves, and of these the mitral valve is perhaps the most accessible. I have been interested for some time in the development of a suitable technique for reaching this valve, and I owe to Dr. Otto Leyton the opportunity presented by the following case for putting my ideas to the test. A description of the case itself will give the clearest indication of the method of approach I adopted and of the technique which I devised.

DESCRIPTION OF CASE. L. H., aged 15, was admitted to the London Hospital in January, 1921, suffering from chorea and mitral stenosis. Her subsequent history was one of many relapses, with steadily increasing failure of compensation. In September, 1924, she was admitted with haemoptysis, vomiting, and severe dyspnoea. She was cyanosed, her feet were swollen, and her liver was enlarged and tender. After three weeks in hospital she had greatly improved and was sent to a convalescent home, whence three weeks later she was discharged.

Early in March, 1925, she appeared at the London Hospital with cough, dyspnoea, and pain in the limbs. She was sent home to bed and given digitalis and aspirin, but she did not improve. After a severe attack of epistaxis and precordial pain she was again admitted as an in-patient.

She was a thin girl with a bright malar flush. Her pulse rate was 128, and respirations 32. Cardiac pulsation was visible over a large area of the left chest, and the rib cartilages in this area were very soft and had a forward bulge. The apex beat was in the fifth space, outside the mid-clavicular line, and the area of cardiac dullness extended to the second space above. In the mitral area there was a long rumbling diastolic murmur, followed by a soft blowing systolic murmur, the latter being conducted out into the axilla. A presystolic murmur was present, but was not very marked. The liver was not obviously enlarged, but was slightly tender on palpation.

After a week's rest in bed her pulse fell to 80 and her respirations to 24, while her general condition greatly improved. Her pulse was now small but perfectly regular with a systolic pressure of 95 mm. There was no presystolic murmur or thrill, but a long diastolic murmur of low pitch was followed by a soft blowing systolic murmur.

In view of her many relapses it appeared that her heart was unable to establish compensation for the combined stenosis and regurgitation

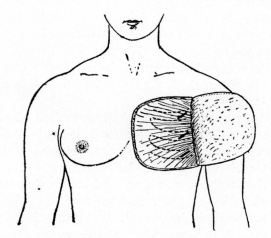

Fig. 1.—Skin and subcutaneous tissue reflected, with ribs exposed prior to division.

from which she suffered, and it was therefore decided to attempt to relieve the stenosis by surgical means.

OPERATIONS. On May 6th, 1925, under intratracheal anesthesia, a curved incision was made along the fourth left intercostal space, up along the middle of the sternum, and outwards along the first left intercostal space. The skin and subcutaneous tissues, with the left breast, were turned outwards, exposing an area of the chest wall about five inches square. On the outer side of this area a short horizontal incision was made along each of the three ribs exposed (Fig. 1), and through these incisions the ribs were in turn divided. The chest wall was now divided a little within the line of the original incision by cut-

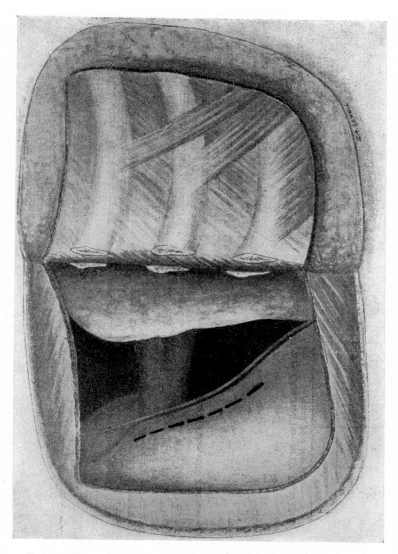

FIG. 2.—Ribs divided, and flap, formed by cutting through muscles and costal cartilages, turned back; left side of pericardium exposed.

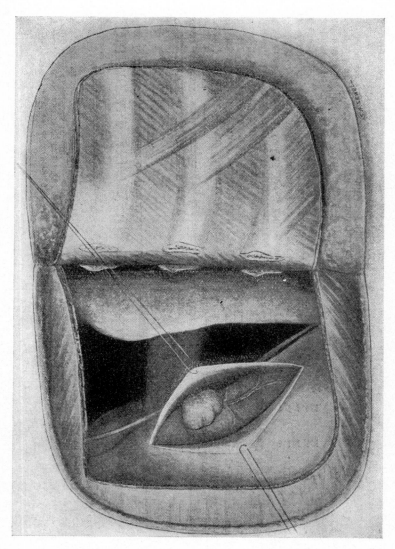

Fig. 3.—Vertical incision in pericardium, exposing left auricular appendage.

ting through the muscles and costal cartilages, and the flap so formed was turned outwards, the pleura being included in the flap (Fig. 2).

A very full exposure of the left side of the pericardium was thus obtained, while with an intratracheal pressure of 15 mm. Hg there was only moderate collapse of the left lung. The action of the heart now became extremely hurried, the pulse rising to 150 and it was evident that until it settled down nothing further could be attempted. After five minutes' delay the beats became slower and steadier, and it was decided that we could safely proceed. The pericardium was

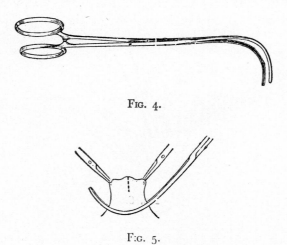

FIG. 4.

FIG. 5.

opened by a vertical incision three inches long, in the centre of which the left auricular appendage came prominently forward (Fig. 3). Two sutures were passed through the upper and lower margins of the appendage, so that it could be readily drawn forward. As the heart was still beating very rapidly the wound was covered with hot saline pads and a subcutaneous injection of $\frac{1}{100}$ grain of strophanthin was given. After a delay of ten minutes the heart had steadied down to a rate of 120, and the blood pressure, which had fallen to 60 mm., had returned to 90 mm.

The auricular appendage was now drawn forward, a soft curved clamp (Fig. 4) was applied to its base, and it was incised in an antero-posterior direction with scissors (Fig. 5). Into this opening the left forefinger was inserted (Fig. 6), the clamp was withdrawn, and

the appendage was drawn over the finger like a glove by means of
the sutures. The whole of the inside of the left auricle could now be
explored with facility. It was immediately evident from the rush of
blood against the finger that gross regurgitation was taking place, but
there was not so much thickening of the valves as had been expected.
The finger was passed into the ventricle through the orifice of the
mitral valve without encountering resistance, and the cusps of the
valve could be easily felt and their condition estimated.

The finger was kept in the auricle for perhaps two minutes, and
during that time, so long as it remained in the auricle, it appeared to
produce no effect upon the heart beat or the pulse. The moment,

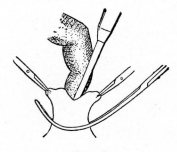

Fig. 6.

however, that it passed into the orifice of the mitral valve the blood
pressure fell to zero, although even then no change in the cardiac
rhythm could be detected. The blood stream was simply cut off by the
finger, which presumably just fitted the stenosed orifice. As, however,
the stenosis was of such moderate degree, and was accompanied by
so little thickening of the valves, it was decided not to carry out the
valve section which had been arranged, but to limit intervention to
such dilatation as could be carried out by the finger. It was felt that
an actual section of the valve might only make matters worse by increasing the degree of regurgitation, while the breaking down of adhesions by the finger might improve the condition as regards both regurgitation and stenosis.

It was now decided to withdraw the finger and close the appendage.
Unfortunately, at the critical moment of withdrawal the lower retaining suture cut through, the appendage slipped back into the

pericardium, and there was a sudden gush of blood, which, however, was instantly checked by pressing the appendage against the heart. With a little manipulation the tip of the appendage was now grasped between the finger and thumb, which held it securely closed while an assistant passed a silk ligature round it and tied it off. The pericardium was closed, and a certain amount of blood, which in this contretemps had escaped into the pleural cavity, was removed with moist gauze pads. The wound was closed in layers, the ribs being accurately sutured in position. Before the flap was actually closed a small quantity of 60 per cent alcohol was injected into the intercostal nerves just outside the point at which the ribs had been divided.

Immediately the chest was closed the heart's action returned to normal, and on the conclusion of the operation the general condition of the patient was indistinguishable from that at the beginning. She had a bright color and an excellent pulse. Except at the moment when the suture cut out her condition had never caused the slightest anxiety, and even then there was only a momentary drop in the blood pressure. The whole operation took precisely sixty minutes.

She made an uninterrupted recovery, the freedom from pain or any disturbance which might have been expected to result from the operation being remarkable. Her general condition appeared to be greatly improved, but the physical signs showed little or no change. She was sent to the country and kept in bed for six weeks, but as at the end of that time her pulse rate had remained constant at about 90 she was gradually allowed to get up. At the end of three months, she declared that she felt perfectly well, although she still became somewhat breathless on exertion.

REMARKS. I believe that this is the first occasion upon which an attempt has been made to reach the mitral valve by this route in the human being, or to subject the interior of the heart to digital examination. The value of the method cannot possibly be judged on a single case, but I think that I may claim to have shown that the method is practicable and that it is reasonably safe. Indeed, the features which most struck all who were present at the operation were the facility and the absolute safety of the whole procedure, while even on a first attempt the amount and precision of the information to be gained by digital exploration were very remarkable. I had intended to divide the aortic cusp by passing a thin hernia bistoury along my finger (Fig. 7) and thus to relieve the stenosis, and this could have been done with perfect facility had it been considered advisable.

The problem of cardiac surgery has frequently attracted the attention of both physicians and surgeons, and two years ago the *British Medical Journal* summed up, in an admirable article, its history and position at that time. It is now being attacked with characteristic energy by several American surgeons from various points of view. On the experimental side Duff Allen, by means of a most ingenious optical device, has succeeded in actually seeing the mitral valve in the cat and in dividing a cusp, using the approach through the auricular appendage. On the clinical side Cutler, after an elaborate experimental

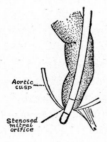

Fig. 7.

investigation, succeeded in excising portions of stenosed mitral valves in human beings by means of an ingenious valvulotome, working through the ventricle. The operation was, however, necessarily blind and proved to be somewhat dangerous.

It appears to me that the method of digital exploration through the auricular appendage cannot be surpassed for simplicity and directness. Not only is the mitral orifice directly to hand, but the aortic valve itself is almost certainly within reach, through the mitral orifice. Owing to the simplicity of the structures, and oddly enough, to their constant and regular movement, the information given by the finger is exceedingly clear, and personally I felt an appreciation of the mechanical reality of stenosis and regurgitation which I never before possessed. To hear a murmur is a very different matter from feeling the blood itself pouring back over one's finger. I could not help being impressed by the mechanical nature of these lesions and by the practicability of their surgical relief.

ROBERT EDWARD GROSS (*1905–*)

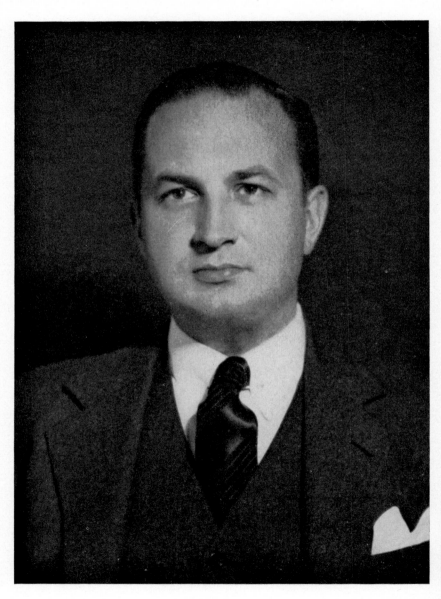

Robert Edward Gross was born in 1905 in Baltimore. He received his M.D. degree from Harvard in 1931. He was an intern in pathology and a resident in surgery at the Children's Hospital in Boston and subsequently completed his surgical residency at the Peter Bent Brigham Hospital. In 1937 he was a Peters Travelling Fellow to European clinics. He has been Professor of Children's Surgery at Harvard since 1947.

Dr. Gross has been a pioneer in the development of many diversified phases of children's surgery. His fundamental contributions have been applicable to adult surgery as well. His works on the patent ductus arteriosus and on blood-vessel grafts are reproduced in this volume. His text-book, with Ladd, on The Surgery of Infancy and Childhood *stands as a classic which is revered by all students of the subject. Although he has contributed far more than can be expected from any one man, it is our feeling that his greatest work is yet to come.*

SURGICAL LIGATION OF A PATENT DUCTUS ARTERIOSUS

Report of First Successful Case

BY ROBERT E. GROSS, M.D., AND
JOHN P. HUBBARD, M.D.

*Surgical and Medical Services of the Children's Hospital and the
Departments of Surgery and Pediatrics of the Harvard Medical School*

The continued patency of a ductus arteriosus for more than the first few years of life has long been known to be a potential source of danger to a patient for two reasons: First, the additional work of the left ventricle in maintaining the peripheral blood pressure in the presence of a large arteriovenous communication may lead eventually to cardiac decompensation of severe degree. Second, the presence of a patent ductus arteriosus makes the possessor peculiarly subject to fatal bacterial endarteritis. While it is true that some persons have been known to live to old age with a patent ductus of Botalli, statistics have shown that the majority die relatively young because of complications arising from this congenital abnormality. Dr. Maude Abbott presented a series of ninety-two cases which came to autopsy in which it was shown that the patient had had a patent ductus arteriosus without any other cardiovascular abnormality. Of these patients, approximately one fourth died of bacterial endarteritis of the pulmonary artery and an additional one half died of slow or rapid cardiac de-

From the *Journal of the American Medical Association,* 112:729, 1939. Reprinted by permission.

compensation. The average age of death of patients in this series was 24 years.

The complications arising from the persistence of a patent ductus arteriosus would seem to make surgical ligation of this anomalous vessel a rational procedure, if such a procedure could be completed with promise of a low operative mortality. Dramatic results have previously been obtained in persons with cardiac enlargement and decompensation resulting from a peripheral arteriovenous aneurysm when the short-circuiting vessels have been ligated or excised. On similar theoretical grounds, future cardiac embarrassment should be averted if a shunt between the aorta and the pulmonary artery could be removed. It would also seem plausible to expect that the shutting off of the anomalous stream of blood pouring into the pulmonary artery would lessen the formation of the thickened endothelial plaques within the pulmonary artery, which are so likely to be the seat of later bacterial infection. The surgical approach to the aortic arch and pulmonary conus having been studied previously in animal experimentation, it seemed within reason that a patent ductus could be adequately exposed in man and possibly ligated without undue danger. It was therefore decided to undertake the operation in a child who presented the classic signs of a patent ductus arteriosus. At the age of 7 years she already had cardiac hypertrophy, which developed presumably from the embarrassment resulting from the anomalous communication. It was to be expected, therefore, that she would have increasingly severe disability in the future, aside from the danger of having bacterial endarteritis develop.

REPORT OF CASE

History.—L. S., a girl aged 7½ years, entered the hospital Aug. 17, 1938, for study of her cardiac condition. The family history was irrelevant. She was born normally at full term. No cyanosis was noted at birth or during the postnatal period. The records of the hospital where she was born give no information about an examination of the heart at that time. At the age of 3 years she was seen in the cardiac clinic of another hospital, where it was found that she had physical signs suggesting congenital malformation of the heart. At that time she had a precordial thrill and a loud murmur. The carotid pulsations were abnormally marked, and pistol shot sounds could be heard over the brachial and femoral arteries. The blood pressure was recorded in both arms as 104 mm. of mercury systolic and 0 diastolic. There was definite cardiac enlargement, as shown by teleoroentgenograms. The diagnosis made at that time was "congenital malformation of the heart with a patent ductus arteriosus."

During the next four years she was seen in several different hospitals, where the same diagnosis was made. At no time had cyanosis been observed. Dyspnea developed after moderate exercise, and her physical activities had been limited accordingly. She had never had peripheral edema or other evidence of cardiac decompensation. Frequently the child had been conscious of "something wrong in the chest" and her mother spontaneously offered the information that she had heard a "buzzing noise" in her daughter's chest when standing nearby.

Physical Examination.—At the time of admission, the patient was slender and undernourished. The pulsations of the carotid arteries were abnormally forceful. The radial pulse was of the Corrigan type, and a capillary pulsation was readily seen. The veins over the chest were somewhat prominent. There was a precordial bulge. The heart was definitely enlarged by percussion, the enlargement being for the most part to the left. Over the entire precordium there was a prominent coarse thrill which was most intense in the third interspace to the left of the sternum. This thrill was continuous but was accentuated during systole. There was a rough "machinery" murmur heard with maximal intensity over the pulmonic area to the left of the sternum in the second and particularly in the third interspace. It was continuous throughout the cardiac cycle but like the thrill was greatly accentuated during systole. It was transmitted to the left along the third interspace and into the axilla with only slightly diminished intensity. The systolic element was heard faintly over the vessels of the neck and could be heard clearly in the right axilla and over the mid-thoracic region posteriorly. Blood pressure readings were respectively right arm 115/40, left arm 110/50, right leg 150/55, left leg 140/40 mm. of mercury. There was no clubbing of the fingers and no evidence of peripheral edema. The liver edge was palpable at the costal margin. The examination in other respects was negative.

Laboratory Data.—A 7-foot x-ray film of the chest showed the transverse diameter of the heart to be 11.7 cm., compared to an internal diameter of the chest of 20 cm. There appeared to be definite enlargement of the left ventricle. There was questionable prominence of the pulmonary artery. A mottled increased density around the lung hili was interpreted as representing circulatory congestion. Fluoroscopic examination showed a "hilar dance." An electrocardiogram was normal, showing no deviation of the axis. The red blood count was 5,080,000 cells per cubic millimeter and the hemoglobin was 85 per cent (Sahli). Circulation time with dehydrocholic acid was 10 and 8 seconds, respectively, on two tests.

Operation.—August 26, operation was undertaken (by R. E. G.) under cyclopropane anesthesia. The approach to the mediastinum was made through the left pleural cavity anterolaterally. Incision was made through the left third interspace, cutting the third costal cartilage, and the third rib was retracted upward. As the left lung was allowed to collapse infer-

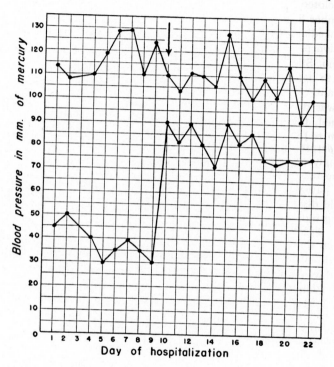

Fig. 1.—Daily blood pressure readings of the patient with a patent ductus arteriosus before and after operation. Prior to operation the large ductus opening from the aorta produced a low diastolic pressure. Following operative closure of the ductus, the diastolic pressure rose to twice its former level. The average daily diastolic pressure preoperatively was 38 mm. of mercury. The average diastolic pressure postoperatively was 80 mm. of mercury. The arrow points to the time of operation.

iorly, an excellent view was gained of the lateral aspect of the mediastinum. The parietal pleura covering the aortic arch and left pulmonic artery was then incised and these structures were directly exposed. A large patent ductus arteriosus was found, which was from 7 to 8 mm. in diameter and from 5 to 6 mm. in length. A palpating finger placed on the heart disclosed a continuous and very vibrant thrill over the entire organ, which was increasingly prominent as the finger reached up over the pulmonic artery. A sterile stethoscope was employed and an extremely loud continuous murmur was heard over the entire heart. When the stethoscope was placed on the pulmonary artery there was an almost deafening, continuous roar, sounding much like a large volume of steam escaping in a closed room.

A number 8 braided silk tie was placed around the ductus with an aneurysm needle, and the vessel was temporarily occluded for a three minute observation period. During this time the blood pressure rose from 110/35 to 125/90. Since there was no embarrassment of the circulation, it was decided to ligate the ductus permanently. The ductus was too short to tie double and divide, so that ligation alone was resorted to. When the thread was drawn up tight the thrill completely disappeared. The chest was closed, the lung being reexpanded with positive pressure anesthesia just prior to placing the last stitch in the intercostal muscles.

Postoperative Course.—The child underwent the operative procedure exceedingly well and showed no signs of shock. Prior to operation blood had been taken from a donor in order to have it ready whenever needed, but the patient's condition was so good that it was not given. There was only mild discomfort on the afternoon of the day of operation, and on the following morning the child was allowed to sit up in a chair. By the third day she was walking about the ward. When the skin sutures were removed on the seventh day the wound was well healed, but because of the interest in the case the child was detained in the hospital until the thirteenth day. After the dressing was removed and the chest could be examined adequately the thrill had completely disappeared, there was a faint systolic murmur in the left third interspace which was not transmitted over the precordium, and no murmur could be heard in the axilla, in the neck or over the back. The daily blood pressures which had been taken prior to operation and subsequent thereto showed a striking change in the diastolic levels, as is shown by the accompanying chart. The average of the daily pressures prior to operation had been 114 systolic and 38 diastolic as contrasted with a postoperative daily average of 108 systolic and 80 diastolic.

SUMMARY

A girl aged 7½ years had a known patency of the ductus arteriosus and beginning cardiac hypertrophy. In the hope of preventing subsequent bacterial endarteritis and with the immediate purpose of reducing the work of the heart caused by the shunt between the aorta and the pulmonary artery, the patent ductus was surgically explored and ligated. The child stood the operative procedure exceedingly well. The most objective finding, which indicated that the serious loss of blood from the aorta into the pulmonic artery had been arrested by operation, was a comparison of the preoperative and postoperative levels of the diastolic blood pressure. Prior to operation the daily blood pressure showed an average diastolic level of 38 mm. of mercury as compared with a postoperative diastolic level of 80 mm. of mercury. This is the first patient in whom a patent ductus arteriosus has been successfully ligated.

METHODS FOR PRESERVATION AND TRANSPLANTATION OF ARTERIAL GRAFTS

Observations on Arterial Grafts in Dogs.
Report of Transplantation of Preserved Arterial
Grafts in 9 Human Cases

BY ROBERT E. GROSS, M.D., F.A.C.S.,
ALEXANDER H. BILL, Jr., M.D., AND
E. CONVERSE PEIRCE, 2ND, M.D.
*Department of Surgery of the Harvard Medical School and the Surgical
Services of The Children's Hospital and the Peter Bent Brigham Hospital*

In certain operative procedures it would be of great value to be able to bridge an arterial defect with a graft, provided the method of grafting is reliable and is not cumbersome. Vein grafts (from the same individual and from other humans) have been used with some success, and are reasonably satisfactory if one is repairing arteries which are not of great size. There has been no safe method for permanently replacing a segment of a very large artery, especially the aorta, and it is to this problem that we have turned our attention.

Veins and arteries have been grafted into animals from the same animal (autografts), from the same species (homografts), and from other species (heterografts). It has been generally reported that autografts or homografts are more satisfactory than heterografts. Many substitutes for blood vessels have been suggested. Various inert substances have been suggested or tried for bridging blood vessel defects, including tubes of glass, of aluminum, of gold plate, and of silver

From *Surgery, Gynecology and Obstetrics,* 88:689, 1949. Reprinted by permission of *Surgery, Gynecology and Obstetrics.*

lined with paraffin. All of these substances have led to thrombosis. Recently, lucite channels for intubation of vessels has led to more promising results. Rigid rings (vein lined) for the nonsuture method of joining vessels have been made from ivory, magnesium, and vitallium.

TABLE I. RESULTS OF IMPLANTATION OF HOMOGRAFTS (PRESERVED BY QUICK FREEZING TO −72 DEGREES C.) INTO DOG AORTAS

Recipient dog No.	Atmosphere in storage tube	Length of time vessel preserved	Length of life of dog post-operatively	Cause of death	Fate of graft
135-47	Air	7 days	5 days	Hemorrhage	Graft broke down
136-47	Air	8 days	5 days	Hemorrhage	Graft broke down and completely thrombosed
137-47	Air	13 days	30 days	Hemorrhage	Graft broke down
139-47	Air	15 days	7 days	Hemorrhage	Graft broke down and completely thrombosed
122-47	Air	33 days	6 months	Sacrificed	Intimal sclerosis
124-47	Air	35 days	8 days	Hemorrhage	Graft broke down
125-47	Air	36 days	5 days	Hemorrhage	Graft broke down. Two thrombi
173-47	Helium	2 days	20 days	Hemorrhage	Graft broke down. Some thrombosis
174-47	Helium	3 days	19 days	Pneumonia	Tubular mural thrombus 2.0 mm. thick
166-47	Helium	7 days	8 days	Hemorrhage	Graft broke down and completely thrombosed
168-47	Helium	8 days	12 days	Hemorrhage	Graft broke down
180-47	Helium	14 days	6 months	(Still alive)	Considerable mural thrombus by aortogram

A wholly satisfactory solution to the problem of bridging a gap in large arteries or in the aorta would seem to lie in the direction of providing a vascular graft which is viable, which would resemble the normal vessel after implantation, which could withstand intra-arterial pressures, which would not cause thrombosis, and which would not set up serious reaction in the regional tissues. Knowing that transplantation of fresh arterial grafts from one animal to another had shown varying degrees of survival in the hands of Carrel and Guthrie and others, we undertook to repeat and extend some of their work, and to investigate extensively methods for preservation and storage of arterial grafts. As a preliminary part of our investigations, a study was made of the effects of transplantation of fresh aorta from one dog to another; this is being reported elsewhere by Gross and Hurwitt.

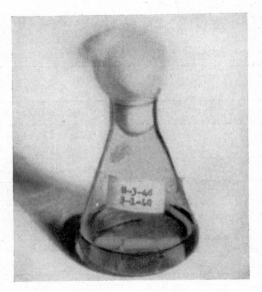

Fig. 1.—Blood vessel in Ehrlenmeyer flask containing nutrient medium, ready for storage in refrigerator.

Preservation of blood vessels has been studied previously by other surgeons. Carrel preserved arteries by storage in a refrigerator at temperatures above freezing, in various media, including vaseline, salt solution, defibrinated blood, and humid air. With these methods he had some degree of success in survival of the grafts following their implantation into other dogs. His results are rather difficult to evaluate because of the relatively few experiments in each method of study. Recently Blakemore and Lord and also Hufnagel have reported the successful preservation of arteries and veins by quick freezing and storage at temperatures well below freezing. The successful transplantation of an artery after preservation in formalin was reported by Levin and Larkin, but they were apparently unable to repeat this in later experiments. This was later successfully repeated by Guthrie.

Based on knowledge of the above previously published data, we outlined and completed three sets of animal experiments. In the first series of experiments an attempt was made to duplicate the work of Blakemore and Lord, and of Hufnagel, in quick-freezing the grafts and storing them at about −70 degrees centigrade. The second series was to investigate further the feasibility of preservation and use of heterografts (from one species to another). The third series was designed to investigate the preservation and use of homografts (from an animal of the same species); storing the grafts at temperatures just above freezing in appropriate media, the constituents of which were based on formulas developed by others interested in the field of tissue culture techniques and which were suggested to us by J. H. Hanks of the Department of Bacteriology of the Harvard Medical School. We thought that it would be of interest to determine whether various methods of preservation would allow the tissues of a vessel to remain alive; hence, it was decided to parallel our animal experimentations with tissue culture studies of specimens of the preserved vessels. Microscopic studies of implanted grafts were also planned; these were conducted (and will be reported) by Alan R. Moritz.

EXPERIMENTAL GRAFTS IN ANIMALS

Grafting into the abdominal aortas of dogs was selected as the method for the operative work. In such a large vessel, anastomoses are easily performed, and it is possible to evaluate the grafts without being hampered by thromboses which are apt to be troublesome when working with small vessels. The arteries to be preserved and tested were taken under sterile conditions from animals which had been sacrificed. The aorta was removed and its branches were tied with fine silk. It was cut into 3.0 centimeter lengths.

When a segment of aorta was to be implanted into a recipient animal the technique used was as follows: The dog was anesthetized with intravenous nembutal and the abdomen was opened through a left rectus incision. The abdominal aorta, between the renal arteries and the inferior mesenteric artery, was exposed and freed of branches for a distance of about 5.0 centimeters. It was then occluded in two places, either by the use of aortic clamps such as described by Gross and Hufnagel, or by the use of tape tourniquets, and severed between the two occluded points. A generous cuff was left beyond each clamp or tourniquet. After an aorta was thus divided, its cut ends retracted for a distance of approximately 3.0 centimeters; the graft to be tested was sutured into place between those ends (Fig. 4). The anastomoses were made by a single, continuous everting mattress stitch, using 5–0 Deknatel silk on an atraumatic needle. The insertion of such a graft took an average of 45 minutes, following which the clamps or tourniquets were removed. The peritoneum was then brought together over the aorta and the abdomen was closed. No chemotherapy or anticoagulants were used. No damage to the spinal cord or hind limbs was observed as a result of the occlusion of the aorta during these operations.

Series A: implantation of aorta homografts (preserved at −70 degrees centigrade). Twelve grafts were carried out with vessels which had been preserved at −70 degrees centigrade. The segments of aorta were obtained from donor dogs and placed in sterile test tubes which were hermetically sealed. Seven of these contained room air. In the five remaining tubes, the air in the tube was replaced by an atmosphere of helium under pressure of 20 to 40 millimeters of mercury above atmospheric level. This was done in an attempt to repeat the work of Hufnagel (20) who felt that helium (particularly under pressure) was a better conductor of heat than was air and hence would allow quicker freezing of the vessel.

When sealed, the test tube containing an aortic segment was immersed in a beaker containing 300 cubic centimeters of 95 per cent alcohol in which was floating one-half its volume of carbon-dioxide ice. The temperature of this mixture was −72 degrees centigrade. The tubes were kept in this for 15 minutes, and were then stored in a carbon-dioxide ice refrigerator at a temperature of about −70 degrees centigrade. The vessels were stored in this manner for lengths of time varying between 2 and 35 days. When a vessel was to be implanted into a recipient dog, it was thawed by immersing its test tube for 10 minutes in a bath of water at 35 degrees centigrade, after which it was removed from the tube and placed in a bowl of Ringer's solution at the operating table. It was then sutured into the abdominal aorta of a recipient dog, as described previously. Table I shows the results.

It will be seen that of 12 dogs, 1 dog died of pneumonia in 19 days, 2 dogs survived for at least 6 months with fairly good arterial pathways, and 9 died of breakdown of one of the anastomoses. The grafts which broke down did so between 2 and 12 days in 7 cases, and at 20 and 30 days in the other 2. Examination of these 9 autopsy specimens showed that the grafts themselves were friable and necrotic to the point of allowing the sutures to pull out before fibrous union had taken place. In our hands, this method of preservation by freezing gave highly unsatisfactory results.

TABLE II. RESULTS OF IMPLANTATION OF HETEROGRAFTS (PRESERVED IN 10 PER CENT DOG SERUM IN BALANCED SALT SOLUTION AT 1 TO 4 DEGREES C.) INTO DOG AORTAS

Recipient dog No.	Source of graft	Length of time vessel preserved	Length of life of dog postoperatively	Cause of death	Fate of graft
198-47	Hog	5 hours	5 months	(Still alive)	Aneurysmal dilatation of graft by aortogram
204-47	Hog	7 days	90 days	Sacrificed	Completely thrombosed
209-47	Hog	14 days	4½ months	Sacrificed	Excellent
215-47	Hog	21 days	30 days	Pneumonia	Excellent
223-47	Baboon	4 days	4 months	Sacrificed	Marked intimal sclerosis
230-47	Baboon	12 days	22 days	Hemorrhage	Disintegrated
6-48	Baboon	33 days	3½ months	(Still alive)	Completely thrombosed as shown by aortogram
49-48	Human	38 days	2 months	(Still alive)	Great dilatation of graft as shown by aortogram

Series B: implantation of aortic heterografts (preserved in balanced salt solution and 10 per cent dog serum at 1 to 4 degrees centigrade). A small number of heterografts were transplanted into dogs, to study the effects of transfer of arteries from one species to another. Four vessels from a hog, 3 from a baboon, and 1 vessel from a human were grafted into abdominal aortas of dogs. These vessels were obtained within 2 to 3 hours of death and were stored, at from 1 to 4 degrees centigrade, in a balanced salt solution to which 10 per cent dog serum was added. (The method of preservation is fully described in Series C.) The vessels were stored for varying periods of time before being implanted into recipient animals, as recorded in Table II.

Examination of Table II shows that the use of baboon aorta was uniformly unsatisfactory, while 3 of the hog vessels and the one piece of human vessel were partially successful in carrying blood for protracted periods of time. This small series of experiments in transplanting vessels from one species to another would seem to indicate that success or failure will depend upon the immunological reaction between the two species involved in the transfer. In some combinations, heterografts seem to live, whereas, other combinations of heterografts cause an intense reaction which leads to rapid degeneration or thrombosis of the implanted vessels.

Series C: implantation of aortic homografts (preserved in balanced salt solution and 10 per cent dog serum at 1 to 4 degrees centigrade). Twenty-five experiments were carried out with segments of aorta which had been stored in a medium which would supply minerals and nutrient elements to keep the tissue of the vessel alive. Each segment was obtained in a sterile manner and was then placed in a sterile 25 or 50 cubic centimeter Ehrlenmeyer flask which contained enough of the nutrient medium to just cover the graft. The medium was composed of 10 per cent homologous (dog) serum in "balanced salt solution"[1] which was maintained at a fairly constant pH by means of a buffer. To this medium was added enough of the salts of penicillin and streptomycin to give a concentration of 50 units of each drug per cubic centimeter of fluid. The flask was closed with a sterile cotton stopper and placed in an electric refrigerator of the hospital's blood bank, which is maintained with great care between the tem-

---

[1] The balanced salt solution is a modification of Tyrode's solution prepared and supplied to us by J. H. Hanks. It is made as follows:

Stock solution, contents 250 c.c.: NaCl 20 gm.; KCl, 1 gm.; $MgSO_4.7H_2O$, 0.2 gm.; $MgCl_2.6H_2O$, 0.2 gm.; $CaCl_2$, 0.35 gm. (dissolved separately); Na_2HPO_4, 0.15 gm. (0.38 gm. of $Na_2HPO.12H_2O$); $KHPO_4$, 0.15 gm.; glucose 2.5 gms.; 0.4 per cent phenol red, 12.5 c.c.

Buffer: 1.4 per cent $NaHCO_3$.

The stock solution is stored at room temperature with 1 c.c. chloroform.

The final solution is made by diluting the stock 1:10, autoclaving, and adding 0.5 c.c. buffer (previously autoclaved) per 20 c.c. This is stored in cotton-stoppered containers in the ice-box; it has an equilibrium at about pH 7.6.

peratures of 1 and 4 degrees centigrade. (A cotton stopper was used originally to allow free diffusion of carbon dioxide and oxygen, but subsequent studies show that a rubber cap is equally satisfactory and is probably more efficient in maintaining a suitable pH range in the flask contents.) After preservation in this manner, and before grafting, a segment of vessel has physical qualities very similar to those of a fresh vessel. This is in contrast to the frozen vessels of Series A, which were often quite friable when thawed out.

We do not mean to imply that the temperature range of 1 to 4 degrees centigrade is necessarily the most optimum one for storage of blood vessels. Indeed we have not extensively studied the preservation of tissue at many ranges of temperature above freezing because there seems to be little practical value in pursuing such investigations. We believed it to be worth while to study methods of preservation only at the low temperatures of refrigeration which are available to us and to many surgeons, such as that commonly used in blood bank storage systems where the range is usually 1 to 4 degrees centigrade.

As we have used it, this method has proved extremely satisfactory. It will be seen that among the 25 dogs with implanted grafts we had no deaths from disruption of the graft. There were 3 instances of complete thrombosis. In 1 of these, a vessel which had been preserved for 1 day, the graft was larger in diameter than the recipient aorta when implanted, giving an effect like that of a slight aneurysm. In the 2 others the grafts had been preserved for 56 days and 98 days respectively, which is considerably longer than we can now recommend for reliable preservation of grafts. In the remaining 22 dogs the grafts were known to be carrying blood at intervals from 4 days to 10 months after operation (Table III).

When viewed grossly at postmortem examination, the vessels were quite satisfactory save for the 3 which were wholly thrombosed. There was very little reaction in the retroperitoneal tissues around the grafts. Inspection of the intima of the grafts in the sacrificed animals has shown 4 which had small, insignificant, mural thrombi. One animal, which died of hepatitis 20 days after implantation of a 34 day preserved graft, showed a thickened, irregular suture line. One graft, sacrificed 3 months after implantation of a 5 day preserved specimen, showed considerable intimal sclerosis. All of the remaining grafts which have been examined after sacrifice have been in excellent condition by gross examination (Fig. 6). A few of the grafts seemed to be thinned somewhat. In several specimens the grafted portion of aorta was much less elastic than were the neighboring portions of host aorta.

TABLE III. RESULTS OF IMPLANTATION OF HOMOGRAFTS (PRESERVED IN 10 PER CENT DOG SERUM IN BALANCED SALT SOLUTION AT 1 TO 4 DEGREES C.) INTO DOG AORTAS

Recipient dog No.	Length of time vessel preserved	Length of life of dog after operation	Cause of death	Fate of graft
157-47	1 day	43 days	Sacrificed	Thrombosed. (Graft larger than host aorta when implanted)
149-47	2 days	3 months	Sacrificed	Good. Small mural thrombus
156-47	2 days	45 days	Sacrificed	Good. Small mural thrombus
30-48	2 days	5 months	(Still alive)	Excellent by aortogram
142-47	3 days	3 months	Sacrificed	Good. Tubular mural thrombus
159-47	4 days	3 months	Sacrificed	Excellent
143-47	5 days	3 months	Sacrificed	Good. Considerable intimal sclerosis
144-47	6 days	6 months	Sacrificed	Good. Slight dilatation
151-47	6 days	6 months	Sacrificed	Excellent
162-47	7 days	15 days	Sacrificed	Excellent
183-47	7 days	6 months	Sacrificed	Excellent
148-47	10 days	10 months	(Still alive)	Excellent by aortogram. ? Small mural thrombus
153-47	10 days	10 months	(Still alive)	Excellent by aortogram
187-47	14 days	12 days	Sacrificed	Excellent
191-47	19 days	8 months	(Still alive)	Excellent by aortogram. ? Tiny mural thrombus
170-47	20 days	6 months	Sacrificed	Excellent
178-47	28 days	11 days	Pneumonia	Excellent
61-48	30 days	5 months	(Still alive)	Excellent by aortogram. ? Tiny mural thrombus at the suture line
25-48	34 days	20 days	Hepatitis	Fair. Small mural thrombi. Graft poor color
80-48	40 days	3 months	(Still alive)	Excellent by aortogram
44-48	42 days	5 months	(Still alive)	Excellent by aortogram
55-48	56 days	35 days	Sacrificed	Completely thrombosed
67-48	70 days	4 months	(Still alive)	Excellent by aortogram
79-48	84 days	4 days	Intussusception	Excellent
78-48	98 days	20 days	Sacrificed	Completely thrombosed

Eight of the 25 dogs have not yet been sacrificed. Their grafts will be examined after longer periods of time. In each of these 8 animals the graft has been studied during life by means of aortography, employing roentgen visualization of the abdominal aorta (Fig. 5). In

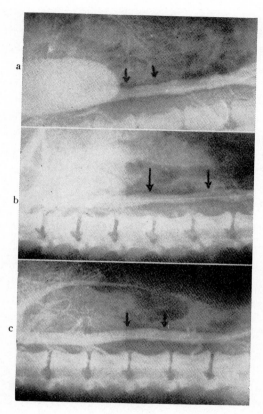

Fig. 5.—Aortograms of homografts in abdominal aortas of dogs, made during life by diodrast injection through a catheter which had been threaded up from the femoral artery. All of the grafts had been previously stored in 10 per cent dog serum in balanced salt solution at 1 to 4 degrees C. The graft is the segment between the two arrows. In each instance the graft is patent. *a.* Dog 170-47. Graft stored for 20 days. Aortogram made 6 months after insertion of graft. *b.* Dog 44-48. Graft stored for 42 days. Aortogram made 2 months after insertion of graft. *c.* Dog 67-48. Graft stored for 70 days. Aortogram made 1 month after insertion of graft.

all of these 8 dogs the aortic graft is patent and has the same caliber as the adjacent host aorta. In 3 of them there are one or several tiny irregularities at anastomotic lines, which probably are insignificant mural thrombi, and which do not diminish the caliber of vessel lumina to any important degree.

Inspection of Table III will show that storage of the grafts for more than 50 days appears to be unsatisfactory. Of the 4 vessels kept for more than 50 days before grafting, 1 was not available for study because the animal died on the fourth day from intestinal obstruction, 2 vessels were thrombosed, and only 1 was wholly satisfactory. Of the 21 grafts stored less than 50 days before implantation, 20 were satisfactory and only 1 was unsatisfactory. It is noteworthy that in this whole series not one animal died from breakdown of a graft.

TISSUE CULTURE EVALUATION OF METHODS OF ARTERIAL PRESERVATION

The vessels which were used in all three experimental series were examined by making tissue cultures of them at appropriate intervals to determine their viability (Fig. 2). These tissue cultures were made

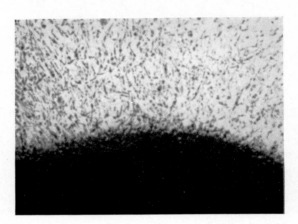

Fig. 2.—Photomicrograph of tissue culture of piece of dog aorta after 28 days of storage in 10 per cent homologous serum in balanced salt solution. The black mass in the lower third of the picture is the border of the original piece of aorta. The lacy substances in the upper two-thirds of the photograph are viable and growing cells, indicating that the specimen of aorta is alive after the 28 days of storage.

under the guidance of J. H. Hanks and John Enders. The work will be described in greater detail elsewhere, but the principal results are summarized herewith.

In the first part of this work 8 pieces of tissue were cultured from each of 12 dog aortas, the pieces of vessel being obtained within 2 to 5 hours after death of the animals. Of the 96 pieces of vessels which were so planted, 91 grew out fibroblastic cells.

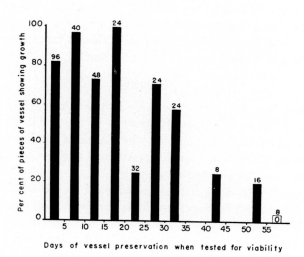

Fig. 3.—Results of tissue culture studies to test viability of pieces of dog blood vessels which had been stored in 10 per cent homologous serum in balanced salt solution at 1 to 4 degrees C. The number above each column indicates the number of tissue culture tests which were made. Most of the vessels appeared to be viable for 35 to 40 days.

Study of portions of dog aorta which had been stored at —70 degrees centigrade (Series A) showed that planting of 34 such specimens led to growth in only 2 instances. The freezing and thawing process doubtless had killed the tissue cells in most instances.

Studies of baboon aortas, hog aortas, and human aortas, each of which had been stored in the cold in balanced salt solution containing 10 per cent dog serum (Series B), showed that most of the vessels were living after more than a month.

Detailed studies were made of dog aortas, each of which had been stored at 1 to 4 degrees centigrade in balanced salt solution containing 10 per cent dog serum (Series C). Samples of the vessels were planted at varying times after initial storage of them, to determine how long the vessels were in a viable state. Figure 3 summarizes the data which were obtained. It will be seen that most of the vessels were living and could be grown out on tissue culture for as long as a month or more. After 30 or 35 days there was a marked diminution in the number of aortas which were still living. After 55 days all vessels were found to be dead. These studies lead us to believe that arteries can be stored and kept viable for a little more than a month by the technique which is described in detail under Series C.

DISCUSSION

We believe that there are three main factors which might influence the success or failure of an arterial graft: (1) the viability of the vessel at the time of implantation; (2) the degree of the immunological reaction between the host and the graft; and (3) the technique employed in making the anastomoses.

In our work with dogs, we have had good results with the transplantation of arterial homografts which had been stored at low temperature in 10 per cent homologous serum in balanced salt solution. We have set certain time limits for obtaining the blood vessel segments after death of the donor; a period of 3 or 4 hours is satisfactory, but it probably should not exceed 6 hours. Vessels removed as long as 6 hours after death were found to be still viable by tissue culture studies, and successful transplants could be carried out with them. Beyond 6 hours we felt that there was a likelihood of rapid appearance of postmortem change and of bacterial contamination.

From animal experimentation we found that vessels could be stored (at low temperature and in 10 per cent homologous serum in balanced salt solution) and subsequently used for grafting into other animals of the same species. The upper limits of safety for storing vessels under these conditions is probably in the region of 35 or 40 days. We have selected this limit because aortic grafts in dogs were successful up until this time, and thereafter began to fail. Furthermore, tissue culture studies also indicated that viability of vascular segments is maintained for approximately 35 or 40 days and then rapidly declines.

If we include the preliminary series of fresh homografts transplanted into dog aortas, reported by Gross and Hurwitt, we have now observed in this laboratory the results of four categories of aortic grafts. They are: (1) fresh homografts; (2) homografts from tissue preserved by quick freezing to about —70 degrees centigrade; (3) heterografts (hog to dog, baboon to dog, and human to dog) from

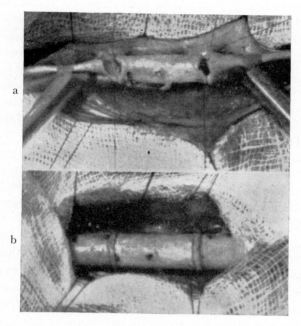

FIG. 4.—Preserved aortic graft being implanted into abdominal aorta of a dog. *a*. Above, graft in place. *b*. Completion of anastomoses (everting, continuous, mattress suture employed).

tissue preserved in 10 per cent dog serum in balanced salt solution; and (4) homografts from tissue preserved in 10 per cent dog serum in balanced salt solution. In our hands, the three series in which the grafts could be shown to be viable up to the time of implantation were much more successful than the series of homografts preserved by quick freezing, in which life could seldom be demonstrated by tissue culture. It is important to note that the homoplastic tissue preserved in a living state (up to 42 days) in the balanced salt and 10 per cent serum mixture was as satisfactory as fresh tissue for grafting. From our various observations we believe that a graft is more apt to be successful if it is viable[2] when implanted.

The factor of immunological reaction between graft and host is exceedingly difficult to evaluate. Our series of heterografts is small, and no conclusions can be drawn therefrom. However, it was a distinct surprise to find that any of the grafts from one species to another would survive. Indeed, the microscopic structure of the grafts which were transferred from hog to dog showed better preservation of the media than was the case in any of the dog to dog homografts. The grafts from baboon to dog, on the other hand, were very poor, both grossly and microscopically. This raises the interesting possibility that the transplantation of heterografts between certain species may be practical. If it could be proved, for example, that vessels of sheep, dog, or hog could be used successfully in human beings, we could have available a relatively convenient source of blood vessel grafts. The successful transplantation of fresh dog arteries to the femoral artery in 3 human beings is being reported by Oudot, from Paris. He stated in a personal communication that dog vessels were used rather than human arteries because French law prohibits autopsy (and any chance of procuring vessels from a dead body) until 24 hours postmortem. He was able to demonstrate, by arteriography, that the dog vessel grafts were patent, but he did not state how long after operation these roentgenographic studies were made.

While our laboratory experiences convinced us of the dependability of homografts—as far as dog to dog is concerned—there is, of course, considerable doubt regarding the possibility of safely transferring arteries from one human to another. While it is true that there might be no correlation between what occurred in dogs and what might happen to homografts in humans, our laboratory experiences did give us some courage to attempt grafts in patients for bridging gaps in large arteries or in the aorta when the circumstances at the operating table demanded such therapy.

[2] We have had some measure of success with a small series of 15 grafts which were definitely known to be nonviable. These grafts were stored in 4 per cent neutral formalin for from 10 to 25 days, were then rinsed thoroughly in buffered salt solution, and implanted into recipient animals. All grafts carried blood well for several months, but roentgenograms of some of these show calcification in the graft walls.

ARTERIAL GRAFTS IN HUMAN CASES

Segments of large arteries, or aorta, have been accumulated from human subjects who have died in automobile accidents and from whom we were able to get the material by the courtesy and co-operation of the medical examiner. In all instances the vessels were removed within a few hours after death of the individual, and in no

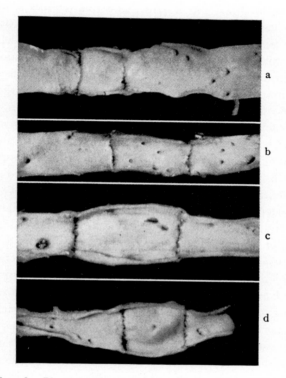

Fig. 6.—Photographs of homografts in abdominal aortas of dogs. Prior to their implantation, all grafts had been preserved in 10 per cent dog serum in balanced salt solution at 1 to 4 degrees C. *a.* Dog 159-47. Graft stored 4 days; animal sacrificed 3 months after implantation. *b.* Dog 187-47. Graft stored 14 days; animal sacrificed 12 days after implantation. *c.* Dog 183-47. Graft stored 7 days; animal sacrificed 6 months after implantation. *d.* Dog 170-47. Graft stored 26 days; animal sacrificed 6 months after implantation.

instance was the time lapse greater than 5 hours. The body was always opened under aseptic conditions (operator with cap, mask, sterile gown, and gloves; skin preparation with tincture of iodine; sterile drapes, instruments, etc.). The acquired segments of vessel—iliac, carotid, subclavian, and aortic—were preserved in individual flasks and just covered with the balanced salt solution described previously under Series C, except that the 10 per cent serum was human in origin. These flasks were then stored in a carefully regulated refrigerator (of the hospital's blood bank) at 1 to 4 degrees centigrade.

Eight of these human grafts have been implanted into patients who had a cyanotic type of congenital heart disease, and in whom it was desirable to make some sort of a shunt of blood (the Blalock-Taussig principle) from the aorta or one of its branches into the pulmonary artery. Ordinarily it is possible to bring such vessels together for a direct anastomosis by the Blalock or the Potts techniques, but under some circumstances it is very difficult to establish such shunts without excessive tension on the suture lines. While we hasten to express the opinion that direct anastomoses will in the majority of cases prove to be superior to any method which employs an interposed vessel, it is also probably true that the use of a graft in an occasional case (which will allow arterial junctions to be made without the slightest tension) will give a result which is better than that which would have been obtained from a poor, direct anastomosis. These same general principles also will probably hold true for treatment of coarctation of the aorta. Excision of a constricted segment and anastomosis of the remaining ends of aorta give a very satisfactory result in most cases, but in some instances a very long portion of aorta must be excised, or else the remaining aortic ends are inelastic and cannot be easily apposed. Under either set of circumstances the use of an interposed graft may prove to be the most satisfactory method of re-establishing an aortic pathway of normal size. The validity of this statement is suggested by the pleasing result obtained in Case 9, wherein a graft was used to repair an aortic defect after excision of a coarctation. A brief summary of each case follows:

CASE 1. D. E., a 5 year old boy, had been cyanotic since birth and had great limitation of physical activity. On physical examination there was marked cyanosis, clubbing of the fingers and toes, and a harsh systolic murmur in the pulmonic area. Roentgenograms of the chest gave findings typical of a tetralogy of Fallot. Electrocardiograms showed a right axis deviation. The red blood count was 7.6 million. At operation on February 6, 1948, a 3 centimeter segment of (adult) iliac artery, which had been preserved for 2 weeks, was sutured into place between the left pulmonary artery and the proximal end of the left subclavian artery. During the 5 months since operation the child has had great alleviation of his cyanosis and has had a marked increase in his tolerance for exercise. The red blood count has fallen to 5.5 million. There is a continuous murmur in the pulmonary area of the precordium.

CASE 2. W. P., a 4½ year old child, deeply cyanotic since birth, had had a right-sided hemiplegia since the age of 2, this neurological damage being presumably on the basis of thrombosis of intracranial vessels. A faint systolic murmur was audible in the pulmonary area. The red blood count was 9.8 million and the hematocrit was 87 per cent. He had insufficient strength to do more than sit in bed. Roentgenograms and electrocardiograms were typical of a tetralogy of Fallot; the aortic arch was on the right. At operation on February 11, 1948, a human arterial graft, 2.5 centimeters long, which had been preserved for 14 days, was sutured in place between the proximal end of the left subclavian artery and the side of the left pulmonary artery (Fig. 7). During the 5 months that the boy has been followed since operation his general condition has been dramatically improved. The red count has fallen to 5.8 million. He can now walk considerable distances and has a marked alleviation of his cyanosis. A continuous murmur is audible in the left second intercostal space anteriorly.

CASE 3. S. F., a 10½ year old girl, had been cyanotic since birth, and was able to walk only 75 yards at a time. Auscultation revealed a pulmonic systolic murmur of moderate intensity. Roentgenograms, electrocardiograms, and cardiac catheterization all gave findings which were compatible with a tetralogy of Fallot. The aortic arch was on the right. At operation on March 2, 1948 a human arterial graft, which had been preserved 1 day, was placed between the right subclavian artery and the side of the right pulmonary artery. Dicumarol therapy was given postoperatively; on the tenth day bleeding began from the nose, mouth, gastrointestinal tract, into the right pleural cavity, and manifestations of intracranial neurological disturbances appeared. Because the blood in the right side of the chest could not be satisfactorily aspirated, a thoracotomy was performed on March 16, 1948, to remove clots. The child died the following day, largely from the neurological complications of the anticoagulation therapy. Postmortem examination showed the graft and shunt to be patent and in good condition, without evidence of leakage or

thrombosis. The thoracic bleeding had apparently come from the muscu-
lature of the chest wall.

CASE 4. L. B., a 12 year old girl, had been cyanotic since the age of
3 to 4 months. She was barely able to climb one flight of stairs. On physical examination there was marked cyanosis, advanced clubbing, and a

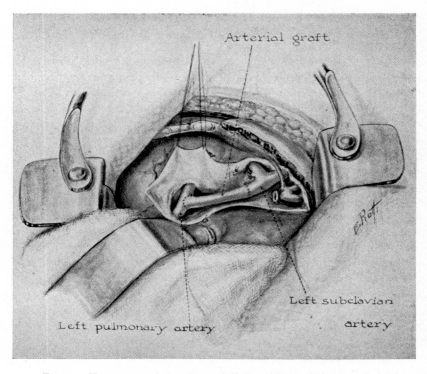

FIG. 7.—Treatment of tetralogy of Fallot (Case 2) by insertion of
a human arterial graft between the left pulmonary artery and the
proximal end of the left subclavian artery. (Patient had a right aortic
arch and an innominate artery on the left.) The graft had been secured from another human and had been preserved for 14 days before
insertion into the recipient patient.

systolic murmur of considerable intensity in the pulmonic area. Roentgenograms and electrocardiograms were consistent with a tetralogy of
Fallot. The red blood count was 8.7 million. At operation on May 1,
1948 a graft, which had been preserved for 4 days, was implanted between the proximal end of the left subclavian artery and the side of

the left pulmonary artery. The child's color was greatly improved for about 24 hours but she then developed congestive heart failure, and died on the second postoperative day. A continuous murmur was heard until death occurred. At autopsy the graft was found to be intact and also to be free of thrombosis.

CASE 5. H. B., a 13 year old boy, was first noted to have persistent cyanosis at the age of 6 years. He was forced to squat and rest after short periods of walking. Physical examination showed moderate cyanosis, well marked clubbing of the fingers and toes, and a loud systolic murmur over the pulmonic area. Roentgenograms of the chest and electrocardiograms were consistent with a diagnosis of tetralogy of Fallot. The red blood count was 6.2 million. At operation on May 3, 1948, a segment of human aorta, 2 centimeters long (from a 5 year old child) which had been preserved 16 days, was sutured into place between the side of the descending aorta and the side of the left pulmonary artery. Postoperatively, a continuous murmur is audible over the pulmonic area. In the 2 months since operation was performed, this boy has progressed extremely well; his color is greatly improved, his physical activity is strikingly increased, and the red blood count has fallen to 5.2 million.

CASE 6. R. D., an 11 year old boy, had been intensely cyanotic since birth. His activity had been so severely limited that he was barely able to ascend one flight of stairs. Physical examination showed marked cyanosis, advanced clubbing of the fingers and toes, and a systolic murmur over the pulmonic area. Roentgenograms, electrocardiograms, and cardiac catheterization were interpreted as indicating that the patient had a stenosis of the tricuspid valve with an associated large interauricular septal defect. The pulmonary blood flow was believed to be insufficient. At operation on May 6, 1948 a segment of human aorta (from a 5 year old child), which had been preserved 19 days, was interposed as a shunt between the side of the descending aorta and the side of left pulmonary artery. Postoperatively, there is a continuous murmur in the pulmonary area. In the 2 months since operation the boy has had an excellent improvement in color and in tolerance for physical activity.

CASE 7. A. H. was a 7 year old boy who had exhibited rather constant cyanosis since birth and had had frequent spells of fainting, without definite evidence of cerebral thrombosis. He had a low tolerance for exercise, and frequently assumed a squatting position. On examination there was marked cyanosis, clubbing, a thrill and a loud systolic murmur in the third left interspace. Electrocardiograms showed a marked right axis deviation, and fluoroscopic findings were not those consistently found with a tetralogy of Fallot. At operation on May 17, 1948, the pressure in the left pulmonary artery—although not actually measured—was obviously much greater than in most cases of tetralogy and it was very doubtful if an aorta-pulmonary artery shunt would be of value. However, it was decided to attempt such an anastomosis. Because the vessels lay in positions which precluded a direct anastomosis, a graft 2 centimeters in length (which had been preserved 20 days) was sutured into the side of the descending aorta, and its opposite end sewed end-to-side into the pulmonary artery. Only a questionable thrill could be felt in the graft when the clamps were removed; the pulmonary artery pressure was so high that probably little, if any, blood flowed through the shunt. Following operation the boy showed no important changes in color or activity; only a systolic murmur could be heard, in the pulmonary area. He was discharged home unimproved. We believe that the failure to produce beneficial changes in this case was due, not to thrombosis of the graft, but to the fact that the child has some sort of a cyanotic state (such as an Eisenmenger complex) which is not benefited by an aorta-pulmonary shunt.

CASE 8. R. A. was a 12 year old boy who had been cyanotic since birth. There had been moderate limitation of activities, "spells of weakness" and frequent "squatting on his haunches." On examination there was moderate cyanosis, a very loud systolic murmur in the pulmonic area, and mild clubbing. The hemoglobin was 25.8 grams and the hematocrit was 71 per cent. The electrocardiogram showed a right-axis shift. Cardiac catheterization and fluoroscopy gave findings indicative of a tetralogy of Fallot. At operation on May 19, 1948 the left subclavian artery was turned downward but in spite of the fact that the left pulmonary artery was divided (and its distal end turned upward), these two ends of vessel could not be brought together for anastomosis. Therefore, a graft 4 centimeters long (which had been preserved 32 days) was inserted end-to-end between the left subclavian artery and the distal end of the left pulmonary artery. Following operation the boy made an excellent recovery; by the time of hospital discharge the hemoglobin had fallen to 16 grams. Since the operation was carried out there has been a loud, continuous murmur in the pulmonary area, the boy's color has greatly improved, and even though the period of postoperative observation is only 7 weeks it is already obvious that his exercise tolerance is increased.

CASE 9. D. S. was a 7 year old boy who entered the hospital for treatment of coarctation of the aorta. Examination showed a pressure in the arms varying on multiple readings from 130 to 150 millimeters of mercury systolic. No femoral pulsations could be felt, and no blood pressure readings could be obtained in the legs. A systolic murmur of moderate in-

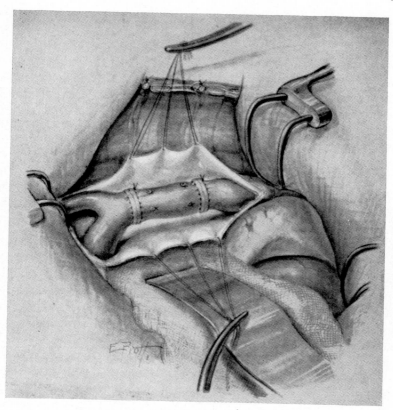

FIG. 8.—Treatment of coarctation of the aorta (Case 9) by removal of narrowed segment of aorta and insertion of a human aortic graft. The graft had been procured from a human who had died in an automobile accident; it had been preserved for 28 days in 10 per cent human serum in balanced salt solution at 1 to 4 degrees C. before insertion into the recipient patient. The graft was 5 centimeters in length.

tensity was heard in the precordium. By fluoroscopy the heart was slightly enlarged. At operation on May 24, 1948 a coarctation of the aorta was found about 1.5 centimeters below the origin of the left subclavian artery. The narrowed portion was excised and it was found to have a lumen of only 2 millimeters in diameter. The remaining ends of the aorta could be brought together only with great tension; it was therefore decided to insert a graft. This graft was a segment of aorta removed from a human

28 days previously; it measured 5 centimeters in length. The anastomoses to the aorta above and to the aorta below were made with continuous mattress stitches of silk, piercing the entire thickness of the vessel walls and everting the ends of the vessels (Fig. 8). The anastomoses could be made without the slightest tension. The patient had an uninterrupted convalescence. Following operation there was an excellent pulsation in the arteries of the legs. By the end of the second postoperative week the arm pressures had fallen to 108 millimeters of mercury systolic and the leg pressures had risen to 135 millimeters of mercury systolic.

SUMMARY

A method for the preservation of arterial segments is described. This consists in the storage of vessels at temperatures just above freezing and immersed in a mixture of 10 per cent homologous serum in a balanced salt solution to which are added a buffer, a pH color indicator, and streptomycin and penicillin. Vessels to be stored in this manner have been removed from donor animals between 1 and 6 hours after death and have been kept for periods of as long as 42 days before they were successfully transplanted into other dogs. Tissue culture studies have shown that viability is maintained for 35 to 40 days in blood vessels stored in this way.

On the basis of these laboratory investigations, segments of arteries or aortas have been secured from humans who have died suddenly and without sepsis. These vessels have been stored in the manner described, and have subsequently been used for human patients when the need arose to bridge gaps in large arteries. Segments of such preserved arteries or aortas have been grafted into 9 human subjects with results which are very promising and which certainly merit further trial and study.

Since completion of this manuscript, 6 more grafts have been inserted into humans. One of these has been used in the treatment of a tetralogy of Fallot and the other 5 were inserted into the aorta after removal of coarctations. These have been in place from 3 to 9 months and all are still patent.

12. The Soul of the Surgeon

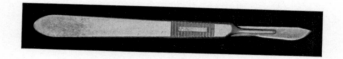

PREFATORY COMMENTS

The present trend towards superradical surgery in the treatment of cancer can be justified only on the basis that the disease is confined to the area of extirpation. Unfortunately this determination is based on gross examination only, since at the present time it is impossible to ascertain the biologic predeterminism of the lesion. It is the hope of many that within a few years there will be available a biochemical test which will help elucidate this problem. In the meantime, we must resort to timeworn surgical procedures which all too frequently fail to achieve a happy outcome. It is in the approach to this problem that a surgeon should become truly humble. What satisfaction can he enjoy if, after he has performed a brilliant operation, the patient dies because of complications secondary to his operation or because of an accelerated spread of the cancer? How many times will he have occasion to ask himself whether the patient wouldn't have been better off if he had refrained from performing such an extensive operation? In other instances he may even upbraid himself for having been too timid in his approach.

The results of surgery are considered under the headings of morbidity and mortality rates. Usually there is no indication of the number of patients who are made worse by the operation and who would have rejected the procedure if they had been aware of its consequences. A patient may survive an extensive operation without a complication but become distraught because of his digestive difficulties following a total gastrectomy, or because of the frustrating experience of managing a "wet" colostomy. A critical article should contain data concerning the number of patients who have been totally unhappy

453

with the changes wrought by surgery. How much more contributory our surgical literature would be if it included a determination of the *aggravation rate* as well as the *mortality* and *morbidity rates*. Dunphy's ensuing article not only reveals some of these misgivings but it also represents a sober evaluation of the physician's responsibility to the patient. For a better understanding of these and other concepts, we urge every physician to read the chapter entitled "The Nature of Conscience" in Sperry's *The Ethical Basis of Medical Practice*.

In our present system of residency training, the emphasis may be wrongly placed on turning out well-trained technicians instead of on the more fundamental attributes that make a surgeon truly great. As educators, our most sacred obligation to society is to develop surgeons with a conscience, men who bow their heads in humility and who treat all patients as they would desire their own brothers or sisters to be treated. This would be a far better world if every surgeon would heed Shakespeare's words in *Measure for Measure:* "Go to your bosom, knock there and ask your heart what it doth know." Vannevar Bush criticized the present medical-school system when he stated, "The medical man deals with his patient in a highly impersonal way. This is not a matter of test tubes or microscopes; it is a matter of human understanding. Many facets of human relationships are absent or distorted in the artificial atmosphere of a hospital or a consulting room. The doctor, above all men, needs to be a full man.

"The finest of the old-time country doctors had something rare and subtle that was without price. We can recapture some of this without sacrificing anything of moment in scientific rigor or detail."

J. ENGLEBERT DUNPHY (1908–)

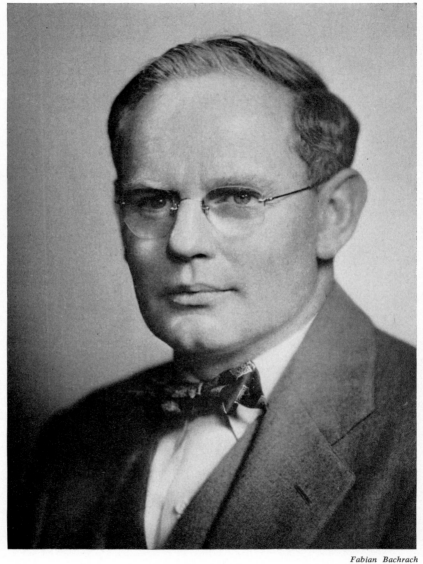

John Englebert Dunphy was born on March 31, 1908, at Northampton, Massachusetts. He was trained at the Harvard Medical School and at the Peter Bent Brigham Hospital. He became Professor of Surgery at Harvard in 1955, after 17 years as a member of the faculty. He served with distinction in World War II and received several decorations.

Dr. Dunphy's contributions to the literature cover a wide variety of topics, particularly wound healing, gastrointestinal tract surgery and surgery of cancer. His sound evaluation of the role of surgery in the treatment of malignant disease is extremely thought-provoking. He is senior author of a textbook on physical diagnosis and a member of the editorial boards of the New England Journal of Medicine *and the* Annals of Surgery. *He is currently Director of the 5th Surgical Service and the Sears Surgical Laboratory at the Boston City Hospital and a member of numerous honorary organizations.*

CHANGING CONCEPTS IN THE SURGERY OF CANCER

BY J. ENGLEBERT DUNPHY, M.D.

Clinical Professor of Surgery, Harvard Medical School; Surgeon,
Peter Bent Brigham Hospital, Boston

In estimating the limitations of surgery we find none except they be set by ourselves. How shall they be set? By conservative judgment opposed to rashness." This estimate of "The Future of Surgery without Limit" was made by David W. Cheever in his presidential address to the American Surgical Association before the turn of the century. Sixty-four years later it has a singular applicability to the surgery of cancer.

The surgeon of today, as Cheever foresaw, is enabled by virtue of the technical advances of his art to carry out an operation of almost unlimited extent. In dealing with cancer, however, he is seriously handicapped in setting the extent of a procedure by an almost total ignorance of the biologic propensities of the lesion he is attempting to treat. The most radical operation on a seemingly early lesion may be followed by widespread, rapidly progressive metastases and, contrariwise, a palliative resection undertaken with no hope of permanent cure may result in an extraordinarily long period of well-being for the patient. Until an accurate appraisal of the growth potentialities of any given tumor can be made, the surgeon must continue to grope in comparative darkness. In this darkness, however there are rays of light, the perception of which will be enhanced by a distinct change

From the *New England Journal of Medicine, 249:1,* 1953. Reprinted by permission.

in the traditional concept of the nature of cancer. This change in concept is of more than philosophic importance to the surgeon.

THEORETICAL CONSIDERATIONS

Traditional notions regarding cancer, which have become so ingrained that they seriously hamper the judgment of the surgeon in its treatment, may be summarized as follows: first, cancer is a lawless, autonomous growth that spreads constantly and progressively throughout the life of the host and is dependent upon the host for its blood supply alone; secondly, early treatment is synonymous with cure and, conversely, late treatment is of little or no avail; finally, there is a close correlation between the histologic structure and the biologic behavior of neoplasms.

Evidence against the Autonomy and Constant Progressive Growth of Cancer

The wild, destructive, continuous and purposeless growth of many tumors has led to the belief that neoplasia is an autonomous process. In this sense a cancer is a parasite that destroys the host on which it depends only for its blood supply. This view was supported by Ewing and has been widely accepted. From a practical point of view, it allows for no alteration in tumor growth except by its direct destruction.

This thesis has been recognized as untenable by a number of pathologists for many years. The orderly cellular pattern and obvious functional activity of certain cancers, particularly of endocrine glands, is against this view. The rare regression of distant metastases after removal of a primary tumor or after castration in ovarian lesions has been recognized for many years. Such a prolonged quiescence or even regression of malignant growth can hardly be ascribed to inadequate blood supply and suggests dependence upon some metabolic factor derived from the host.

Convincing evidence of the dependence of certain neoplasms on the metabolism of the host has been provided by the studies of Huggins and others on the regression of prostatic carcinoma after orchidectomy and adrenalectomy. The alterations of the growth pattern of cancer of the breast by androgens and estrogens is additional evidence that the metabolism of cancer cells may be altered by indirect measures. Although many years may elapse before similar changes can be induced in other cancers, the implications are obvious, particularly in relation to avenues of research in cancer.

One of the most widely accepted characteristics of cancer is that the rate of growth is constant for each tumor. Part of this belief is based on the histologic structure of particular neoplasms, which tends to remain fairly constant throughout the life of the host. The most convincing evidence, however, is that the life space of the host with an untreated tumor is remarkably similar for lesions in specific organs. Shimkin has collected statistical data from several sources that show, for example, that in cancer of the esophagus nearly all the patients die within three years. In cancer of the breast, on the other hand, over 20 per cent are alive at the end of five years. The rate varies for other lesions such as carcinoma of the bladder, rectum and cervix. But in general, the data indicate that the life span of hosts with tumors in particular locations is sufficiently similar to suggest a true correlation.

These data do not, however, exclude the possibility of great variations in the rate of growth during the career of any particular tumor. Thus, an untreated cancer of the rectum that kills the host at the end of three years falls within the anticipated survival curve of cancer of the rectum, but careful observation of the patient during this period may indicate that for the first two and a half years the tumor had remained comparatively quiet and then had grown at an extraordinarily rapid rate during the last six months of the patient's life. Certainly, clinical observations of patients with advanced cancer strongly suggest that variations in the rate of growth within the life span of the host are extraordinarily common. This is particularly characteristic of recurrent and metastic lesions. Indeed, the vast majority of metastatic lesions that appear several years after the removal of primary tumors must be interpreted as showing evidence of a significant period of quiescence since they must have been present at the time the original lesion was excised. A case has been described in which at reexploration four and a half years after excision of a large recurrent cancer, no evidence of neoplasm could be found within the abdominal cavity. Yet six months later, the patient was dead from extensive abdominal carcinomatosis. A second primary lesion could not be demonstrated. Although the logarithmic character of tumor growth accounts in part for the apparently more rapid progression as a tumor increases in size it does not explain such a long period of quiescence as occurred in this case, in which no evident progression of the lesion could be demonstrated.

It is particularly important to realize that the rate of growth of metastatic lesions varies in different locations. This phenomenon is readily seen in the skin metastases of cancer of the breast. A new lesion may appear and grow with extraordinary rapidity at a time when an earlier adjacent lesion remains exactly the same size or is regressing. Scott described a patient with cancer of the prostate in whom successive crops of skin metastases appeared and regressed completely without therapy. Cases of metastatic cancer in which the rate of growth varied widely in different locations have occurred.

The most remarkable evidence of fluctuations in the growth of malignant neoplasms is seen in the rare but significant cases of spontaneous regression. In 1918 Rohdenburg collected 100 such cases from the literature. More recently, similar cases have been described by Rae and Dunphy. Duke-Elder believes that there are at least 11 well authenticated cases in which spontaneous cure of malignant retinoblastomas of the eye has occurred. Prolonged quiescence of malignant melanomas are well known, and there are rare but well documented cases of spontaneous regression of this disease.

A significant point to be made about these retrogressions of tumor and variations in the growth of metastatic lesions lies not in the hope that it offers the patient but in the evidence that it provides of the susceptibility of malignant growths to systemic and local factors arising within the host.

Significance of Time in the Treatment of Cancer

The traditional concept of cancer reveals it as a mutation of cells arising in a single microscopic location and steadily expanding in accordance with a specific rate of growth; after reaching a certain size, which varies with different tumors, it spreads through lymphatic channels to regional nodes. After being temporarily arrested by lymph nodes, the neoplastic lesion extends into neighboring structures and finally enters the blood stream, where it produces distant metastases. Accordingly, effective treatment merely should be carried out early enough, which means before the lesion metastasizes to distant areas, preferably before it spreads to regional nodes and ideally while it is still a microscopic nest of cells. According to this theory, time is the essence of cancer therapy. In rapidly growing, undifferentiated lesions there is little time during which successful therapy may be accomplished; in slowly growing lesions there is more time, but theoretically, if all cancers were detectable early, the cure rate would approach 100 per cent.

Apart from the fact that this traditional concept cannot be supported by the available evidence, it has one serious and dangerous consequence. Overemphasis of the importance of early treatment is blinding clinicians to the fact that many large, so-called "late cases" are amenable to successful treatment. This is particularly true of cancer of the gastrointestinal tract in patients in the older age group. I have heard it argued in view of the recognized poor salvage rate in gastric cancer, that resection of a large gastric tumor in an old man was unwarranted, because in the particular case under discussion "the story was of such long duration and the tumor so large that it must have metastasized." How many patients have been deprived of the benefit of a surgical opinion on this basis is a matter of conjecture.

Although there are tumors that in their behavior adhere faithfully to the traditional ideas of cancer, the spectrum of growth is so wide and variable that a radical revision of this concept is essential.

In the first place it is of more than theoretical importance for the surgeon to know that the unicentric, microscopic, single-focus, one-cell or two-cell origin of cancer is no longer tenable. There is abundant evidence that neoplasia arises from fields of tissues and enlarges not merely by cellular proliferation but also by progressive neoplastic conversion of tissue within these fields. Multicentric or large field origin of cancer is particularly characteristic of cancer of the skin, breast, pancreas, prostate and gastrointestinal tract.

Regardless of the mode of initial carcinogenesis the variations in growth potential are extraordinary. Some tumors must begin to metastasize while the initial focus of tumor is still microscopic. Others may be confined to a local area for months or years. The extremes of the spectrum are familiar to every experienced clinician. A huge, solitary metastasis from a small focus of tumor in the thyroid gland or in the kidney may be contrasted with the prolonged local invasion of a comedo cancer of the breast. Although these extremes are recognized, the frequency with which the biologic propensities of the cancer outweigh any advantage to be gained by early treatment is not appreciated. It is a discouraging fact that with the exception of certain cancers, notably of the cervix and the skin, there is little difference in five-year survival rates in groups of patients treated within the first few months of the onset of symptoms and in those treated after delays as long as a year. This has been demonstrated in studies of cancer of the stomach and ovary, certain series of cancer of the breast and in osteogenic sarcoma.

One must not conclude from these data that time is of no importance. It is quite obvious that a patient who is cured after a resection of a large carcinoma of the rectum that has been present for two years would have been better and more effectively treated with less risk to life had the operation been performed one and a half years earlier. Moreover, although it is unlikely that the earliest possible treatment will alter the ultimate cure rate in highly malignant neoplasms, it unquestionably increases the months or years of salvage given to that patient. Early treatment will always be a desideratum, but it is not the *sine qua non* of successful therapy. The same emphasis that is placed upon the factor of time must also be given to a better understanding of the complex biologic nature of this disease, particularly the wide variations in growth patterns, the great disparity in behavior of different tumors and of the same tumor in different locations and the possible role of natural defenses arising within the host.

HISTOLOGY AS AN INDEX OF BIOLOGY

Morbid histology has helped so much to place surgery on a rational basis that surgeons are apt to accept the interpretation of a pathologist at more than its face value. The penultimate classification of tumors undertaken by some pathologists is particularly misleading because it implies a close correlation between the histologic appearance of a tumor and its biologic behavior. Actually, no such correlation exists. When the pathologist looks at a section from a particular tumor and classifies it as "highly malignant" or "carcinoma simplex, Grade 3," he knows nothing about the biologic propensities of the tumor in question. He merely means that, in his experience or according to what he has read, a majority of tumors, conforming more or less to this histologic appearance, have proved to be highly malignant in the past. There is no doubt that generally the more anaplastic a tumor appears histologically, the more highly malignant it is likely to be. However, there as so many exceptions to this general rule that no precise predictions are warranted. The discrepancy is so great that treatment should never be withheld or altered solely on the histologic appearance of a tumor. Thus, the pathologist who looks at a section of a metastatic thyroid tumor with well differentiated follicles might be hard pressed to make a diagnosis of malignant growth; conversely, when confronted with a benign melanoma from a child, he might advocate amputation if he were not familiar with all the related circumstances. Histology is a guide to the probable biologic potentialities of a tumor, but it must be carefully correlated with the origin of the tumor, its size and the known duration of its presence. In planning the therapy of cancer the surgeon is largely involved in balancing probabilities, and the histologic appearance of the tumor should be given no more than its proper weight.

PRACTICAL CONSIDERATIONS

Up to the present moment changing concepts of the nature of cancer have produced no advance of revolutionary significance in the surgery of this disease, but several avenues of research that have opened should be mentioned. The first of these is a renewed interest in the old idea that there are natural defenses against the growth of tumors. A second is a search for a biologic indicator of the growth potentialities of tumors, and a third is the study of the hormonology of neoplasia, particularly the relation between pituitary-adrenal function and the growth of cancer of the breast and prostate. No attempt to cover the voluminous literature that has sprung up in this field is made in this review. Suffice it to say that from the point of view of the surgeon the most acute need is a rapid method of assaying the growth characteristics of each tumor before operation. The advantages to be gained are so obvious that they require no elaboration, but what a boon it would be to know that in a particular cancer multiple distant metastases had already occurred or were inevitable and that a limited surgical procedure was indicated—or to know that a radical resection of the chest wall and mediastinal lymph nodes was fully justified because the nature of a particular cancer of the breast was such that if a radical extirpation of the nodal spread could be accomplished, a cure would be assured! Indeed, by this means the place of all superradical resections for cancer could be pin-pointed, and their permanent place in the surgeon's armamentarium established. Until this kind of knowledge becomes available, however, the surgeon must continue to balance probabilities in his selection of operative procedures for cancer, and it is to a consideration of this problem that the rest of this review is directed.

According to the traditional concept of cancer, surgery, if it is to be effective, must only be applied early and be sufficiently radical to encompass the spread of the disease. "How radical?" is the question that continually besets the surgeon, and a growing dissatisfaction with the results of surgery is leading to the development of more and more extensive procedures. In fact, the current trend in the surgery of cancer may be compared with the behavior of a savage who has learned how to extract nails with a hammer. He knows that the larger the nail, the harder he must pull. He has had no experience with screws, however, and so long as he is dealing with nails, the results are quite satisfactory, but when he is confronted with a screw, his efforts succeed only by shattering the wood. The surgeon is in fact a step worse off since too frequently he shatters the patient but fails to extract the cancer.

How, then, should the limitations of surgery for cancer be set? Until more accurate means of appraising the biologic propensities of a particular tumor become available, the answer can only be "by conservative judgment opposed to rashness." The subject is considered under several headings.

Place of Established Operations in the Treatment of Cancer

An increasing awareness of the inadequacy of surgery in the treatment of cancer has led to much criticism and revision of established operations.[1] There are those who would replace radical subtotal gastrectomy with total gastrectomy for carcinoma of the stomach. Others would revise the Miles operation to include a pelvic-lymph-node dissection, ligation of the inferior mesenteric artery at its origin and re-

[1] An established operation for cancer is defined as one that has been employed with only minor variations for many years so that the morbidity, mortality and percentage of arrested cases that follow its use are fairly well known. Examples are the Halsted operation for cancer of the breast, abdominoperineal resection for cancer of the rectum and radical subtotal resection for cancer of the stomach.

moval of the entire descending colon. The Halsted operation for cancer of the breast is being extended to include dissection of the supraclavicular and mediastinal lymph nodes with removal of a portion of the chest wall. Hindquarter and forequarter amputations have been advocated for the treatment of malignant melanoma of the extremities.

There has been a tendency to misinterpret many of these recommendations as an advocation of wholesale adoption of superradical operations. A careful study of the original contributions indicates that this is not the intent of the authors. Most of these are carefully controlled studies of what may be accomplished by widening the scope of the established operations. Excellent presentations of the temperate view of the more radical operations in the treatment of cancer have been made by Allen, Gatch, Carey and Kirklin, Lahey and Marshall and Baker.

To date there is no evidence to justify any general or routine extension of the established operations for cancer. A judicious widening of the scope of the resection in particular cases is fully warranted, but before the superradical operations can be expected to replace the established ones, it must be shown that they can be performed with a reasonably comparable mortality and morbidity, and whatever disadvantages they may have in this or other respects must be compensated for by a distinctly superior cure rate. Not only will it take some years to establish this fact but also, if one considers the wide range in the biologic behavior of cancer, it appears quite unlikely that further extension of the areas of excision routinely applied will materially affect the over-all survival rate.

There are no natural boundaries to the growth of cancer. There is no reason to suppose that a tumor that has spread from the rectum to the hypogastric, iliac and the mesenteric lymph nodes will be miraculously blocked at the level of origin of the inferior mesenteric artery. Nor in cancer of the breast is it to be expected that a tumor that has spread to the axilla and the supraclavicular and mediastinal lymph nodes is not also extending into the opposite side of the chest and up and down the retropleural lymphatics. And these hypothetical situations take no cognizance of the frequent occurrence of direct spread of cancer through the blood stream, a circumstance that places the lesion beyond extirpation, however wide the regional excision.

It is abundantly clear either that the majority of tumors that respond well to surgical excision are confined to the organ of origin and the immediately adjacent tissues or that the metastases from such tumors are so constituted biologically that long periods of arrest of distant lesions follow removal of the primary growth. The consistently similar results of well performed surgery of the breast, stomach, colon and rectum over the years in the hands of different surgeons (for example, 7 to 10 per cent five-year survival in cancer of the stomach, 50 per cent survival in cancer of the breast and 45 per cent survival in cancer of the colon) suggest that this represents about the number of tumors biologically susceptible to surgical extirpation. It seems unlikely that superradical excision as a routine will materially affect these figures, but in the hands of all but the most gifted surgeons it will significantly increase the mortality and morbidity.

It is also clear that there can be no retreat from the established procedures. The hazard of cutting across a tumor in the process of its removal, the horrors of local recurrences in wounds and the empirical observations of all surgeons of experience that when one gets into tumor in the course of a dissection it is disseminated widely would render anything less than the established radical operations for cancer a regrettable backward step. Moreover, in certain areas there is an obvious need for certain revisions in the so-called "established procedures" in order that they may more adequately meet the demands of a good cancer operation, but without placing them in the superradical classification. An example is the emphasis that has been placed on the restriction of anterior resection of the rectum to tumors for which it provides a reasonably adequate margin of excision. Another is the abandonment of "resection of the sigmoid" in favor of anterior resection or total resection of the descending colon for lesions involving the sigmoid. The emphasis that has been placed on wider margins in cancer of the gastrointestinal tract in general and a trend toward combined oral and neck dissection for cancer of the oral cavity are similar examples of the manner in which a careful review of the established procedures has led to a modification that improves its application but does not place it in the superradical category. The objective of a good cancer operation is a generous en bloc excision of all tumor without significant permanent disturbances of the patient's physiology or well-being and with little or no risk to his life.

Radical and Superradical Surgery

The opinion expressed in the previous section that superradical operations will not replace the established procedures as a routine does not imply that there is no place for the more extensive resections. Total gastrectomy with resection of the pancreas, spleen, colon, adjacent liver and all intervening lymphatic tissues is an acceptable operation for a huge, invasive, apparently slowly growing carcinoma of the stomach that has invaded locally without distant spread. This procedure, however, as a routine for cancer of the stomach is unthinkable, but where to draw the line between it and a wide resection of the stomach with removal of the omentum and ligation of the left gastric artery at its origin is a matter that must be decided in the individual case. Total gastrectomy for all operable gastric carcinomas is not a satisfactory compromise. There are many objections to it. First of all it is evident that it is not always necessary. Secondly, it unquestionably is a more disabling procedure to the patient than a radical subtotal gastrectomy. Thirdly, it is not a good palliative operation, being particularly badly tolerated by older patients with recurrent disease. In the over-all picture it will increase the morbidity and mortality of gastric surgery for cancer, neither of which can be overlooked. Finally, it will not solve the problem of the very poor results in gastric carcinoma. It adds to the total survival period chiefly when it is used for a slowly growing biologically favorable tumor that cannot be encompassed by subtotal gastrectomy. The incidence of such cases is low, but they constitute a brilliant example of the proper application of the more radical operations.

The gross characteristics of an abdominal cancer are a most important determining factor in electing a superradical operation and are a better index to the biology of the lesion than the histologic appearances are. Any tumor that is large and locally invasive but in which there are no demonstrable lymph-node or distant metastases should be regarded as biologically favorable for surgical resection. No matter how large or apparently fixed such a tumor is, a superradical attack is justified. Some of the most gratifying of all long-term arrests follow such operations. On the other hand, diffuse peritoneal seeding in cancer of the stomach or the bowel, although it does not contraindicate a palliative removal of the primary growth, makes a superradical resection preposterous. The presence of liver or other distant metastases has a deterring effect upon the extent of an operation. How far one should go in the presence of such metastases must again be settled by the particular circumstances. In general, primary growths should always be removed. In abdominal lesions, solitary hepatic metastases involving the left lobe of the liver present a challenge that at times must be accepted. Involvement of the liver by direct extension, all other circumstances being favorable, requires excision.

These general principles are applicable to all cancers in all areas of the body. For example, resection of the chest wall for a neglected, slowly growing carcinoma of the breast is fully justified, whereas removal of the chest wall and dissection of the adjacent mediastinal lymph nodes for a small anaplastic carcinoma of the breast in a young pregnant woman with axillary and supraclavicular metastases obviously would be wrong. Between these extremes there can be no rules except the best judgment of the surgeon tempered by his appraisal of the probable biology of the tumor in question.

Carefully and judiciously applied, the superradical operations will contribute in a significant way to an improvement in the over-all survival rate of cancer. The surgical extirpation of huge tumors, biologically favorable but technically difficult, is the precise point at which a widening of surgical excision is indicated. A classic example is the experience with cancer of the upper third of the stomach. Here is a lesion that in the past has been turned down as "inoperable." In many cases, however, it was not associated with widespread metastases and with further improvement in surgical technics, the routine radical resection of such lesions produced a significant improvement in the five-year survival rate.

One of the most pressing problems today is the place of pelvic exenteration for cancer of the uterus, cervix or rectum or for extensive irradiation necrosis. The results of Brunschwig, Parsons and Bell, Bricker and Modlin and others indicate that this procedure is already an established operation with an acceptable mortality and morbidity provided it is properly applied. Undertaken as a surgical feat for a biologically unfavorable tumor, it has nothing to recommend it. The future of the operation should be a restricted one since it is to be hoped that more and more surgically favorable lesions will be dealt with early and the surgically unfavorable lesions are not going to be significantly benefited by superradical surgery anyway. The application of this and all other superradical procedures for extensive cancer might be judiciously applied if the operating surgeon were required to follow all these patients personally regardless of the outcome. A significant share of the emotional and economic burden that such operations produce would have a most salutary influence.

The expressed objection to superradical operations as routine procedures for cancer should not be construed as a criticism of surgeons who have undertaken a carefully controlled study of the results that can be obtained from a routine widening of the scope of the established operations. Such experimental departures are fully warranted, but advocation of general adoption of the procedures as a routine is illogical and certainly is not supported by any available data. If one considers the complex biologic nature of cancer, it seems clear that the place of the superradical resections must be a restricted one. Carefully applied to certain extensive tumors that are biologically susceptible to surgery, these procedures will have a permanent place in the surgeon's armamentarium.

Management of Recurrent or Metastatic Cancer

Despite a general swing toward surgical radicalism in the management of primary cancer, there is a persistent and not entirely warranted pessimism concerning recurrent or metastatic cancer. If one considers the complex behavior of cancer, recurrent and metastatic lesions occasionally must be amenable to surgical ablation. In some cases local recurrences are attributed to seeding of tumor at the time of a primary resection. The hazards of implantation of tumor cells during open anastomosis of the colon or stomach are greater now than the dangers of infection. Washing of the bowel with agents designed to inhibit implantation of cells at the suture line is becoming a common practice. A study of the effects of the antibiotics on the transplantability of shed cells from lesions of the gastrointestinal tract is greatly needed. In other cases local recurrence may represent progressive carcinogenesis in a field of neoplasia rather than a disseminated lesion. In either of these situations reoperation is indicated, and long periods of arrest may follow such secondary operations.

The most aggressive attack on recurrent cancer has been advocated by Lewis and Wangensteen, who advise taking a "second look" after an interval of two or three months in all cases of abdominal cancer with lymph-node metastases. The wisdom of this approach can be questioned. Recurrent tumor within a few weeks or months of a primary operation indicates either failure to extirpate a favorable lesion or very rapidly growing tumor in most cases. The fact that tumor has not recurred after a second look at intervals of three, six or even eighteen months does not ensure against a local recurrence. However, repeated surgical attacks on rapidly growing recurrent lesions may result in the salvage of some patients. The experience of Wangensteen and his associates suggests that this may be so, but more data are needed to decide when second and third operations are indicated.

Time is an important factor in assessing the biologic characteristics of a recurrent tumor. The longer the interval between the time of the operation and the appearance of a recurrence or metastases, the more favorable the secondary lesion is to surgical excision. In my experience, operations for recurrent cancer of the colon have produced long-term arrests only when the lesion recurred a year or more after the original operation. Whenever a locally recurrent or metastatic lesion appears at an interval of a year or more after an initial operation and seems to be solitary and is so located that it can be resected, a secondary surgical attack is indicated. The initial characteristics of the tumor need not be considered when one is appraising the biology of the recurrence. I have seen recurrences successfully operated on when the initial gross and histologic characteristics of the tumor suggested that it was most unfavorable. For example, a moderately anaplastic tumor that had extended into the regional lymph nodes and had involved several adjacent organs was removed. A recurrence occurred eighteen months later and proved to be a mass of undifferentiated cancer cells, but after resection an interval of ten years has elapsed without recurrence. If the unfavorable pathological features of this tumor had been given undue weight, the opportunity to bring about a long-term arrest of cancer would have been lost.

Emphasis must be placed on the extraordinary behavior of metastatic cancer. The case reported by Trimble in which the metastasis was excised three years before the primary tumor was removed is a case in point.

Long-Range Surgical Care of Cancer

The role of the surgeon in the palliative treatment of cancer is a most important one. Because surgery still remains the only hope of permanent arrest of cancer, the surgeon stands in a position of singular significance to the patient. Whether he realizes it or not, he is the knight in shining armor who is going to save the patient from the cancer dragon. His lack of interest or his withdrawal from the case when it is evident to all that the battle is not won, takes all hope away from the patient.

The modern management of advanced cancer places a moral obligation on the surgeon to see his patient through one way or another. The daily care of the patient requires the services of an able and sympathetic physician or of an institution skilled in the management of these problems, but unless the surgeon is somewhere in the background, as the strategist if not the tactician, the patient loses faith and courage and his existence becomes a kaleidoscope of pain, despair and narcosis.

Most important of all, the surgeon is the only one equipped at the present time to evaluate the changing pattern of so-called "hopeless cancer." Once it is generally realized that a great many factors, most of them unknown at the moment, may influence the growth of cancer, a new vista full of hope is open to the patient with what is regarded as an incurable lesion. By taking full advantage of general supportive measures, by intelligent use of sedatives and narcotics, by judicious use of secondary operations, by irradiation both external and through radioactive isotopes, by appropriate administration of hormones and the antitumor drugs and by neurosurgical procedures for the relief of pain the surgeon may provide years of salvage from total disability; the progress attained is so encouraging that an aggressive confidence that something may be done must replace the archaic but still prevalent attitude of sympathetic despair commonly expressed to the patient's family in the words, "Too bad he didn't seek advice sooner; I can do nothing for him."

In this connection there is a need for much greater co-operation between radiologist and surgeon. The surgeon knows not only the patient but also the tumor. He has lived with the former, and he has seen, felt and generally appraised the latter. This background should be incorporated into the radiologist's phase of therapy in a way that no requisition blank can possibly fulfill. Radiation should be employed with the same accuracy and judgment as the scalpel. If there is reasonable expectation of destruction of the tumor, no holds are barred and a cancericidal dose should be given. On many occasions, however, the extent and nature of the lesion indicate that it is as far beyond radiologic arrest as it is beyond the reach of surgery, and under such circumstances the judicious application of radiation to symptomatic lesions may bring about extraordinary regressions without the severe disability that a cancericidal dose would occasion. Unconventional radiology technics must have as important a place in the long-range control of "incurable cancer" as unorthodox operations on recurrent metastatic lesions.

Secondary surgical attacks on recurrent or metastatic lesions are fully justified whenever a specific lesion in question is solitary, especially if it has developed at some time after the original operation. Excision of painful symptomatic lesions in the presence of other metastases is also advisable whenever this can be done without serious disability to the patient and with reasonable promise of a period of significant comfort and well-being. There is no substitute in this situation for the judgment that comes from experience in balancing the probabilities of cancer behavior.

Finally, when various chemotherapeutic measures are invoked, the management of the patient should not be dropped into the lap of the oncologist. It is essential that the care of the patient continue in the hands of a team composed of the surgeon, the radiologist, the oncologist and strong and sympathetic members of the patient's family.

A word of caution regarding palliative treatment and especially palliative surgery for cancer is necessary, however. The primary purpose of palliation is to relieve suffering, not to prolong the life of the patient. One of the greatest errors is to perform a colostomy for the pseudo-obstruction that commonly accompanies advanced abdominal carcinomatosis. Such a colostomy never functions properly, adds nothing to the patient's comfort and greatly complicates his care. Another error is the "anticipatory colostomy" performed for "inoperable cancer" because the surgeon was sure obstruction would ensue. Anticipating the development of obstruction in gastrointestinal cancer is as unreliable and unwise as predicting the duration of life in all forms of advanced cancer. The surgeon must meet these exigencies as they arise, and the final decision whether or not to employ a palliative procedure must be determined by the probability of alleviating suffering, not merely of prolonging existence.

There is much muddled thinking in this regard, and too often the conscientious but misguided surgeon performs a colostomy or a gastrostomy and gives thousands of cubic centimeters of blood to drag out a patient's tortured existence for a few odd days or weeks. The surgeon has no right to take the patient's life, but he is likewise under no obligation to employ fantastic measures to prolong it in the face of intolerable and clearly terminal disease. Under these circumstances all measures should be designed to keep the patient comfortable, to help him face his disease and its probable consequences with courage and equanimity and to support his family, for whom the crisis, if it is well handled, is often more trying than for the patient himself.

In these terminal stages of cancer it is a great boon to all if both patient and all members of the family are fully aware of the nature of the disease. This is no time to dissemble. Patients are rarely afraid to die. They are always afraid if they are being deceived and seem to be abandoned. A good physician, a sympathetic surgeon clearly visible in the background, a united family, an attitude of aggressive optimism and a determination to control pain intelligently can make these tribulations not only bearable but deeply moving and ennobling experiences.

13. Milestones on the Horizon

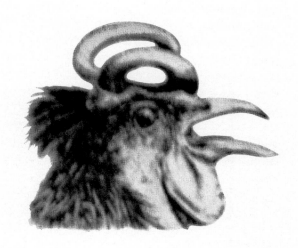

PREFATORY COMMENTS

Along what lines will surgical progress be made in the future? It probably will not result from improvements in technique but from the application of discoveries made by a team of investigators interested in diverse aspects of a complex problem. To reap the harvest, advances made by the members of these groups must be coordinated and applied to the solution of the many unanswered problems that confront us. This approach has been responsible for the great strides made in the field of cardiac surgery. The pharmacologist, the physiologist, the cardiologist, the roentgenologist, the anesthetist and the surgeon have all been important contributors. They must continue to work together not only to ensure the best possible care for the patient but also to open up new horizons.

In 1928, Dale and Schuster and, independently, O. S. Gibbs described the first use of extracorporeal pumps in the experimental animal. Gibbs, a member of the Pharmacology Department of Dalhousie University, Nova Scotia, wrote a most illuminating paper entitled "An Artificial Heart" in the *Journal of Pharmacology and Experimental Therapeutics*. His observations were remarkably prophetic when he stated: "Consideration of the problem indicated certain requirements. First the moving parts must be light or mechanical difficulties both in construction, as well as in the interpretation of the results would be excessive. Secondly, the capacity of the instrument should be such that extra blood is unnecessary. Thirdly, its rate should be dependent on the return blood-flow, the stroke remaining constant (though adjustable at will while the machine is running)." There was a delay of many years before John Gibbon, Jr., of Philadelphia de-

477

veloped the first pump oxygenator to be used in the human. It seems highly probable that if Gibbs' work had been published in a journal widely read by surgeons, it would not have gone unheeded for such a long time. Gibbon deserves renown for his development of an efficient pump–oxygenator which has been emulated but, as yet, not surpassed by many investigators who include Dennis, Lillehei and De Wall.

A second development that rendered open-heart surgery safer was the use of hypothermia. In 1940 Temple Fay of Philadelphia made many observations on the physiological functions of patients undergoing progressive cooling used at that time to curb the rapid spread of carcinoma. Ten years later, a group of surgeons in Toronto headed by Bigelow, and another group at Minneapolis led by Lewis, studied the effects of hypothermia on the experimental animal. Later they applied their knowledge to the correction of intracardiac anomalies in patients. Hypothermia and the pump–oxygenator have enabled surgeons to correct malformations under direct vision with relative safety and with increasing success. At the present time, numerous investigators are working zealously to perfect a simple and efficient pump–oxygenator. When this is accomplished, the scope of open-heart surgery will be extended greatly.

At long last, the heart, the surgical *noli me tangere,* has yielded to the knowledge gained by the enterprising, brilliant studies made in the laboratory combined with the indomitable courage and uncanny skill of the surgeon.

We pondered over the idea of including a "surgical" milestone which had an internist as its lead author, and after careful consideration we feel justified on the basis that the team approach will bring the new era in surgery. Therefore, we have included the article on renal homotransplantation which required the combined talents of an internist, a surgeon, a urologist and a plastic surgeon, sprinkled with innumerable bits of information obtained from the biological scientists.

The problem of transplantation of tissues has captured the imagination of investigators for many years. John Hunter transplanted a cock's spur to its comb. In 1887 William Halsted successfully transplanted the hind leg of a dog from one side to the other by leaving the main artery intact for 10 days. In 1909 Dr. Halsted implanted parathyroid tissue with reported success. Alexis Carrel's interest in organ transplantation led to his description of blood-vessel suturing. Carrel actually succeeded in transplanting kidneys in dogs in 1907, proving that the feat was possible technically. In 1932 Harvey Stone did several experiments on implantation of thyroid and parathyroid tissues with questionable success.

In the past decade there has been increasing interest in organ transplantation. In 1954 Sterling and Goldsmith successfully transplanted the thyroid gland of a 21-day-old infant by preserving its blood vessels together with the carotid artery and jugular vein which were anastomosed to the vessels in the recipient's thigh. A similar method had been employed by Carrel in doing renal homotransplants. The article reproduced in this section describes the first long-term survival of a kidney transplant from one identical homozygous twin to another and emphasizes the biologic problems involved in transplantation. It also serves to indicate that the surgeon has overcome the technical restrictions. Unfortunately, the reason for immunologic rejection of homografts is still unsolved. It remains for the biologist to provide us with material with which to make homografts survive. The work of Medawer, Dempster, Billingham and others, is encouraging. Medawer's optimism is evident in this quotation: "I now feel certain that the clinical homograft problem is soluble: Workers all over the world are discovering gaps in the immunological defences that were unheard of even five years ago, and there seems no reason to doubt that, if the homograft problem continues to be the subject of systematic and careful research, the gaps can be made a great deal wider yet." Rob expresses the importance of the problem as follows: "The transplantation of tissue is the greatest unsolved problem of surgery. If the transplantation of organs from one person to another ever becomes a practical proposition, surgery will change overnight and expand as dramatically as it did after the discovery of antiseptics and anaesthesia."

Rays of light are beginning to filter in. Good and Varco have shown that patients with agammaglobulinemia will tolerate skin homografts. Patients with uremia have increased tolerance to grafts. Siblings with similar lineage tolerate homografts better than others. Can the immunologic response be modified or obliterated? Can the geneticist type us closely enough to predict grafting possibilities? Can desensitization be made practical? We challenge the reader to produce this next milestone which will usher in a new era in surgery.

JOHN H. GIBBON, JR. (*1903–*)

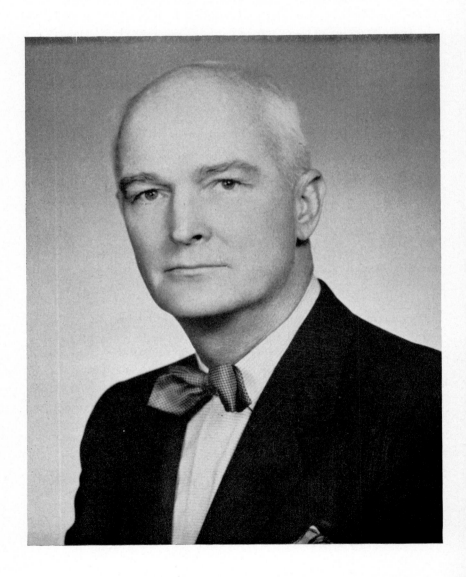

John H. Gibbon, Jr., was born in Philadelphia on September 29, 1903. His early training was at Princeton and at the Jefferson Medical College. At present he is Samuel D. Gross Professor of Surgery at the Jefferson Medical College and Hospital. He is a member of numerous societies and has been President of the American Surgical Society.

Dr. Gibbon was one of the earliest workers on an extracorporeal pump. Many changes have taken place since his original article in 1938, as evidenced by his most recent work.

His four essentials for a satisfactory mechanical heart–lung apparatus have set the standard for future developments.

APPLICATION OF A MECHANICAL HEART AND LUNG APPARATUS TO CARDIAC SURGERY[1]

BY JOHN H. GIBBON, JR., M.D.

Professor of Surgery and Director of Surgical Research,
The Jefferson Medical College, Philadelphia, Pennsylvania

It is a pleasure to be here and to talk about a subject in which I have been interested for many years. The ultimate objective of my work in this field has been to be able to operate inside the heart under direct vision. From the beginning, I have not only been interested in the substitution of a mechanical device for the heart, but also for the lung. We have always considered congenital abnormalities of the heart the most suitable lesions for operative repair. Many of these abnormalities are septal defects. In the presence of a septal defect, shunting the flow of blood around one side of the heart with a pump, will not provide a bloodless field for operative closure of the defect. An apparatus which embodies a mechanical lung, as well as pumps, enables you to shunt blood around both the heart and lungs, thus allowing operations to be performed under direct vision in a bloodless field within the opened heart. Furthermore, an apparatus which embodies a mechanical lung enables you to provide partial support to either a failing heart or failing lung where a major operative procedure is not contemplated. Such an apparatus can also be used as an adjunct dur-

---

[1] Presented in the Symposium on Recent Advances in Cardiovascular Physiology and Surgery, University of Minnesota, Minneapolis, September 16, 1953.

From *Minnesota Medicine,* March, 1954. Reprinted by permission.

ing the course of a major operative procedure. This partial support of
the cardiorespiratory function consists in removing venous blood from
some peripheral vein continuously, oxygenating the blood and getting rid of the carbon dioxide in it and then injecting the blood continuously in a central direction in a peripheral artery. Of course, such
partial circulation, or cardiorespiratory support, requires the use of a
mechanical lung in the circuit.

I shall not describe in detail the entire apparatus. I shall merely
discuss six aspects of the problem which I consider of fundamental
importance. Four of these concern the apparatus itself, and two concern problems which arise on opening the heart and operating within
it under direct vision.

The first feature of a mechanical heart-lung apparatus is a suitable
pumping mechanism to move the venous blood from the subject,
through the apparatus, and back into an artery of the subject. There
is no real problem about a pumping apparatus. There are many
ways of moving blood through tubing without producing significant
amounts of hemolysis. We have used for many years a roller type of
pump which does not contain any internal valves. Such pumps are extremely simple. Because of the absence of valves, the blood circuit is
easy to clean and there are no stagnate regions where fibrin might be
apt to form. There are many other advantages in this type of pump
such as the simple and rapid control of the rate of blood flow. The
pumps cause no significant hemolysis. In human patients in which we
have used the apparatus, hemolysis has always been well below 100
mg. of free hemoglobin per 100 ml. of plasma. In animal experiments,
hemolysis is similarly minimal.

The second main feature of a mechanical heart-lung apparatus is
the mechanical lung itself. This presents far more difficulties than
pumping blood. I am sure that the most efficient apparatus for performing the functions of the lung has not yet been devised. Our present mechanical lung, however, provides a reasonably satisfactory
working solution to this problem. The mechanical lung performs the
gas exchange required for respiratory function by filming blood on
both sides of screens which have a somewhat larger mesh than ordinary fly screens. These screens are made of stainless steel wire and are
suspended vertically and parallel in a plastic chamber. As the blood
flows over these screens, it takes up oxygen and gives off carbon diox-

ide. It should be remembered that it is equally important to remove carbon dioxide from the blood as it is to add oxygen. It is easy to observe that sufficient oxygen is being picked up in the apparatus, as the blue blood entering the oxygenator becomes red as it leaves. This can be determined more accurately, of course, by intermittent sampling or by continuous reading with a Wood cuvette and oximeter. On the other hand, there is no way of estimating the carbon dioxide tension by observing the color of the blood. We have solved this problem by reading continuously the pH of the blood as it leaves the oxygenator. As there is no significant increase in fixed acids in the blood in the course of these experiments, the pH changes are due practically entirely to changes in carbon dioxide tension. We have an automatic control which keeps the carbon dioxide tension at the desired normal level and which is operated by any change in the continuously recorded pH level of the blood.

A third important feature of any apparatus which temporarily performs the function of the heart and lungs is constancy of fluid volume. The apparatus should at all times hold a constant volume of blood at any rate of blood flow. If the apparatus is not designed so as to hold a rigid volume of blood at all rates of blood flow, blood might accumulate in the apparatus with consequent depletion of the subject's vascular system and a dangerous drop in the subject's blood pressure. Similarly, if the apparatus should hold less blood at any time, there would be an excessive amount of blood in the subject's vascular system. Obviously the tubing in the blood circuit will always hold a constant amount of blood. There are two places in the circuit, however, where the blood volume might vary. One is in the blood reservoirs at the bottom of the plastic chambers which draw venous blood from the subject, and the other is in the thickness of the film of blood on the screens in the oxygenator. Rigid control of the volume of blood at the bottom of these plastic chambers has been obtained by an electronic device invented by Dr. B. J. Miller in our laboratory. This electronic device senses the level of the blood in these chambers and automatically operates the pumps which draw blood from the chambers. Thus when the level of blood tends to rise, the pump automatically operates at a faster rate. When the level falls the pump automatically is slowed. This electronic circuit has proven eminently satisfactory and maintains a rigid volume of blood in these chambers.

In the second place where blood might accumulate, on the screens of the oxygenator, a very simple way to avoid such an increase is by inserting an additional pump in the circuit which draws not only from the bottom of the mechanical lung but also from the tubing carrying venous blood from the subject. This additional pump operates at a rate which is always greater than the rate of blood flow from the venae cavae of the subject. As this pump operates at a fixed rate, the thickness of the blood on the screens in the oxygenator does not vary.

The fourth important requirement of any mechanical heart and lung apparatus is that the apparatus should remove all of the blood returning to the heart through the venae cavae and yet should not apply too great a negative pressure to the orifices of the cannulae because the venae cavae would then be collapsed around the orifice of these cannulae. We have found that the simplest way of obtaining such a smooth blood flow from the cavae is to interpose a suction chamber between the pump and the cannulae in the venae cavae. The degree of negative pressure can be easily regulated in this chamber and a smooth uniform flow of blood is easily obtained.

In summary, then, every mechanical heart-lung apparatus devised to take over temporarily the entire functions of the heart and lungs must comprise four essential features. First, there must be a good method of pumping blood through the circuit which does not cause hemolysis, which can be quickly and easily adjusted to varying flow rates and finally which enables the blood circuit to be easily and thoroughly mechanically cleaned. Second, the mechanical lung must not only fully saturate the blood with oxygen but must maintain the carbon dioxide tension of the blood at a normal level. The latter requirement may be taken care of by an automatic apparatus which continuously reads the pH of the blood leaving the mechanical lung and adjusts the carbon dioxide tension accordingly. Third, the apparatus must hold a constant amount of blood at all rates of blood flow. This can be accomplished by electronic control of the pumps removing blood from plastic chambers so that the pumps operate always to maintain a constant level of blood in the reservoirs at the bottom of the chambers. The thickness of the blood film on the screens in the oxygenator is kept constant by an extra pump which always circulates a constant flow of blood over the screens. Fourth such an apparatus must be able to remove smoothly all the venous blood returning to the heart through the venae cavae without collapsing these veins. We have found the simplest way of accomplishing this is to interpose a negative pressure chamber between the pump and the cannulae in the venae cavae.

There are two problems concerning operations upon the open heart which merit discussion. The first consists in the disposal of the blood returning to the chambers of the heart even though all the blood flow from the venae cavae is diverted to the apparatus. The second problem is the avoidance of air embolism when the heart is opened.

The first problem is not difficult to solve. When the entire functions of the heart and lungs are taken over temporarily by the mechanical heart-lung apparatus, the myocardium continues to receive its normal flow of oxygenated blood by way of the coronary arteries. This blood is returned to the interior of the heart by way of the coronary sinus and the Thebesian veins. This blood must be disposed of so that the operative field can be clearly visualized when the heart is opened. We have accomplished this by aspirating this blood into a special plastic chamber in which any air aspirated is dissipated. The blood collects at the bottom of this chamber and is pumped back into the main extracorporeal circuit free of air.

Air embolism must be avoided when the heart is opened. If there is no septal defect, operations upon the right side of the heart can be performed without any great danger from air embolism. It is easy to flood the chamber of the heart with blood or salt solution after the operation is completed so as to avoid air embolism. Small amounts of air in the pulmonary arteries are probably not significant. On the other hand, operations on the left side of the heart, or on the right side of the heart in the presence of a septal defect, present a real problem in the prevention of air embolism into the ascending aorta. The immediate result of such air embolism is usually blockage of the coronary arteries with ventricular fibrillation and death. Our solution of this problem is to insert a small plastic catheter through a stab wound in the apex of the left ventricle. Suction is applied to this plastic catheter during the course of the open cardiotomy so that any air or blood entering the left ventricle takes the path of least resistance out through this plastic catheter instead of being ejected into the aorta. This plastic catheter is also connected to the debubbling chamber which receives the cardiac venous blood aspirated from inside the heart. Thus this blood is also returned to the circuit, and so to the subject, after the air bubbles are removed. After the wound in the heart is closed, and no further bubbles of air appear in the tubing connected to this catheter, it is removed and the small stab wound in the left ventricle closed by suture. Since employing this method in both animals and patients, we have had no instances of air embolism.

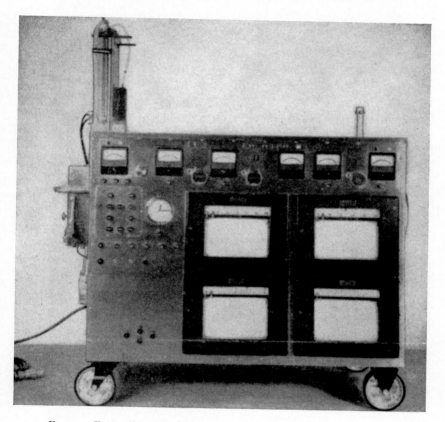

Fig. 1.—Front view of apparatus showing the recording and control instruments and the lung suspended above the cabinet on the left.

Figure 1 shows the front view of the apparatus which I have described, with the recording and control devices on the front panel. Figure 2 shows the rear view with the roller type pumps on top of the cabinet. Two rollers on a revolving arm pass over the rubber tubing which is clamped in a semicircular position. The rollers move

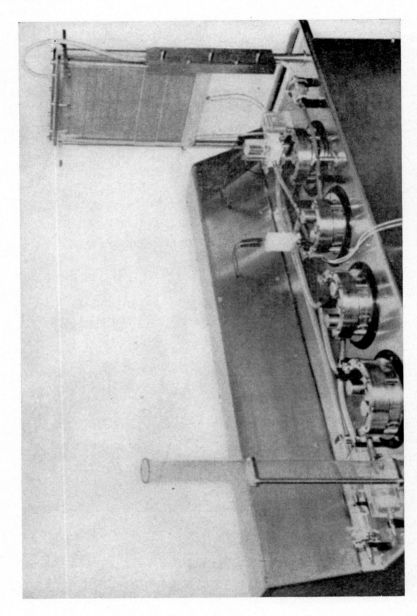

FIG. 2.—Oblique rear view of apparatus showing the rotary blood pumps and the battery-type screen lung suspended above the cabinet on the right side.

the blood through the tubing and the blood cannot flow back because there is always a roller compressing the tube. To the right of Figure 2 is the mechanical lung which consists of vertical screens suspended in parallel in the plastic case. Blood passes onto the screens through slits at the top of the lung. The blood collects in the bottom of the plastic case as it leaves the screens. The pump returning the oxygenated blood to the subject is automatically controlled by the electronic device which senses the level of the blood at the bottom of the plastic case, through which the blood passes. The lucite block near the oxygenator contains glass and calomel electrodes which continuously measure the pH of the blood. The filter consists of a screen with wires 150 microns in diameter and a 300-micron mesh. We do not know whether such a filter is necessary before returning the blood to the subject. However, we regard it as a good safety precaution in human patients. The tube at the end of the apparatus returns the blood to the patient through a cannulae directed in a central direction in an artery. In human patients we employ the central end of the divided left subclavian artery. The other two tubes are connected with cannula which are inserted into the superior and inferior venae cavae.

Oxygen is blown over the screens suspended in the plastic case. Thus the blood film on the screens is exposed to an atmosphere of pure oxygen. The lung shown in Figures 1 and 2 has six screens. We have a larger mechanical lung with eight screens which are of longer length and which we have used on adult patients. An additional pump draws blood both from the bottom of the oxygenator and from the tubing containing the venous blood coming from the patient. The pump maintains a constant rate of flow through the oxygenator so that there is no variation in the thickness of the films on the screens. The electronic control circuit maintains the blood level in the bottom of the plastic case constant at all rates of flow. The pump removing the blood from this chamber is controlled by this electronic device.

There are two plastic negative pressure chambers. One of them collects the blood from the venae cavae and the other (Fig. 3) is the debubbling chamber in which the blood from the cardiac veins and from the left ventricle is collected. As the blood passes down the sides of this plastic chamber any bubbles of air are dissipated. Last spring we reported the successful repair of interatrial septal defects in animals using a flap of pericardium. We have been prepared to use such a flap of pericardium in human patients. We found, however, as Swan has, that it is quite easy to close such defects with a continuous suture in the open heart under direct vision and that consequently a pericardial graft is not needed.

The inferior vena cava is cannulated by a "tygon" tube passed into the inferior vena cava by way of the right atrial appendage. The superior vena cava is cannulated by a "tygon" tube passed through a

CARDIAC VENOUS BLOOD COLLECTING APPARATUS

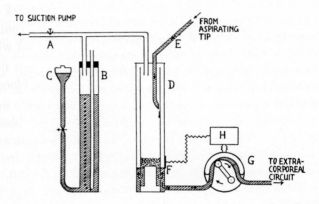

Fig. 3.—Diagram of the cardiac venous blood collecting apparatus. The diagram is self-explanatory. The rotary pump G returns the blood to the main extracorporeal circuit after it has dissipated its bubbles in the inner chamber of cylinder D.

Reprinted from the Medical Clinics of North America (Volume 37, page 1615) with permission of the publishers.

stab wound in the right atrial wall. Oxygenated blood from the apparatus is pumped into the aorta through the divided central end of the left subclavian artery. Ligatures passed around the superior and inferior venae cava are tied over the enclosed cannulae. This diverts all the venous blood to the extracorporeal blood circuit. In addition to closing atrial septal defects in dogs with the pericardial graft, we have successfully closed interventricular defects in dogs by direct suture. The defect is exposed by an incision in the anterior wall of the right ventricle parallel to the left anterior descending coronary artery.

There has been a progressive decline in operative mortality in successive series of animals operated upon in our laboratory. Three years ago we had an 80 per cent mortality. In the most recent series this mortality has declined to 12 per cent. By operative mortality we mean any death which could be attributed to the operation and any death occurring the first month after operation. We have successfully temporarily taken over the entire blood flow through the heart and lungs of a dog for as long as one hour and forty minutes with prolonged survival in a healthy condition.

The average saturation of the venous blood entering the apparatus is 63 per cent. We regard a normal saturation of venous blood with oxygen as the best indication of an adequate blood flow to the tissues. If the saturation of venous blood with oxygen falls to low levels it is obvious that there is an inadequate blood flow to the tissues. We have been successful in maintaining the pH in a normal range. The hemolysis in this group of experiments averaged 35 mg. of free hemoglobin per hundred ml. of plasma. You are all aware that this is an insignificant amount of hemolysis and that a similar degree of hemolysis can occur if blood is forced rapidly through a fine needle. There is only slight increase in the fixed acids, generally in the neighborhood of three millimoles per liter which is within the normal diurnal variation.

Now I suppose what you are all interested in is not how many animals we have successfully operated upon but how many humans we have operated upon. The details of our animal experiments have appeared in two articles recently published. The human patients we have operated upon, using the apparatus, have not yet been reported.

We have used the apparatus to carry temporarily the entire cardio-respiratory functions of four human patients. The first was operated upon a year and one-half ago, and the last in July, 1953, of this year. We have one surviving patient who is quite well in every way with complete closure of an atrial septal defect. The three deaths have all been due to human error and not to failure of the apparatus.

The first patient, who was operated upon a year and one-half ago, was a fifteen-month-old baby that weighed eleven pounds and was in severe congestive cardiac failure. Attempts at cardiac catheterization in this baby were unsuccessful. It was the opinion of everyone who saw this baby that the cardiac abnormality was an interatrial septal defect. We explored the right side of the heart using the apparatus and discovered that no atrial septal defect existed. The child died after operation and at postmortem was shown to have a huge patent ductus arteriosus which had not been recognized at the time of operation. This, of course, illustrates the importance of complete exploration of every heart which is operated upon. We might have saved this child's life if we had closed the ductus.

The second patient was operated upon May 6, 1953. She was an eighteen-year-old girl who had a large interatrial septal defect proved by cardiac catheterization. The patient had been symptom free until about six months before operation, when she began to show symptoms of right-sided heart failure. She was hospitalized three times in these six months. Every time she returned to ordinary activity, she had symptoms of heart failure. Cardiac catheterization revealed an atrial septal defect with a left to right shunt through the defect amounting to nine liters per minute. The patient was connected with the apparatus for forty-five minutes and for twenty-six minutes all cardiorespiratory functions were maintained by the apparatus. She had a large interatrial septal defect which was quite easily closed with a continuous silk suture. The patient's postoperative convalescence was uneventful. She was readmitted to the hospital in July, 1953. At this time, cardiac catheterization showed that the septal defect was completely closed and that there was no evidence of any shunt. The cardiac murmur had completely disappeared and she was in good health. We believe that a transverse incision extending from one axilla to the other opening both pleural cavities through the fourth interspace, and dividing the sternum, gives the best exposure for this type of cardiac operation. The chest wound heals quite solidly and results in an inconspicuous scar beneath the breasts.

The last two patients were operated upon in July, 1953. They were both underdeveloped girls aged five and one-half years. Each of them weighed only about thirty pounds. The first child had a large interatrial septal defect proved by cardiac catheterization. Cardiac arrest occurred after we had opened the chest but before we cannulated any vessels. The heart became blue and dilated as the chest was being explored. We tried for one hour to establish normal cardiac contractions but were unable to do so. We then rather reluctantly cannulated the superior and inferior venae cavae and the left subclavian artery while an assistant massaged the heart. As soon as the patient was connected with the apparatus the heart action became strong and the color of the heart pink. We then opened the right atrium and repaired five separate defects in the interatrial septum. After the defects were closed and the heart wound sutured, the ligatures around the venae cavae were cut allowing the heart to take over part of the circulation. Whenever we stopped the artificial support by the machine, the heart dilated and began to fail. Partial support by the extracorporeal blood circuit was maintained for three or four hours at the end of which time the cannulas were withdrawn and the chest was closed. The patient's heart, however, dilated and cardiac arrest occurred. Death, of course, in the patient cannot be attributed in any way to the use of the heart-lung apparatus as cardiac failure occurred prior to the use of the apparatus. Perhaps the dilatation of the heart and cardiac arrest was the result of a reversal of the shunt through the interatrial defect due to blood transfusion which was given during the early part of the operation.

The second five and one-half-year-old child had a proven interatrial septal defect by cardiac catheterization. It proved impossible, however, to pass the catheter into the right ventricle. On clinical grounds an interventricular septal defect was thought to exist in addition to the interatrial defect. It was known that the patient had a left superior vena cava which was somewhat larger than the right superior vena cava. The child turned out to have not only a huge interatrial septal defect but also a large interventricular septal defect and a small patent ductus arteriosus. Cannulation proceeded normally in this child and when we opened the right atrium we found it to be flooded with bright red blood returning to the atrium through the tricuspid valve. As we could not get a clear field to work and the flow of bright red blood was so excessive, we closed the atrium and removed cannulae. The child died after the operation, which was to be expected due to our failure to correct any of the cardiac defects.

(Motion picture shown)

This motion picture was taken during the course of the operation in which the five separate interatrial defects were sutured. It illustrates the value of being able to visualize the interatrial septum. It seems to me that the four smaller defects might have been missed by the employment of indirect blind methods. The film clearly shows how simple it is to keep the operative field clear of blood and that the heart appears of normal color and is beating well because the myocardium is receiving oxygenated blood from the apparatus through its coronary vessels.

In conclusion, I would like to say that I think the work I have reported is some of the early work in this field and that there is considerably more work to be done. It seems to me that there will always be a place for an extracorporeal blood circuit because it permits a longer safe interval for opening of the heart than can ever be obtained by any of the hypothermia methods.

JOHN PUTNAM MERRILL (*1917–*   )

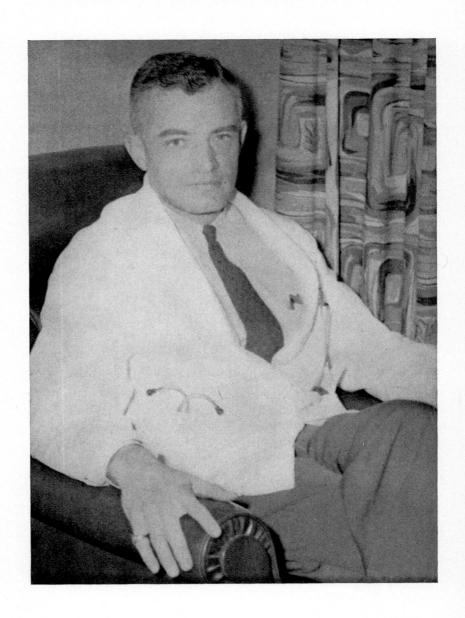

John Putnam Merrill, was born in Hartford, Connecticut, on March 10, 1917. He attended Dartmouth and was graduated from the Harvard Medical School in 1942. During the war he was associated with the atomic bomb project at Kwajalein. His subsequent activities have been at the Peter Bent Brigham Hospital in Boston and as Assistant Professor of Medicine at Harvard.

Dr. Merrill's work on renal homotransplantation followed an extensive experience with the artificial kidney. He has been an integral member of the team with Drs. Murray, Harrison and others, who have been pioneers in human homotransplantation.

SUCCESSFUL HOMOTRANSPLANTATION
OF THE HUMAN KIDNEY
BETWEEN IDENTICAL TWINS

BY JOHN P. MERRILL, M.D.,
JOSEPH E. MURRAY, M.D.,
J. HARTWELL HARRISON, M.D., AND
WARREN R. GUILD, M.D.
Medical and Surgical Services of the Peter Bent Brigham
Hospital and Harvard Medical School

A patient whose illness had begun with edema and hypertension was found to have suffered extreme atrophy of both kidneys. Because of the steady worsening of the condition and the appearance of uremia with other unfavorable prognostic signs, transplantation of one kidney from the patient's healthy identical twin brother was undertaken.

Preparations included collection of evidence of monozygosity and experimental transplantation of a skin graft from the twin. During the transfer of the healthy kidney it was totally ischemic for 82 minutes. Evidence of functional activity in the transplanted kidney was obtained.

The hypertension persisted until the patient's diseased kidneys were both removed. The homograft has survived for 11 months, and the marked clinical improvement in the patient has included disappearance of the signs of malignant hypertension.

This report documents the successful transplantation of a human kidney from one identical twin to another. The function of the homograft remains excellent 12 months after the operative procedure. Pre-

From the *Journal of the American Medical Association*, January 28, 1956. Reprinted by permission.

496

vious attempts at renal homotransplantation, both clinically and experimentally, have been unsuccessful with one exception. In dizygotic cattle twins, a kidney transplant has survived and functioned for at least nine months. Success in this instance, however, presumably resulted from the production of an acquired mutual tolerance to each other's tissues by the mingling of fraternal protein in the common placental circulation. Transplantation of the kidney in dogs and other animals rarely maintains function for more than a 10-to-14-day period in spite of vigorous attempts to modify the presumed antibody response that results in rejection of the homograft. Similarly, permanent function has not been maintained in a human renal homograft, although in one such instance adequate renal function in a transplanted kidney has persisted for five and a half months. The ultimate cause for rejection in such cases is in all probability differences in individual tissue specificity. Since, however, skin homografts between identical human twins have survived permanently, it might be expected that renal homotransplantation might also be successful when performed between identical twins. The following case history describes such an event.

REPORT OF A CASE

A 24-year-old, white, single male was apparently in excellent health until 14 months before his first admission to the Peter Bent Brigham Hospital. Except for scarlet fever at age 5 without apparent complications, the history was noncontributory. A few months prior to his discharge from military service, the patient noticed some puffiness about the eyes on awakening in the morning, and on a routine physical examination some elevation of blood pressure was noted. During a five-month study period while at the Boston Public Health Service Hospital, he remained essentially asymptomatic except for epistaxis. Physical examination was negative except for a consistently elevated blood pressure averaging 170/100 mm. Hg. Pertinent laboratory findings included persistent 2 to 3+ proteinuria. The urinary specific gravity was fixed at 1.010 and microscopic hematuria and cylindruria with occasional red blood cell casts were found in all urine specimens. Blood urea nitrogen level ranged between 75 and 100 mg. per 100 cc. Hemoglobin level varied between 7 to 10 gm. per 100 cc. Phenolsulfonphthalein excretion was less than 1% in two hours, and an intravenous pyelogram revealed no dye excretion on either side. X-ray of the chest showed the lungs to be clear and the heart normal in size and shape. After seven transfusions of whole blood he was discharged improved. Five months later he was readmitted again to the Boston Public Health Service Hospital and appeared pale and chronically ill. The blood pressure now varied between 160/80 and 208/120 mm. Hg. The retinal vessels showed narrowing of the arterioles with changes in caliber and occasional arteriovenous compression. He was discharged after a three-day period and readmitted six weeks later because of nausea, vomiting, headache, and general muscular aches. At this time he appeared more seriously ill, and marked pallor of the skin was evident. The blood pressure was 172/90 mm. Hg; retinal vessels showed narrowing and arteriovenous compression; and lungs were clear. The heart appeared to be slightly enlarged to the left. There was a grade 2 blowing systolic murmur over the entire precordium. The remainder of the physical examination was normal. Pertinent laboratory data follow. Hemoglobin was 6.7 gm. per 100 cc. and hematocrit 20%; urine showed 3+ protein, 2+ sugar, and 5-25 red blood cells per high-power field on spun sediment. There were occasional granular and hyaline casts. The blood urea nitrogen was 185 mg. per 100 cc. His course was characterized by persistent nausea and vomiting and on the third hospital day he had a generalized convulsion. In succeeding days he became increasingly drowsy, disoriented, and irritable and had several convulsions. Since the patient had a twin brother, it was suggested by Dr. David C. Miller of the U. S. Public Health Service that the possibility of homotransplantation of a kidney should be considered. For the investigation of this possibility, he was transferred to the Peter Bent Brigham Hospital on Oct. 26, 1954.

On admission the initial blood pressure was 140/90 mm. Hg. The patient appeared thin, pale, drowsy, and extremely disoriented. The remainder of the physical examination and laboratory data were consistent with that outlined above. Urine culture grew out Escherichia coli and enterococci. The patient continued to be restless and unable to tolerate oral feedings and became overtly psychotic. On the fourth hospital day he was treated by external dialysis with the artificial kidney for a four-hour period. A good chemical response was obtained and 36 hours later the patient's sensorium had cleared and he was cooperative and able to take diet and medicaments by mouth.

On the 15th hospital day, full-thickness skin grafts, 2.5 by 2.5 cm., were exchanged between the twins. A control autograft was placed proximally and the homograft was placed 1 cm. distally, allowing a bridge of normal tissue to intervene between the two grafts. On the following day the patient was discharged feeling well on a diet containing 50 gm. of protein and no added salt. He was followed at weekly intervals in the outpatient clinic, continued to show hypertension, and gradually developed the manifestations of congestive heart failure for which he was digitalized with some improvement. On Dec. 12, 1954, however, he was re-admitted to the Peter Bent Brigham Hospital because of marked increase in signs and symptoms of his congestive heart failure. Physical examination at this time revealed blood pressure of 220/146 mm. Hg. There was 3+ pitting edema of the lower legs up to the knees. Bilateral basal rales were present. The liver edge was tender and was palpated 4 cm. below the right costal margin. There was slight periorbital edema and the optic fundi now showed a 2 diopter papilledema with exudates and hemorrhages. The heart was enlarged to the left with a loud diastolic gallop heard over the entire precordium. A chest film showed marked cardiac enlargement with evidence of fluid at the base of the right side of the chest. During the next three days, 350 cc. of turbid, amber fluid was removed from the right side of the chest and the patient received three units of packed red blood cells. He was started on therapy with parenterally given protoveratrine. On this therapy there was marked clinical improvement.

On Dec. 16, 31 days after the original skin transplant, biopsy study of the homograft was done. In both gross and histological section the transplanted tissue appeared to have survived as normal skin. Because of this evidence of tissue compatibility and ancillary observations suggesting that the twins were monozygotic, on Dec. 23 a normal left kidney was removed from the healthy twin and transplanted to the patient. (Previous hospitalization had disclosed the absence of discoverable disease in the healthy twin and confirmed the presence of two normally functioning kidneys free of infection.)

The postoperative course of the donor was uneventful, and he was discharged on the 14th hospital day. The recipient tolerated the operative procedure well and, soon after the anastomoses were completed, clear urine was noted draining freely from the transplant. Nine days after surgery the intravenous injection of sodium indigotindisulfonate (indigo carmine) showed prompt appearance in good concentration in the urine from the transplanted kidney and no excretion from the patient's own kidneys. During the course of the following month, the homograft appeared to function well and began to hypertrophy. The patient was discharged from the hospital on the 37th postoperative day. He had gained 11 lb. (5 kg.) and was edema free. The blood urea nitrogen was 14 mg. per 100 cc. and the resting blood pressure, 120/60 mm. Hg. The chest was clear and the heart size normal. The serum carbon dioxide combining power was 25 mEq. per liter and the serum concentrations of sodium, chloride, potassium, calcium, and phosphate were all within normal limits. The phenolsulfonphthalein excretion was 18% in 15 minutes and 48% in two hours. Urinalysis at the time of discharge showed a trace of albumin, 4 to 6 white blood cells, and a rare blood cell per high-power field. Urine culture grew out Proteus vulgaris.

After discharge the patient's appetite was good and he had no edema, dyspnea, or orthopnea. Blood pressures ranged from 130/80 to 160/88 mm. Hg. The optic disks were normal, and the retina vessels became normal, although a few old scars persisted in the optic fundi. Because of continued mild bacilluria and pyuria, the patient was begun on methenamine mandelate (Mandelamine) therapy. An excretory urogram performed two months after the renal homotransplantation showed prompt excretion of the injected dye in good concentration from the transplanted kidney but no detectable excretion by the two diseased kidneys.

Because of persistent mild hypertension, the patient was admitted to the Peter Bent Brigham Hospital for the third time three months after renal homotransplantation. At this time the initial blood pressure was 152/90 mm. Hg. The patient appeared healthy and completely asymptomatic. There had been further gain in weight and muscle development. The palpable mass of the homograft in the right lower quadrant had hypertrophied to half again its original size. The electrocardiogram showed disappearance of the changes of left ventricular hypertrophy. The hematocrit was 48%, blood urea nitrogen 14 mg. per 100 cc. and carbon dioxide combining power 23 mM. per liter. On the fifth hospital day a left nephrectomy was performed. The kidney weighed only 49 gm. and was covered by a markedly thickened capsule that was fibrosed and scarred. The cortex was markedly diminished in size and the microscopic section showed the majority of the glomeruli to be completely fibrosed. The renal parenchyma showed diffuse atrophy and fibrosis with disappearance of tubular elements and the appearance was that of diffuse advanced chronic glomerulonephritis. The patient was discharged 12 days after operation feeling entirely well. However, because of the persistence of mild pyuria and mild labile hypertension, he was readmitted for the fourth time on June 14, 1955, five and a half months after renal homotransplantation. On the seventh hospital day the patient underwent an uneventful right nephrectomy. The right kidney weighed only 29 gm. and showed the typical changes of advanced diffuse chronic glomerulonephritis with little functioning parenchyma remaining. On discharge the patient's appetite was good; he had gained more weight and was essentially asymptomatic. At the present time his blood pressure ranges from 125/70 to 146/82 mm. Hg. He weighs 25 lb. (11.3 kg.)

more than his initial preoperative weight. He carries on unlimited activity and has no apparent physical disability. The urinary sediment is negative, although his 24-hour protein excretion is 4.5 gm.

COMMENT

The transplantation of functioning tissue from one individual to another of the same species has, with few exceptions, not been successfully accomplished to date. Successful transplantation has been occasionally reported in the case of embryonic thyroid, parathyroid, and in one instance adrenal tissue. The successful transplantation of bone and blood vessels depends not on their survival as living tissues but on their ability to act as bridges over which recipient tissue may grow. Because of its particular structure and the fact that it is frequently transplanted into an avascular field, corneal transplants in man, however, do survive as living tissues in a large percentage of cases. The immune response leading to the rejection of homografts is incompletely understood. Circulating cytotoxic antibodies cannot be measured in significant amounts. It is probable, however, that antibodies to donor tissue are formed by the recipient and that these are removed by the homograft so rapidly that they cannot be measured in the blood. The fact that an antigen–antibody reaction is responsible for the rejection of homografted tissue and that this response can be modified is suggested by work in which successful skin transplants were made after acquired tolerance to donor tissue resulting from the injection of donor cells into the embryonic recipient. This acquired tolerance by the embryo to foreign cells probably accounts also for the survival of renal homotransplants between dizygotic bovine twins. In the human the role of acquired antibodies is suggested by recent reports of the successful homotransplantation of skin to a recipient with agammaglobulinemia.

Although at the present time permanently successful renal homografts between humans cannot be performed because of this "antigen antibody like" reaction between donor tissue and recipient, skin homografts are known to survive between identical twins. Having established this fact, there were several experimental observations that made the success of a renal homograft seem likely if performed between identical twins and that justified the removal of a normal kidney from a healthy donor.

First, immunologic and genetic similarity accounts for the permanent survival of skin homografts between identical twins. Second, when skin or kidney homografts are carried out between antigenically dissimilar humans, the early function and the histological picture of rejection of each appears similar. Third, skin and kidney homografts possess a common antigen that can sensitize a recipient to a subsequent homograft of either tissue from the same donor. This further suggests that skin and kidney homografts behave similarly. Fourth, we have established to our own satisfaction that renal autografts have normal function indefinitely in animals. This observation is important because, presupposing initial success of the transplant between antigenically similar (identical) twins, a second problem to be weighed was the permanency of such function. There were no reported instances of adequate functional studies in long-term surviving renal autografts.

It thus became imperative to establish beyond a reasonable doubt the fact that the twins were monozygotic (identical). Information that there was a common placenta was obtained from the hospital record of their birth. Blood samples from both twins were tested for all presently known reliable blood groups. These were found to be identical in both instances for each group (table). The two other

RESULTS OF TESTS FOR ANTIBODIES IN BLOOD SAMPLES FROM BOTH TWINS

	A	B	C	D	E	c	e	M	N	S	Kell	Lewis	Lewis	Luther	Duffy	Kidd
Recipient twin...	o	o	+	+	o	+	+	+	+	+	o	o	+	o	+	+
Donor twin......	o	o	+	+	o	+	+	+	+	+	o	o	+	o	+	+

siblings tested did not match. This was considered good but not indubitable evidence that the twins were identical. The twins and two other siblings were studied by Dr. Arthur G. Steinberg, geneticist of the Children's Medical Center, Boston, who felt that, "On the basis of eight blood group systems plus the ability to taste phenylthiocarbamide, the sex similarity, and the a priori probability of dizygotic versus monozygotic twinning, the probability that these boys are identical twins is 0.985. Other data indicating that they are identical are 1) the presence of a single placenta, 2) both twins have the relatively rare Darwin's tubercle on their ears while their sibs do not, 3) the twins have identical eye colors, including iris structure and pigment patterns, and their eyes are markedly different from their sibs' eyes in color and in iris structure, 4) there are no data suggesting they are not identical. My conclusion is that the twins are identical." Final decision to operate, however, was based on the most closely applicable evidence for antigenic similarity, that is the survival of transplanted skin between the two twins (Fig. 1).

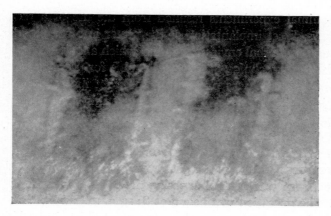

Fig. 1.—Sites of skin autograft (left) and homograft (right). Photograph taken three and a half months after grafting. There is no discernible difference between the patient's own transplant and that of his twin brother (scarred areas are biopsy sites).

Evaluation of several factors determined the site for transplantation. The natural site for the homograft, the renal fossa, has two disadvantages. First, it requires simultaneous nephrectomy, thus increasing the magnitude of the operation. Secondly, it necessitates a ureteroureteral anastomosis with the possibility of subsequent stricture formation because the length of the transplanted ureter vascularized by the renal pedicle is too short to reach the bladder. The upper thigh, the site of 13 previous homotransplants, was not used because it requires a skin ureterostomy with the possibility of subsequent ascending infection. In addition, it creates a problem in the collection of urine. The site selected, utilizing the iliac vessels for an anastomosis and placing the homograft retroperitoneally within the pelvis, allows implantation of the short ureteral segment directly into the bladder and places the kidney in its natural thermal environment. Furthermore, gravity drainage of the renal pelvis and ureter approaches normal physiological conditions. The observations mentioned above, that renal autografts in animals maintain normal function indefinitely, appear important because of the previous opinion of other investigators that renal autografts so capable of survival soon develop impaired function manifested by abnormal renal dynamics and electrolyte excretion. We surmised that the permanently successful function observed in our animal experiments resulted from the use of a recipient site that allows direct implantation of the ureter into the bladder, which has a normal thermal environment and which allows gravity drainage. This laboratory technique proved adaptable for use in man, provided that the left kidney was placed into the right iliac area or the right kidney into the left iliac fossa, thus reversing the normal anteroposterior relationship of the artery, vein, and ureter.

With this background, a nephrectomy was begun on the donor simultaneously with the operation on the recipient in an adjacent operating room. Through a right lower quadrant incision, the retroperitoneal area was entered exposing the right iliac vessels in the recipient. The operation was begun at 8:15 a. m., and the vessels were prepared for the anastomoses by 9:50 a. m. The donor kidney was brought into the room at 9:53 a. m. At this time the common iliac artery was occluded for the duration of the anastomosis. An end-to-end anastomosis between the free end of the hypogastric artery and the renal artery was completed at 10:40 a. m., and an end-to-side anastomosis between the renal vein and the common iliac vein was finished at 11:15 a. m. Total ischemia of the donor kidney was one hour and 22 minutes. Both arterial and venous anastomoses were satisfactory, and the entire kidney became turgid and pink immediately on release of the arterial clamp. Therefore, a small artery in the renal pedicle that appeared to be an accessory renal artery was ligated rather than anastomosed. The last clamp was removed from the common iliac artery 10 minutes later, and pulsation was noted in the right foot immediately. At this point a suprapubic cystotomy was made in the medial and superior portion of the bladder and a small tunnel dissected in the submucosa. The ureter was let in through the muscular wall of the bladder and through the submucosal tunnel, and a mucosa-to-mucosa suture was carried out (Fig. 2). A polyethylene ureteral catheter had been inserted in the ureter to the renal pelvis and carried out through the cystotomy at this time. The incisions in the bladder were then closed after a mushroom catheter had been inserted from a suprapubic site. At this time clear urine was flowing copiously from the ureteral catheter. The kidney now lay rather neatly in its new site except that it projected forward where the lower pole

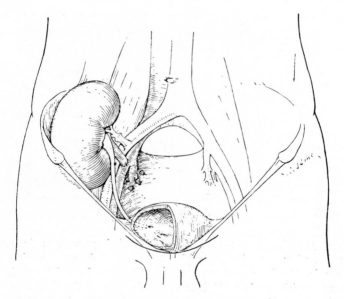

Fig. 2.—Schematic diagram of renal homograft in situ showing vascular anastomoses completed and ureter implanted in bladder. Renal artery end-to-end with hypogastric; renal vein end-to-side with common iliac; ureter mucosa-to-mucosa anastomosis with bladder.

impinged upon the iliac crest. The kidney was fixed by sutures to prevent its rotation, and the overlying oblique muscles and fascia were sutured together over it. The total operating time was three hours and 30 minutes. The postoperative course was smooth, and the incision healed per primam. The ureteral catheter was removed on the ninth postoperative day after evidence of function had been confirmed by the prompt excretion of injected sodium indigotindisulfonate.

The patient's subsequent course was characterized by continued improvement. Renal function improved; and, as it did so, acidosis and nitrogen retention disappeared (Fig. 3). There was a marked decrease in blood pressure, and with this decrease the evidence of cardiovascular disease disappeared (Fig. 4). Marked cardiomegaly (Fig. 5) disappeared, and the abnormalities in the electrocardiogram vanished. The significance of these changes by the addition of a normally

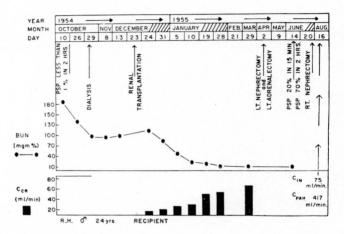

Fig. 3.—Disappearance of azotemia and improvement in renal function after renal homotransplantation. There is a progressive decrease in blood urea nitrogen and an increase in serial creatinine clearances (shown in solid bars at the bottom of the diagram). In October, 1954, there was almost no discernible phenolsulfonphthalein excretion. On June 14, 1955, phenolsulfonphthalein excretion was normal. In August, 1955, filtration rate and renal plasma flow as measured by the clearances of inulin and *p*-aminohippurate were at near normal values.

functioning kidney in the presence of two badly damaged kidneys will be discussed in a future publication.

During the follow-up visits, however, the patient continued to show evidence of some elevation of blood pressure. This elevation was labile and in some instances directly related to the presence of the examining physician. A persistent tachycardia (pulse rate of 90 to 100 per minute) continued in spite of normal blood chemistry and hemoglobin values. The urine continued to show 6 to 8 white blood cells, a rare cast, and 1+ protein. Clean voided urine specimens grew out a variety of organisms, which included P. vulgaris and Esch. coli. In vitro sensitivity tests showed these organisms to be resistent to most of the antibiotics except chloramphenicol. Colony counts varied from 100 colonies per milliliter on a pour plate to 2,000 colonies. After a consideration of the foregoing facts, it was decided to remove the two

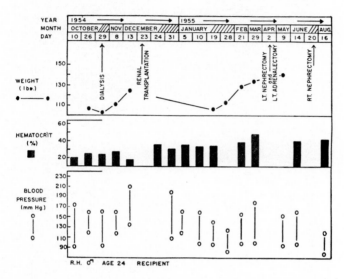

Fig. 4.—There is striking decrease in blood pressure immediately after renal transplantation and some tendency for this to rise again with improved levels after left nephrectomy and return to normal values after removal of the second diseased kidney. Increase in hematocrit and gain in weight reflect improvement in general clinical condition.

damaged kidneys for the following reasons. 1. Intravenous pyelography and renal function tests had shown that the renal homograft was functioning well. 2. The data indicated almost total lack of function in the two diseased kidneys. 3. The possibility existed that infection of the graft might occur from the two remaining diseased kidneys. 4. Experimental evidence suggests that a nonfunctioning or infected kidney may ultimately interfere with the function of a normal kidney, particularly with regard to its role in preventing renal hypertension.

After the second nephrectomy the patient's blood pressure stabilized at lower, and almost normal, levels. Frequent urine examinations since that time have shown clearing of the evidence of urinary tract infection. Some proteinuria, however, persists. The renal function of the homograft as measured by the clearance of inulin and *p*-aminohip-

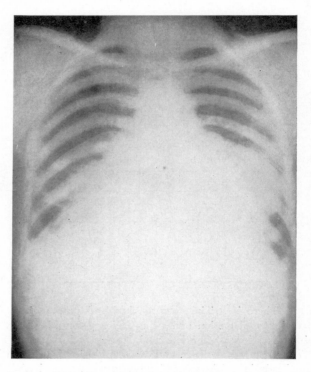

Fig. 5.—Chest film taken nine days before operation shows marked cardiomegaly and pulmonary congestion. Three weeks after operation lung fields were clear and heart size decrased to within normal limits.

purate closely approximates that of its fellow, which remains in the donor twin. Intravenous urography shows prompt excretion of dye in good concentration (Fig. 6). The ureter appears somewhat dilated and tortuous, but this appearance might be expected in view of the fact that it lacks innervation.

The survival of the renal homograft for this period of time with continuing good function indicates the complete lack of a rejection response by the host and demonstrates that renal transplantation is a technically feasible procedure. It stresses further that, as indicated in previous studies, total anoxia of the kidney (in this case for a period of one hour and a half) does not mitigate against resumption of adequate function. The implications of the dramatic response in malignant hypertensive disease to the transplantation of a normal kidney should carry considerable weight in future thinking about the renal mechanism in human hypertension. Why one identical twin and not

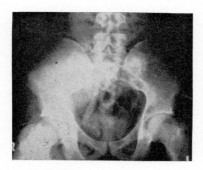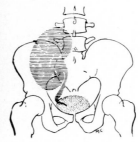

Fig. 6.—There is prompt excretion of the opaque medium in good concentration. Renal pelvis shows no extrarenal dilatation but there is definite dilatation of ureter, attributed to complete denervation of the kidney. No evidence of ureterovesicle obstruction is seen and prompt emptying of ureter into bladder occurs. Bladder is seen to be partially filled on this exposure and more so on subsequent exposures.

the other should develop glomerulonephritis and whether the kidney of the unaffected twin transplanted into the diseased recipient will be susceptible to further attacks is a question still to be answered. Unanswered also is the question of whether the transplanted kidney in its unusual position with a short and abnormally innervated ureter will escape eventual infection.

SUMMARY

Homotransplantation of a healthy kidney from one identical twin to another was performed. The homograft has survived for a 12-month period, and renal function is apparently normal despite the fact that both of the recipient's diseased kidneys were removed. A striking sequel to the marked clinical improvement that was observed was the disappearance of the signs of malignant hypertension. Tissue transplantation including that of a functioning kidney appears to be a feasible procedure in identical twins, but to date successful permanently functioning homografts appear to be limited to such individuals.

Index

INDEX

513

Set in Intertype Baskerville
Format by Norma Stahl
Manufactured by The Haddon Craftsmen, Inc.
Published by PAUL B. HOEBER, INC.
Medical Book Department of HARPER & BROTHERS